Springer-Verlag Berlin Heidelberg GmbH

32nd Hemophilia Symposium

Hamburg 2001

Editors: I. Scharrer, W. Schramm

Presentation:

Epidemiology
Genetic Diagnosis of Clotting Disorders
Hemophilia
Pediatric Hemostaseology
Free Lectures

Scientific Board:
I. Scharrer, Frankfurt/Main
W. Schramm, Munich

Chairmen:
G. Auerswald (Bremen); H.-H. Brackmann (Bonn); L. Gürtler (Greifswald)
W. Kreuz (Frankfurt/Main); H. Lenk (Leipzig); E.O. Meili (Zurich)
I. Scharrer (Frankfurt/Main); R. Seitz (Langen); A.H. Sutor (Freiburg)
R. Zimmermann (Heidelberg)

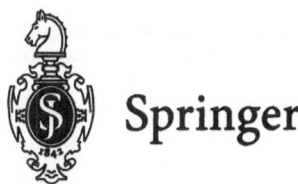 Springer

Professor Dr. med. INGE SCHARRER
Hemophilia Center, Dept. of Internal Medicine
University Hospital
Theodor-Stern-Kai 7
D-60590 Frankfurt am Main
Germany

Professor Dr. med. WOLFGANG SCHRAMM
Dept. of Hemostasiology
University Hospital
Ziemssenstr. 1a
D-80336 München
Germany

Mit 128 Abbildungen

ISBN 978-3-540-43884-7

Library of Congress Cataloging-in-Publication Data

Hämophilie-Symposion (32nd : 2001 : Hamburg, Germany)
    32nd Hemophilia Symposium : Hamburg, 2001 / editors, I. Scharrer, W. Schramm ;
    chairman, G. Auerswald ... [et al.].

    Includes bibliographical references and index.
    ISBN 978-3-540-43884-7   ISBN 978-3-642-18150-4 (eBook)
    DOI 10.1007/978-3-642-18150-4

    1. Hemophilia-Congresses. I. Title: Thirty-second Hemophilia Symposium. II.
    Scharrer, I. III. Schramm, W., 1943- IV. Title.
    [DNLM: 1. Hemophilia A--diagnosis--Congresses. WH 325 H228z 2003]
    RC642 H355 2001
    616.1'572--dc21

                              2002030317

http://www.springer.de/medizin

© Springer-Verlag Berlin Heidelberg 2003
Originally published by Springer Verlag Berlin Heidelberg in 2003

The use of general descriptive names, registered names, trademarks, etc. in this publication does not imply,
even in the absence of a specific statement, that such names are exempt from the relevant protective laws and
regulations and therefore free for general use.

Product Liability: The publisher cannot guarantee the accuracy of any information about dosage and application contained in this book. In every individual case the user must check such information by consulting
the relevant literature.

Typesetting: cicero Lasersatz, Dinkelscherben

Printed on acid-free paper   SPIN 10874809   21/3130   5 4 3 2 1 0

Contents

V. Free Lectures

VI. Poster

a) Clinic and Casuistic

b) Hemophilia and Hemorrhagic Disorders

List of Participants

ANDERS, O., Prof. Dr.
Klinik und Poliklinik für Innere Medizin der Universität Rostock, D-Rostock

AUERSWALD, G., Dr.
Professor-Hess-Kinderklinik, Zentralkrankenhaus St.-Jürgen-Str., D-Bremen

AUMANN, V., Dr.
Klinik für Pädiatrische Hämatologie und Onkologie,
Otto-von-Guericke-Universität, D-Magdeburg

AVOLEDO, P., Dr.
Universitätskinderspital, Hämatologie/Onkologie, CH-Basel

AYGÖREN-PÜRSÜN, E., Frau Dr.
Zentrum der Kinderheilkunde, Johann-Wolfgang-Goethe-Universität,
D-Frankfurt/Main

BALLEISEN, L., Prof. Dr.
Abteilung Hämatologie u. Onkologie, Innere Medizin,
Evangelisches Krankenhaus, D-Hamm

BARTHELS, M., Frau Prof. Dr.
D-Hannover

BAUMGARTNER, CH., Dr.
Facharzt für Kinder und Jugendliche, spez. Hämatologie, CH-Gossau

BECK, CH., Frau Dr.
Ärztin für Kinderheilkunde, D-Berlin

BECK, E.A., Prof. Dr.
Arzt für Hämatologie, CH-Lugano

BECK, K.H., Dr.
Medizinischer Dienst der Krankenkassen, D-Freiburg

BECKER, TH., Dr.
Interessengemeinschaft Hämophiler, D-Bonn

BEESER, H.P., Prof. Dr.
Institute for Quality Management and Standardization in Transfusion Medicine
and Hemostaseology, D-Teningen

BENEKE, H., Dr.
Sektion Hämostaseologie, Abteilung Innere Medizin III,
Medizinische Universitätsklinik, D-Ulm

BERGMANN, F., Frau Dr.
Gemeinschaftslabor Dr. Keeser und Prof. Arndt, D-Hamburg

BERGSTRÄSSER, E., Frau Dr.
Universitätskinderspital, Hämatologie, CH-Zürich

BERNER, F., Dr.
Zentrum für Kinderheilkunde und Jugendmedizin, Hämatologie/Onkologie,
Universitätskliniken, D-Gießen

BERTHOLD, B., Dr.
Hämophiliezentrum, Klinik für Innere Medizin I, Klinikum Neubrandenburg,
D-Neubrandenburg

BEUTEL, K., Frau Dr.
Abteilung Hämatologie/Onkologie, Universitätskinderklinik Eppendorf,
D-Hamburg

BLAZEK, B., Dr.
FNsP Ostrava, Childrens Dept. – Hematology, CZ-Ostrava-Poruba

BLICKHEUSER, R., Dr.
DRK-Kinderklinik, D-Siegen

BÖHM, M., Frau
Hämostaseologie, Medizinische Klinik I,
Klinikum der Johann-Wolfgang-Goethe-Universität, D-Frankfurt/Main

BÖKER, M.
Annastift, Orthopädie, D-Hannover

BÖTTCHER, D., Prof. Dr.
Abteilung Innere Medizin, Krankenhaus Bethesda, D-Wuppertal

BRACKMANN, CH., Frau
Institut für Experimentelle Hämatologie und Transfusionsmedizin
der Universität, D-Bonn

BRACKMANN, H.-H., Dr.
Institut für Experimentelle Hämatologie und Transfusionsmedizin
der Universität, D-Bonn

BRAUN, A., Dr.
DRK-Kinderklinik, D-Siegen

BRAUN, U., Frau Dr.
Deutsche Hämophiliegesellschaft, D-Hamburg

BREUER, W.
Interessengemeinschaft Hämophiler, D-Bonn

BROCKHAUS, W., Dr.
Abteilung für Hämostaseologie, Hämatologie und Angiologie, D-Nürnberg

BROCKMANN, M.
Abteilung Neurochirurgie, Universitätsklinik Eppendorf, D-Hamburg

BRUHN, H.D., Prof. Dr.
I. Medizinische Klinik, Klinikum der Christian-Albrechts-Universität, D-Kiel

BUDDE, U., Prof. Dr.
Gemeinschaftslabor Dr. Keeser und Prof. Arndt, D-Hamburg

CALATZIS, A., Dr.
Abteilung Hämostaseologie, Medizinische Klinik Innenstadt
der Ludwig-Maximilians-Universität, D-München

CARLSSON, L.E., Frau Dr.
Institut für Immunologie und Transfusionsmedizin
der Ernst-Moritz-Arndt-Universität, D-Greifswald

CHRAST, B., Dr.
Hematology Department, Nemocnice Ceske Budejovice, CZ-Ceske Budejovice

CHRISTOPH, V., Frau Dr.
Krankenhaus im Friedrichshain, Innere Medizin II, D-Berlin

CLAUSEN, N., Dr.
Department of Pediatrics, University Hospital of Aarhus, DK-Aarhus N

CSABANE, Frau Dr.

CVIRN, G., Mag.
Allgemeines Österr. Landeskrankenhaus Graz,
Universitätsklinik für Kinder- und Jugendheilkunde, A-Graz

DITTMER, R., Frau Dr.
  Gemeinschaftslabor Dr. Keeser und Prof. Arndt, D-Hamburg

DULICEK, P., Dr.
  Hämatologische Abteilung, I. Medizinische Klinik, Universitätskrankenhaus,
  CZ-Hradec Králové

EBERL, W., Dr.
  Kinderklinik, Städtisches Klinikum Holwedestraße, D-Braunschweig

EICKHOFF, H.H., Dr.
  Orthopädische Klinik, St.-Josef-Hospital, D-Troisdorf

EIDHER, U., Frau Dr.
  Wilhelm-Hospital, A-Wien

EIFRIG, B., Frau Dr.
  Abteilung Onkologie/Hämostaseologie, Medizinische Klinik,
  Universitätskrankenhaus Eppendorf, D-Hamburg

EIS-HÜBINGER, A.M., Frau PD Dr.
  Institut für Medizinische Mikrobiologie und Immunologie der Universität,
  D-Bonn

ESCURIOLA-ETTINGSHAUSEN, C., Frau Dr.
  Zentrum der Kinderheilkunde,
  Klinikum der Johann-Wolfgang-Goethe-Universität, D-Frankfurt/M.

ETZLER, J., Frau
  D-Hamburg

FÄSSLER, H., Dr.
  FMH Medicina interna, CH-Chiasso

FRANK, J., Dr.
  Abteilung Transfusionsmedizin, Medizinische Klinik Innenstadt der Ludwig-
  Maximilians-Universität, D-München

FRANKE, D., PD Dr.
  Schwerpunktpraxis für Gerinnungsstörungen und Gefäßkrankheiten,
  D-Magdeburg

FRANKE, ST., Frau
  Hämostaseologie, Medizinische Klinik I,
  Klinikum der Johann-Wolfgang-Goethe-Universität, D-Frankfurt/M.

FUNK, M., Dr.
Zentrum der Kinderheilkunde,
Klinikum der Johann-Wolfgang-Goethe-Universität, D-Frankfurt/Main

GALLISTL, S., Prof. Dr.
Allgemeines Österr. Landeskrankenhaus Graz,
Universitätsklinik für Kinder- und Jugendheilkunde, A-Graz

GEHLHAAR, K.D.
Blutspendedienst, Zentralinstitut Springe, D-Springe

GEIDEL, K., Frau
Abteilung für Transfusionsmedizin, Chirurgische Klinik und Poliklinik,
Universitätsklinik Eppendorf, D-Hamburg

GEISEN, U., Dr.
Zentrallabor, Medizinische Universitätsklinik,
der Julius-Maximilians-Universität, D-Würzburg

GERHARDT, A., Frau Dr.
Abteilung für Transfusionsmedizin,
Medizinische Einrichtungen der Heinrich-Heine-Universität, D-Düsseldorf

GILBERG, E., Dr.
Kinderklinik, Klinikum Neubrandenburg, D-Neubrandenburg

GÖHAUSEN, M., Frau
Praxis für Diagnostik und Therapie von Blutgerinnungsstörungen,
Ambulanzzentrum der Raphaelsklinik, D-Münster

GRAW, J., Prof. Dr.
GSF-Forschungszentrum für Umwelt und Gesundheit GmbH,
Institut für Säugetiergenetik, Neuherberg, D-Oberschleißheim

GROSS, J., Dr.
Institut für Transfusionsmedizin und Immunhämatologie,
Universitätsklinikum, D-Magdeburg

GROSS, W., Prof.Dr.
Franz-von-Prümmer-Klinik, D-Bad Brückenau

GRÜNINGER, M., Frau
Krankenhaus Dornbirn, A-Dornbirn

GRUNSKE, A.
Klinik für Kinder- und Jugendmedizin, Carl-Thiem-Klinikum, D-Cottbus

GÜLDENRING, H., Dipl.-Med.
Städtisches Krankenhaus Dresden-Neustadt, Kinderklinik, D-Dresden

GÜRTLER, L., Prof. Dr.
Institut für Mikrobiologie, Ernst-Moritz-Arndt-Universität, D-Greifswald

GUTENSOHN, K., PD Dr.
Chir. Universitätsklinik und Poliklinik, Abteilung für Transfusionsmedizin,
Universitätskrankenhaus Eppendorf, D-Hamburg

HALIMEH, S., Frau Dr.
Abteilung für Hämostaseologie, Kinderklinik, Medizinische Einrichtung
der Westfälischen-Wilhelms-Universität, D-Münster

HASSENPFLUG, W., Dr.
Abteilung Hämatologie/Onkologie, Kinderklinik, Universitätsklinik Eppendorf,
D-Hamburg

HAUSHOFER, A., Dr.
Allgemeines Österr. Krankenhaus der Landeshauptstadt St. Pölten,
Zentrallabor, A-St. Pölten

HAWLINA, H.A., Frau Dr.
Institut für Experimentelle Hämatologie und Transfusionsmedizin
der Universität, D-Bonn

HEINRICHS, CH., Frau Doz. Dr.
Krankenhaus im Friedrichshain, Abteilung Klinische Hämostaseologie,
Hämophiliezentrum, D-Berlin

HEINTEL-REBSTOCK, D., Frau Dr.
Paul-Ehrlich-Institut, FG711, D-Langen

HELLSTERN, P., Prof. Dr.
Institut für Transfusionsmedizin und Immunhämatologie,
Klinikum der Stadt Ludwigshafen, D-Ludwigshafen

HEMPELMANN, L., Dr.
Klinik für Kinder- und Jugendmedizin, Krankenhaus Lichtenberg, D-Berlin

HERBINIAUX, U., Frau
Institut für Experimentelle Hämatologie und Transfusionsmedizin
des Universitätsklinikums, D-Bonn

HERRMANN, F.H., Prof. Dr. Dr.
Institut für Humangenetik, Medizinische Fakultät
der Ernst-Moritz-Arndt-Universität, D-Greifswald

HESS, L., Dr.
Institut für Experimentelle Hämatologie und Transfusionsmedizin
der Universität, D-Bonn

HILGENFELD, E., Frau Dr.
D-Berlin

HILLER, U., Frau Dr.
Abteilung für Angiologie, Zentrum der Inneren Medizin,
Klinikum der Johann-Wolfgang-Goethe-Universität, D-Frankfurt/Main

HOCHMUTH, K., Frau Dr.
Orthopädische Universitätskliniken, Frankfurt/Main

HOFMANN, H., Dr.
Facharzt für Transfusionsmedizin, D-Töplitz

HOFMANN, U., Frau
Klinikum Ernst-von-Bergmann, D-Potsdam

HOHMANN, D.
Interessengemeinschaft Hämophiler, D-Bonn

HORNEFF, S., Frau Dr.
Klinik für Kinderheilkunde der Martin-Luther-Universität, Halle-Wittenberg,
D-Halle

HOVY, L., Prof. Dr.
Annastift, Orthopädie, D-Hannover

HUTH-KÜHNE, A., Frau Dr.
Kurpfalzkrankenhaus Heidelberg und Hämophiliezentrum gGmbH,
D-Heidelberg

IMAHORN, P., Dr.
Kinderspital Luzern, CH-Luzern

JONES, N., Dr.
Landeskrankenhaus Salzburg, Kinderspital, A-Salzburg

JULEN, E., Dr.
FMH, Allgemeine Medizin, CH-Zermatt

KALNINS, W., Dr.
Deutsche Hämophiliegesellschaft, D-Marmagen

KÄSE, M., Frau
Abteilung Hämatologie/Onkologie, Kinderklinik, Medizinische Einrichtung
der Westfälischen-Wilhelms-Universität, D-Münster

KÄTZEL, R., PD Dr.
Abteilung für Transfusionsmedizin und Hämostaseologie,
Städtisches Klinikum St.Georg, D-Leipzig

KESSLER, C.M., Dr.
Georgetown University, Med. Center, Lombardi Cancer Center,
USA-Washington DC

KIESEWETTER, H., Prof. Dr. Dr.
Institut für Transfusionsmedizin und Immunhämatologie,
Campus Charité Mitte, D-Berlin

KIRCHMAIER, C.M., PD Dr.
Deutsche Klinik für Diagnostik, D-Wiesbaden

KLAMROTH, R., Dr.
Krankenhaus im Friedrichshain, Abteilung Klinische Hämostaseologie,
Hämophiliezentrum, D-Berlin

KLARE, M., Dr.
II. Innere Klinik, Klinikum Berlin-Buch, D-Berlin

KLARMANN, D., Dr.
Abteilung Hämatologie und Gerinnung, Zentrum der Kinderheilkunde,
Klinikum der Johann-Wolfgang-Goethe-Universität, D-Frankfurt/Main

KLEMPAU, K., Frau Dipl.-Biol.
Institut für Experimentelle Hämatologie und Transfusionsmedizin
des Universitätsklinikums, D-Bonn

KNÖBL, P., Prof. Dr.
Allgemeines Krankenhaus der Stadt Wien,
Abteilung für Hämatologie und Hämostaseologie, A-Wien

KNÖFLER, R., Dr.
Klinik und Poliklinik für Kinderheilkunde
Universitätsklinikum Carl-Gustav-Carus, D-Dresden

KOBELT, R., Dr.
FMH Kinder- und Jugendmedizin, CH-Wabern

KÖHLER-VAJTA, K., Frau Dr.
Ärztin für Kinderheilkunde, D-Grünwald

KONRAD, H., Prof.Dr.
Arzt für Innere Medizin und Hämatologie, D-Rostock

KOSCH, A., Frau Dr.
Pädiatrische Hämatologie/Onkologie der Medizinischen Einrichtung
der Westfälischen-Wilhelms-Universität, D-Münster

KOSCIELNY, J., Dr.
Institut für Transfusionsmedizin und Immunhämatologie,
Campus Charité Mitte, D-Berlin

KÖSTENBERGER, M., Dr.
Allgemeines Österr. Landeskrankenhaus Graz,
Universitätsklinik für Kinder- und Jugendheilkunde, A-Graz

KÖSTERING, H., Prof. Dr.
D-Lemgo

KOTITSCHKE, S., Frau
Zentrum der Kinderheilkunde,
Klinikum der Johann-Wolfgang-Goethe-Universitätskliniken,
D-Frankfurt/Main

KRAUSE, M., Frau
Hämostaseologie, Medizinische Klinik I,
Klinikum der Johann-Wolfgang-Goethe-Universität, D-Frankfurt/Main

KREBS, H., Dr.
Abteilung Hämostaseologie, Medizinische Klinik Innenstadt
der Ludwig-Maximilians-Universität, D-München

KREUZ, W., PD Dr.
Zentrum der Kinderheilkunde,
Klinikum der Johann-Wolfgang-Goethe-Universität, D-Frankfurt/M.

KRONBERGER, Frau Dr.
St.-Anna-Kinderspital, A-Wien

KÜHNE, TH., Dr.
Universitätskinderspital, Hämatologie/Onkologie, CH-Basel

KURNIK, K., Frau Dr.
Kinderklinik im Dr. von Hauner'schen Kinderspital
der Ludwig-Maximilians-Universität, D-München

KURNIK, P., Dr.
Allgemeines Österr. Landeskrankenhaus,
Abteilung für Kinder- und Jugendheilkunde, A-Klagenfurt

KYANK, U., Frau Dr.,
Universitätskinderklinik, Medizinische Fakultät, Universität Rostock,
D-Rostock

LANDMANN, T.
Klinikum der Stadt Ludwigshafen, D-Ludwigshafen

LECHLER, E., Prof.Dr.
D-Esslingen a. N.

LEHMANN, I., Frau
Medizinische Klinik und Poliklinik I, Hämophiliezentrum, Universität Leipzig,
D-Leipzig

LENK, H., PD Dr.
Universitätsklinik und Poliklinik für Kinder- und Jugendliche,
Universität Leipzig, D-Leipzig

LESCHNIK, B.,
Allgemeines Österr. Landeskrankenhaus Graz,
Universitätsklinik für Kinder- und Jugendheilkunde, A-Graz

LESTIN, H. G., Prof. Dr.
Institut für Labormedizin, Klinikum Schwerin, D-Schwerin

LIESE, M., Frau
Ltd. MTA, Labor, Medizinische Hochschule Hannover, D-Hannover

LIGHEZAN, D., Dr.
Universitatea de Medicina si Farmacie Timisoara, Clinica Medicina Interna II,
Spital Municipal, R-Timisoara

LOSONCZY, H., Frau Doz. Dr.
I. Medizinische Klinik, Medizinische Universität, H-Pécs

LÜHR, C., Frau
Abteilung Hämophilie, Medizinische Poliklinik,
Medizinische Hochschule Hannover, D-Hannover

LUTZ, W., Dr.
Gerinnungslabor D-Lab 28, Universitätsspital, CH-Zürich

LUTZE, G., Prof. Dr.
Institut für Klinische Chemie und Pathobiochemie,
Otto-von-Guericke-Universität, D-Magdeburg

MAAK, B., Prof. Dr.
Thüringen-Klinik, Georgius Agricola Saalfeld, D-Saalfeld

MAGENS, M.
Abteilung Transfusionsmedizin, Transplantationsimmunologie,
Universitätskrankenhaus Eppendorf, D-Hamburg

MALE, CH., Dr.
Universitätsklinik für Kinderheilkunde, A-Wien

MANNHALTER, CH., Frau Prof. Dr.
Allgemeines Krankenhaus der Stadt Wien,
Klinisches Institut für Medizinische und Chem. Labordiagnostik, A-Wien

MAREK, R., Dr.
Wiener Gebietskrankenkasse, A-Wien

MARTINKOVÁ, I., Frau Prim. Dr.
odd. Hematologie, Fakultni nemocnice v Plzni, CZ-Plzen-Bory

MATZDORFF, A., PD Dr.
Abteilung für Hämatologie und Onkologie,
Zentrum für Innere Medizin, Klinikum der Justus-Liebig-Universität, D-Gießen

MAURER, M., Prof. Dr.
D-Bernau, Chiemsee

MEILI, E.O., Frau Dr.
Universitätsspital, Gerinnungslabor, CH-Zürich

METZEN, Frau
Abteilung für Transfusionsmedizin,
Medizinische Einrichtungen der Heinrich-Heine-Universität, D-Düsseldorf

MEYER, V., Frau
Hämostaseologie, Medizinische Klinik I,
Klinikum der Johann-Wolfgang-Goethe-Universität, D-Frankfurt/M.

MIESBACH, W., Dr.
Hämostaseologie, Medizinische Klinik I,
Klinikum der Johann-Wolfgang-Goethe-Universität, D-Frankfurt/Main

MIHAILOV, D., Frau Dr.
University of Medicine, Clinica I-a Pediatrie, R-Timisoara

MONDORF, W., Dr.
Haemostas-Frankfurt, D-Frankfurt/Main

MÖSSELER, J., Dr.
Arzt für Kinderheilkunde, D-Dillingen

MOSLER, K., Frau Dr.
Medizinische Einrichtungen der Heinrich-Heine-Universität, Kinderklinik,
Allgemeine Pädiatrie 2, D-Düsseldorf

MÜNCHOW, N., Frau Dr.
Ostschweizer Kinderspital, CH-St.Gallen

MUNTEAN, E.W., Prof. Dr.
Allgemeines Österr. Landeskrankenhaus Graz,
Universitätsklinik für Kinder- und Jugendheilkunde, A-Graz

MUSS, N., Dr.
Salzburger Gebietskrankenkasse, A-Salzburg

NEIDHARDT, B., Dr.
Abteilung für Transfusionsmedizin, Chirurgische Universitätsklinik,
D-Erlangen

NIEKRENS, C., Frau Dr.
Pädiatrie, Städtische Klinik Delmenhorst, D-Delmenhorst

NOHE, N., Frau Dr.
Kinderklinik im Dr. von Hauner'schen Kinderspital
der Ludwig-Maximilians-Universität, D-München

NOWAK-GÖTTL, U., Frau Prof. Dr.
Abteilung Hämatologie/Onkologie, Kinderklinik,
Medizinische Einrichtung der Westfälischen-Wilhelms-Universität, D-Münster

OLDENBURG, J., Dr.
Institut für Experimentelle Hämatologie und Transfusionsmedizin
der Universität, D-Bonn

PETRITSCH, M., Frau Dr.
Allgemeines Österr. Landeskrankenhaus Graz,
Universitätsklinik für Kinder- und Jugendheilkunde, A-Graz

PLENDL, H., Dr.
Institut für Humangenetik, Klinikum der Christian-Albrechts-Universität,
D-Kiel

PODEHL-KLOSE, J., Dr.
Annastift, Orthopädische Klinik, D-Hannover

POEK, KL.
Deutsche Hämophiliegesellschaft, D-Berlin

POLLMANN, H., Dr.
Praxis für Diagnostik und Therapie von Gerinnungsstörungen,
Ambulanzzentrum der Raphaelsklinik, D-Münster

RABENSTEIN, C.
Hämostaseologie, Medizinische Klinik I,
Klinikum der Johann-Wolfgang-Goethe-Universität, D-Frankfurt/Main

RAUCH, R., Dr.
Klinik der Eberhard-Karls-Universität, Kinder- und Jugendmedizin,
D-Tübingen

REHBERGER, G., Dr.
Ordination, A-Frastanz

REITER, W.W., Dr.
Facharzt für Innere Medizin, Hämatologie, D-Viersen

RICHTER, H.
Praxis für Diagnostik und Therapie von Blutgerinnungsstörungen,
Ambulanzzentrum der Raphaelsklinik, D-Münster

RIESS, H., Prof. Dr.
Medizinische Klinik mit Schwerpunkt Hämatologie und Onkologie,
Campus Virchow-Klinikum, D-Berlin

RINGKAMP, H., Frau
Praxis für Diagnostik und Therapie von Blutgerinnungsstörungen,
Ambulanzzentrum der Raphaelsklinik, D-Münster

ROSCHITZ, B., Frau Dr.
Allgemeines Österr. Landeskrankenhaus Graz,
Universitätsklinik für Kinder- und Jugendheilkunde, A-Graz

RUSICKE, E., Frau
Zentrum der Kinderheilkunde,
Klinikum der Johann-Wolfgang-Goethe-Universität, D-Frankfurt/Main

SCHARRER, I., Frau Prof. Dr.
Hämostaseologie, Medizinische Klinik,
Klinikum der Johann-Wolfgang-Goethe-Universität, D-Frankfurt/M.

SCHEEL, H., Dr.
D-Leipzig

SCHELLE, G.
Interessengemeinschaft Hämophiler, D-Bonn

SCHLENKRICH, U., Dr.
D-Großlehna

SCHMELTZER, B., Frau Dr.
Ärztin für Kinderheilkunde, D-Potsdam

SCHMIDT, O., Dr.
Praxis für Gefäßkrankheiten, D-Magdeburg

SCHMUTZLER, R., Prof. Dr.
D-Wuppertal

SCHNEPPENHEIM, R., Prof. Dr.
Abteilung Hämatologie/Onkologie, Kinderklinik, Universitätsklinik Eppendorf,
D-Hamburg

SCHOBESS, R., Frau Dr.
Klinik für Kinderheilkunde der Martin-Luther-Universität, Halle-Wittenberg,
D-Halle

SCHÖN, A., Frau cand. med.
Abteilung für Transfusionsmedizin, Universitätskrankenhaus Eppendorf,
D-Hamburg

SCHRAMM, K., Frau
D-München

SCHRAMM, W., Prof. Dr.
Abteilung Hämostaseologie, Medizinische Klinik Innenstadt
der Ludwig-Maximilians-Universität, D-München

SCHRÖDER, J.
Institut für Humangenetik, Biozentrum, Universität Würzburg, D-Würzburg

SCHRÖDER, W., Frau Dr.
Institut für Humangenetik, Medizinische Fakultät
der Ernst-Moritz-Arndt-Universität, D-Greifswald

SCHULTE-OVERBERG, U., Frau Dr.
Kinderklinik, Campus Virchow-Klinikum, D-Berlin

SCHULZ, M., Frau Dr.
Abteilung Blutspende- und Transfusionsmedizin
der Ernst-Moritz-Arndt-Universität, D-Greifswald

SCHULZE-SCHEITHOFF, E., Frau Dr.
Institut für Experimentelle Hämatologie und Transfusionsmedizin
der Universität, D-Bonn

SCHUMACHER, R., Dipl. Med.
Kinderklinik, Klinikum Schwerin, D-Schwerin

SCHWAAB, R., Dr.
Institut für Experimentelle Hämatologie und Transfusionsmedizin
der Universität, D-Bonn

SEDLAK, M., Dr.
Allgemeines Krankenhaus der Stadt Linz, Interne II, A-Linz

SEIFERTOVA, N., Frau Dr.
Haematology Department, Nemocnice Ceske Budejovice, CZ-Ceske Budejovice

SEITZ, R., Prof. Dr.
Paul-Ehrlich-Institut, Abteilung Hämatologie und Transfusionsmedizin,
D-Langen

SELKE, K., Dr.
Abteilung Nephrologie, Kinderklinik,
Klinikum der Albert-Ludwigs-Universität, D-Freiburg

ŞERBAN, M., Frau Prof. Dr.
University of Medicine, IIIrd Pediatric Clinic, R-Timisoara

SEREBROWA, I., Frau Dr.
Abteilung Hämatologie/Onkologie, Kinderklinik, Universitätsklinik Eppendorf,
D-Hamburg

SEUSER, A., Dr.
Kaiser-Karl-Klinik, Fachklinik für Orthopädie, D-Bonn

SEVERIN, TH., Dr.
Abteilung Hämatologie u. Hämostaseologie, Kinderklinik,
Klinikum der Albert-Ludwigs-Universität, D-Freiburg

SIEGEMUND, A., Frau Dr.
Institut für Klinische Chemie, Gerinnungslabor Innere Medizin,
Universität Leipzig, D-Leipzig

SIEMENSEN, M., Frau
Abteilung für Transfusionsmedizin und Transplantationsimmunologie,
Universitätskrankenhaus Eppendorf, D-Hamburg

SILLER, M.
Deutsche Hämophiliegesellschaft e.V., D-Berlin

SROUR, M., Dr.
Institut für Experimentelle Hämatologie und Transfusionsmedizin
der Universität Bonn, D-Bonn

STOLL, H., Frau
Zentrum der Kinderheilkunde, Johann-Wolfgang-Goethe-Universität,
D-Frankfurt/Main

STRASSER, E., Dr.
Abteilung für Transfusionsmedizin, Chirurgische Universitätsklinik,
D-Erlangen

STRUVE, S., Frau Dr.
Abteilung für Transfusionsmedizin,
Medizinische Einrichtungen der Heinrich-Heine-Universität, D-Düsseldorf

SUBERT, R., Frau Dr.
Abteilung für Hämatologie u. Onkologie, Klinik für Innere Medizin II,
Klinikum Schwerin, D-Schwerin

SULOVSKA, I., Frau Dr.
Hämatologische Klinik, Fakultätskrankenhaus, CZ-Olomouc

SUTOR, A.H., Prof. Dr.
Abteilung Hämatologie u. Hämostaseologie, Kinderklinik,
Klinikum der Albert-Ludwigs-Universität, D-Freiburg

SUTTORP, M., Prof. Dr.
Universitätsklinik Carl-Gustav-Carus, Klinik und Poliklinik
für Kinderheilkunde, Hämatologie/Onkologie, D-Dresden

SYKORA, K.W., PD Dr.
Zentrum Kinderheilkunde, Medizinische Hochschule Hannover, D-Hannover

SYRBE, G., PD Dr.
Innere Abteilung, Landesfachkrankenhaus Stadtroda, D-Stadtroda

TONN, T., Dr.
Institut für Transfusionsmedizin und Immunhämatologie, Blutspendedienst
DRK-Hessen, D-Frankfurt/Main

TÜRK-KRAETZER, B., Frau Dr.
Ärztin für Kinderheilkunde, D-Oldenburg

ÜN, C.
GSF-Forschungslabor für Umwelt und Gesundheit GmbH,
Institut für Säugetiergenetik, Neuherberg, D-Oberschleißheim

UNKRIG, CH., Dr.
Medizinische Universitätspoliklinik, D-Bonn

VARVENNE, M., Dr.
Abteilung Hämophilie/Med. Poliklinik, Medizinische Hochschule Hannover,
D-Hannover

VAVRA, V., Dr.
II. Detska Klinika, FN Motol, CZ-Praha

VIGH, TH.
Hämostaseologie, Medizinische Klinik I,
Klinikum der Johann-Wolfgang-Goethe-Universität, D-Frankfurt/Main

VOERKEL, W., Dr.
Gemeinschaftspraxis für Labormedizin,
Mikrobiologie und Transfusionsmedizin, D-Leipzig

VOGT, B., Frau
Universitäts-Kinderklinik Leipzig,
Abteilung für ambulante und soziale Pädiatrie, D-Leipzig

VON DEPKA PRONDZINSKI, M., Dr.
Abteilung Hämophilie, Medizinische Poliklinik,
Medizinische Hochschule Hannover, D-Hannover

VON DER WEID, N., Dr.
Medizinische Kinderklinik, Inselspital, CH-Bern

VONDRYSKA, F., Dr.
Czech Hemophilia Society, CZ-Praha

VORLOVA, Z., Frau Dr.
Institut für Hämatologie und Bluttransfusion, CZ-Praha

WALLNY, TH., PD Dr.
Orthopädische Klinik, Medizinische Einrichtungen
der Rheinischen Friedrich-Wilhelms-Universität, D-Bonn

WALZER, I., Frau Dr.
Landeskrankenhaus Salzburg, Kinderchirurgie, A-Salzburg

WANKE, Dr.
St.Anna-Kinderspital, A-Wien

WATZKE, H., Prof.
Allgemeines Krankenhaus der Stadt Wien, Hämatologie-Hämostaseologie,
A-Wien

WEBER, Dr.
Abteilung Onkologie/Hämostaseologie, Medizinische Klinik,
Universitätskrankenhaus Eppendorf, D-Hamburg

WEISSBACH, G., Prof. Dr.
D-Dresden

WEISSER, J., Dr.
Kinderarzt, Rehabilitation, Fachkrankenhaus Neckargemünd gGmbH,
D-Neckargemünd

WENZEL, E., Prof. Dr.
Abteilung Klinische Hämostaseologie und Transfusionsmedizin,
Universitätskliniken d. Saarlandes, D-Homburg

WERMES, C., Frau Dr.
Abteilung Hämophilie / Medizinische Poliklinik,
Medizinische Hochschule Hannover, D-Hannover

WERNI, A., Frau Dr.
Abteilung Hämostaseologie, Medizinische Klinik Innenstadt
der Ludwig-Maximilians-Universität, D-München

WIEDING, J.U., Dr.
Abteilung Transfusionsmedizin, Universitätskliniken, D-Göttingen

WIEGAND, G., Frau Dr.
Universitätsklinik für Kinderheilkunde und Jugendmedizin, D-Tübingen

WINDYGA, J., Dr.
Institute of Hematology and Blood Transfusion, P-Warsaw

WOLF, H.H., Dr.
Klinik u. Poliklinik f. Innere Medizin IV, Medizinische Fakultät, Martin-Luther-
Universität, Halle-Wittenberg, D-Halle

WOLLINA, K., Frau Dr.
Klinik Innere Medizin II, Friedrich-Schiller-Universität, D-Jena

WULFF, K., Frau Dr.
Institut für Humangenetik,
Medizinische Fakultät der Ernst-Moritz-Arndt-Universität, D-Greifswald

ZANIER, U., Frau Dr.
Allgemeines Österr. Krankenhaus Dornbirn,
Abteilung für Kinder- und Jugendheilkunde, A-Dornbirn

ZEN RUFFINEN, Frau Dr.
CH-Visp

ZIEGER, B., Frau PD Dr.
Kinderklinik, Klinikum der Albert-Ludwigs-Universität, D-Freiburg

ZIMMERMANN, R., Prof. Dr.
Kurpfalzkrankenhaus Heidelberg und Hämophiliezentrum gGmbH,
D-Heidelberg

ZUPANCIC-SALEK, S., Dr.
Lug Samoborski, Croatia

ZWIEAUER, K., Prim. Dr.
Abteilung für Kinderheilkunde, Allgemeines Österr. Krankenhaus,
A-Pölten

I. Epidemiology

Chairmen:

R. Seitz (Langen)
L. Gürtler (Greifswald)

HIV Infection and Causes of Death in Patients with Hemophilia in Germany (Year 2000/2001 Survey)

W. Schramm and H. Krebs, on behalf of the GTH Hemophilia Committee

Basic Facts on the Surveys

Already in the late 1970s Professor Landbeck began to survey annually hemophiliacs living at that time in West Germany for causes of death and the prevalence of diseases. The early questionnaires used in the surveys focused on basic data were later expanded by additional information particularly about HIV infection and AIDS-related death. Since 1998 more specific data on hepatitis and antiretroviral therapies have been included. Future surveys will be strengthened by data derived from the German Hemophilia Registry that is currently being established on behalf of the GTH Hemophilia Commission.

Participating Centers

Since the first survey the number of participating centers has increased every year with a particularly rise in 1991 when the hemophilia treatment centers of the former East Germany joined in. Today these centers contribute a significant portion of the overall data (Fig. 1). Although this year the number of reporting hemophilia centers slightly decreased again from 87 centers last year to 72 centers this year (Table 1 and Fig. 2). In contrary the total number of patients (including patients with von Willebrand disease) reported from all centers has again clearly increased from 7548 to 8055 patients or 6,7% (Table 2).

Patients

In 2001, a total number of 8055 patients (including possible double registrations) have been reported from the participating centers. The distribution of patients with

Table 1. Numbers of participating hemophilia centers

	1991	1992	1993	1994	1995	1996	1997	1998	1999	2000	2001
east	47	62	79								
west	18	18	24								
totals	65	80	103	111	119	119	71	75	93	87	72

I. Scharrer/W. Schramm (Ed.)
32nd Hemophilia Symposium Hamburg 2001
© Springer-Verlag Berlin Heidelberg 2003

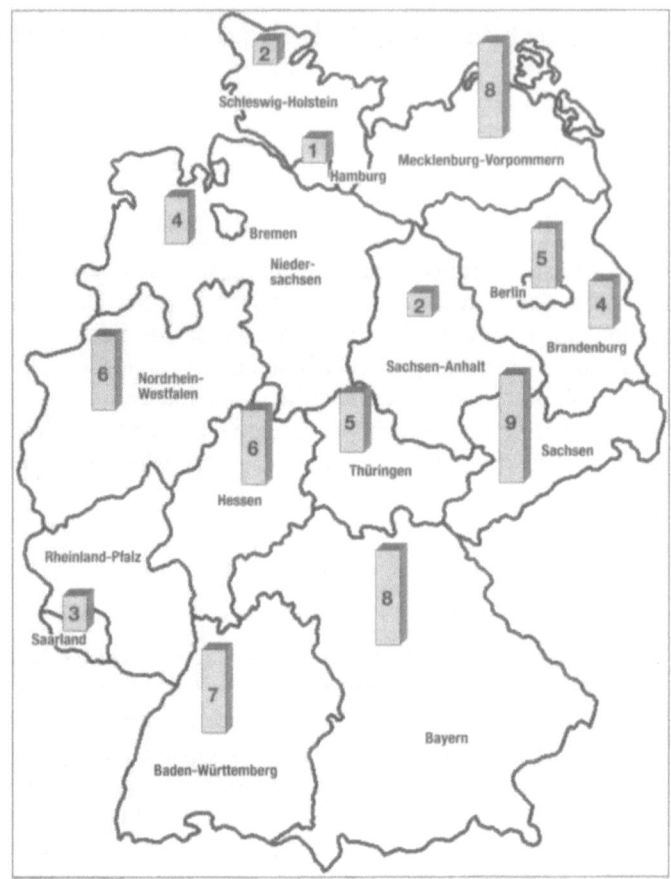

Fig. 1. Distribution of reporting hemophilia centers in Germany

hemophilia A (47.94%), B (8.52%) and patients with von Willebrand disease (43.54%) is given in Figure 3.

When severity of disease is analyzed with a cut-off of 2% factor activity, the distribution between the two subgroups, i.e. below 2% and above 2%, is similar in patients with hemophilia A and B as shown in Figure 4.

In 4.92% of the patients with hemophilia A and in 2.48% of the patients with hemophilia B an inhibitor was found (see Fig. 5 and Table 2). 25% of patients with von Willebrand disease showed ristocetin co-factor levels below 30% as demonstrated in Figure 6 and Table 2.

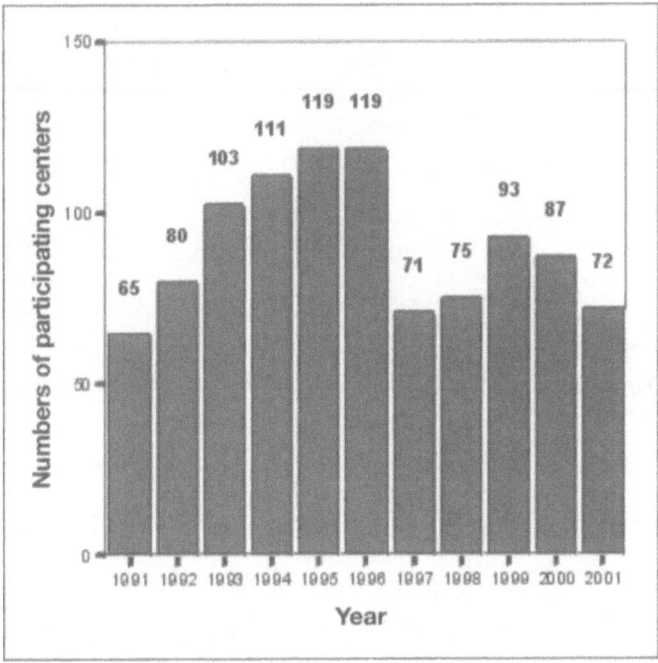

Fig. 2. Numbers of participating hemophilia centers

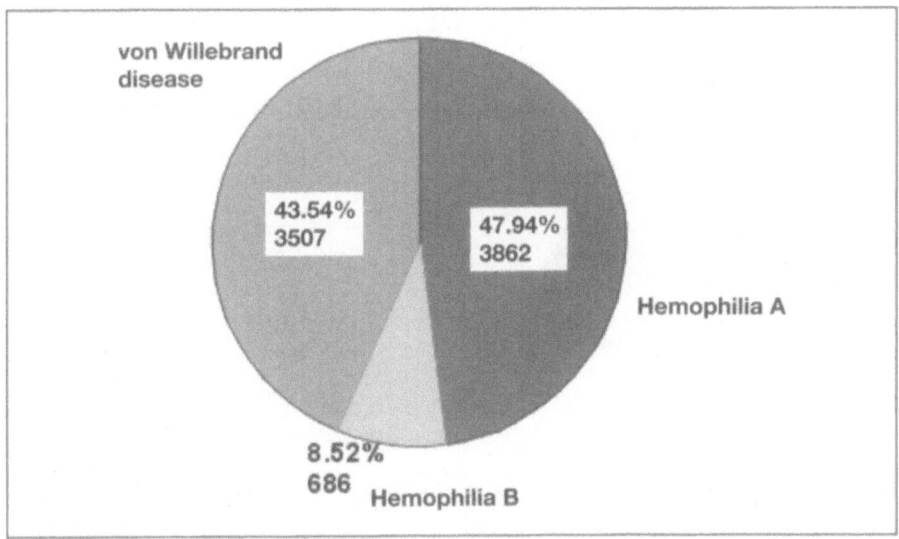

Fig. 3. Overall distribution of diseases

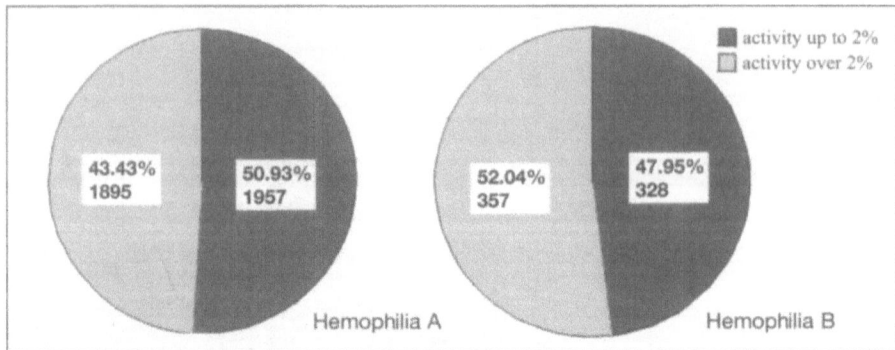

Fig. 4. Distribution of factor VIII/IX activity in patients with hemophilia A and B

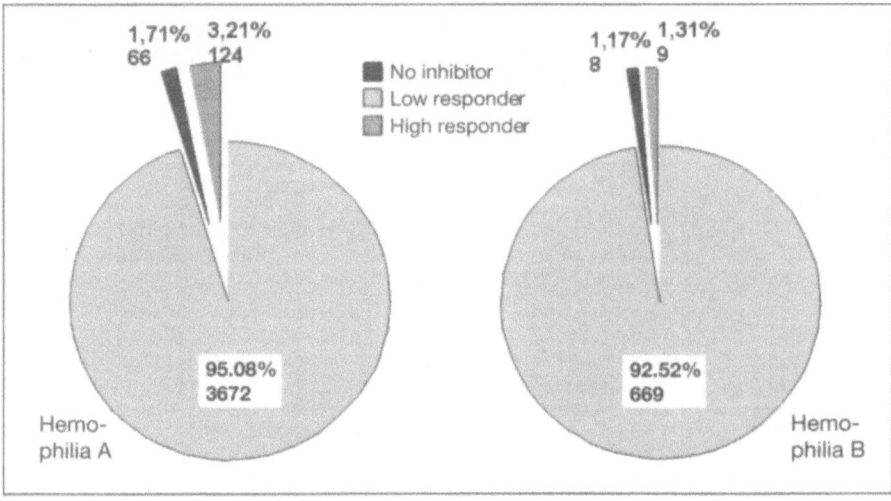

Fig. 5. Distribution of inhibitors in patients with hemophilia A and hemophilia B

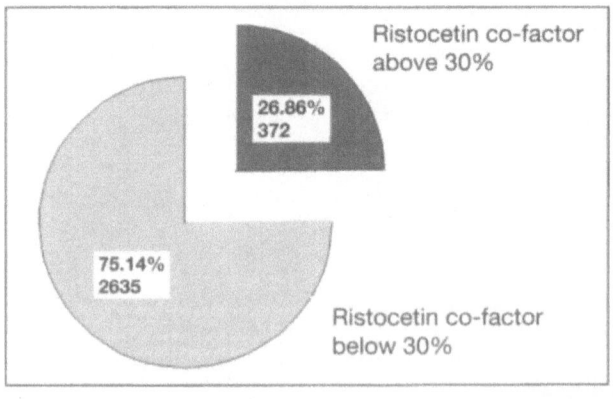

Fig. 6. Distribution of ristocetin co-factor in patients with von Willebrand disease

Table 2. Cumulative data from 72 centers as of 2000/2001

	Hemophilia A		Hemophilia B		von Willebrand disease		Total
	N	%	N	%	N	%	N
Total	3862	47.95%	686	8.52%	3507	43.57%	8055
Factor activity ≤ 2%	1967	50.93%	329	47.96%	–	–	2296
Factor activity > 2%	1895	49.07%	357	53.04%	–	–	2252
Ristocetin Co-factor ≤ 30%	–	–	–	–	872	24.86%	872
Ristocetin Co-factor > 30%	–	–	–	–	2635	75.14%	2635
Inhibitor (low responders)	66	1.71%	8	1.17%	–	–	74
Inhibitor (high responders)	124	3.21%	9	1.31%	–	–	133
Total HIV negative	3227	–	603	–	3291	–	7121
Total HIV positive	589	–	82	–	9	–	680
HIV positive, no AIDS	244	–	46	–	5	–	295
HIV positive, CD4<200 cells/µl	146	–	9	–	1	–	156
HIV positive, full blown AIDS	30	–	3	–	1	–	34
HIV positive, no comment	169	–	24	–	2	–	185

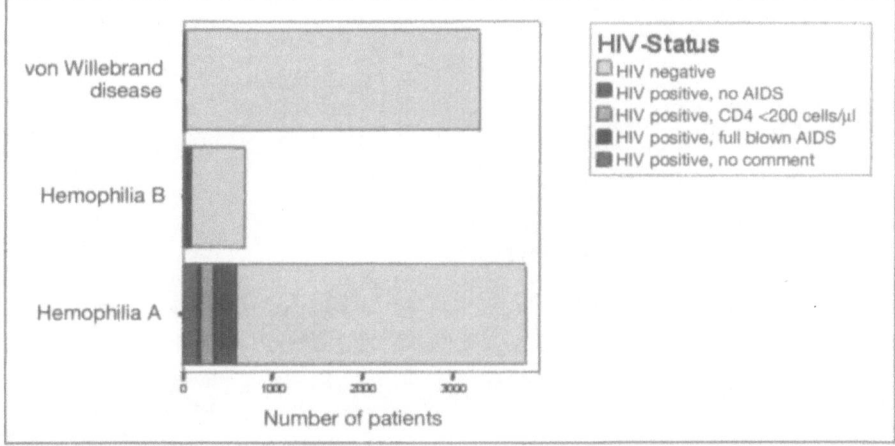

Fig. 7. Distribution of HIV-infected patients

Table 3. HIV status

HIV status	Hemophilia A	Hemophilia B	von Willebrand disease	Total
HIV negative	3227	603	3219	7121
HIV positive, no AIDS	244	46	5	295
HIV positive, CD4+ < 200 cell/μ	146	9	1	156
HIV positive, full-blown AIDS	30	3	1	34
HIV positive, no comment	169	24	2	195
Total HIV positive	589	82	9	680

HIV Status

Of all reported patients a total of 680 were infected with HIV, equivalent to 8.4%. Analyzed for HIV distribution in subgroups 15.2% of all patients with hemophilia A, 12.0% of all patients with hemophilia B, and 0.3% of all patients with von Willebrand disease were HIV-infected (Fig. 7). A total of 34 patients (5.0%) has reached the stage of full-blown AIDS, compared to 244 patients (35.9%) that have up to now not shown severe symptoms of the immune disease (Table 3).

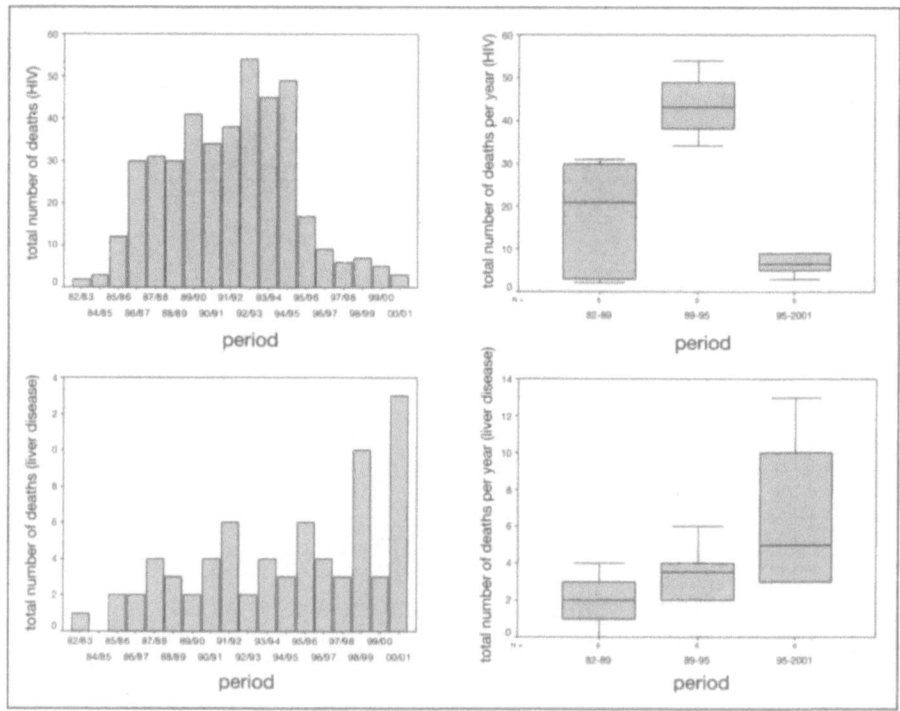

Fig. 8. Total number of deaths of HIV compared to total number of deaths of liver disease

Table 4. Distribution of death causes

Patients	N	%
Died of AIDS	3	8.3
Died of liver disease	13	36.1
Died of bleeding	6	16.7
Died of cancer	3	8.3
Died of other diseases	6	16.7
Died, no comment	5	13.9
Total	36	100.0

Causes of Death

In the 2000/2001 period a total of 36 patients were reported dead with the distribution of causes of death given in Table 4. Since the beginning of the survey in 1982, a total of 690 patients have been reported dead. Unfortunately this year again a noticeable increase of deaths was reported, corresponding to a rise of 80% compared to the last years survey. In particular this is due to the sharp increase of patients died of liver disease. The development of mortality and causes of death since 82/83 are depicted in Figure 9 and Figure 10.

Up to 1995 the number of AIDS-related deaths increased continuously with decline taking place since. AIDS-related deaths again receded this year. The main reason for this development can probably attributed to improved antiretroviral therapies.

When analyzing the data (Table 4) it is striking that liver disease has become the far most important cause of death in this survey. The reason for this may be the increasing number of liver cirrhosis due to Hepatitis C. Arranging data for greater periods one can see this effect obviously, although not yet statistically significant (Fig. 8). The future development of a possible correlation should be observed carefully.

No indications for Creutzfeld-Jakob disease in our patient collective has been reported since 1978.

GTH Hemophilia Registry

The German Society of Thrombosis and Hemostasis (GTH) is currently establishing a central registry accessible to all German centers treating patients with bleeding disorders. The goal is to set up a suitable and easy to use system for acquiring and analyzing epidemiologic data of diseases related to bleeding disorders, HIV and hepatitis infection. An offline- and online-version of the registry was established (Fig. 11). For both systems a data security concept was developed and approved by official authorities. This project is supported by an unrestricted grant from Wyeth Pharma GmbH.

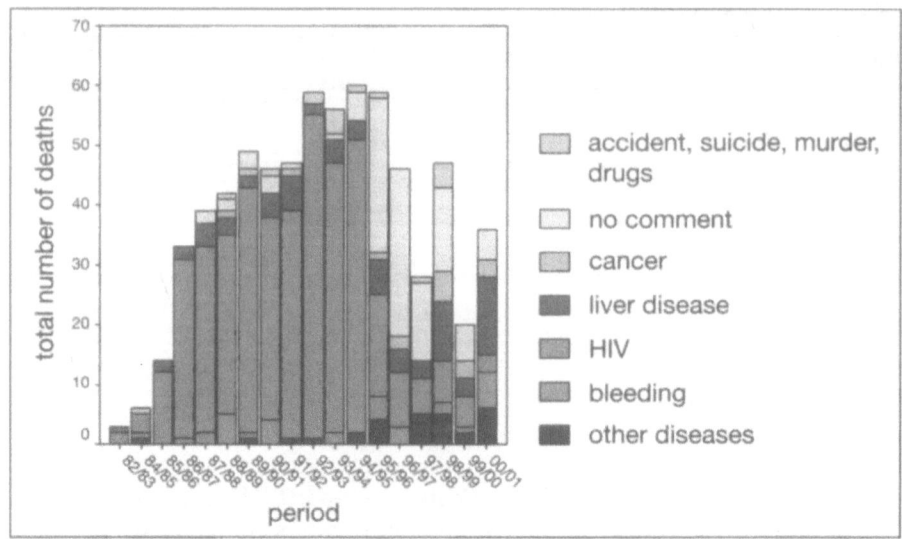

Fig. 9. Causes of death since the beginning of the survey

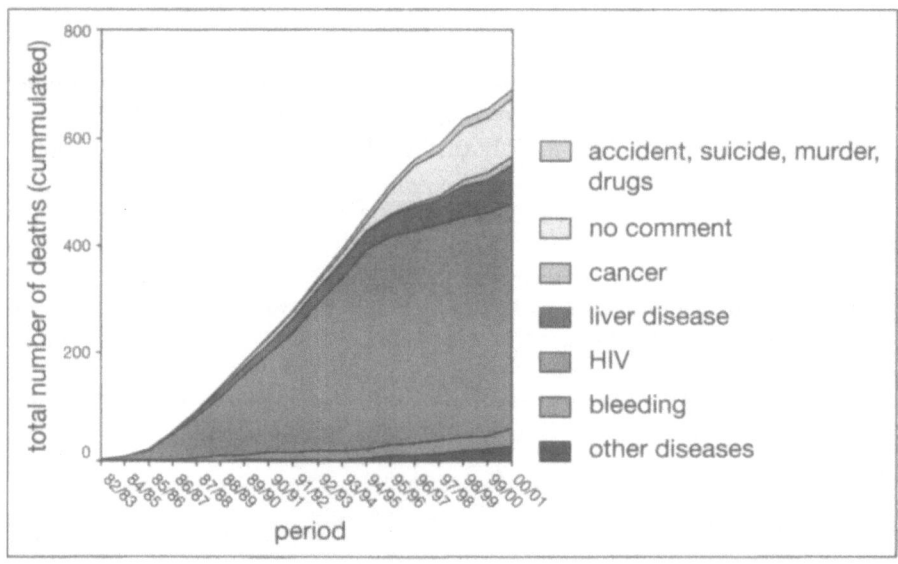

Fig. 10. Cumulative chart of deceased patients, separated for causes of death

Acknowledgment. Peter Heidemann, Astrid Heidemann, Augsburg; Schlimok, Linné, Augsburg; K. Rager, Bad Mergentheim; Lothar Hempelmann, Berlin; Günter Henze, Frau U. Schulte Overberg-Schmidt, Berlin; Christiane Beck, Dorothea Kroll, Berlin; Ch. Heinrichs, Frau Stumpe, Berlin; H. Koop, M. Klare, Berlin; H. Kiesewetter, Koscielny, Berlin; H.H. Brackmann, Bonn; Wolfgang Eberl, Braunschweig; G. Auers-

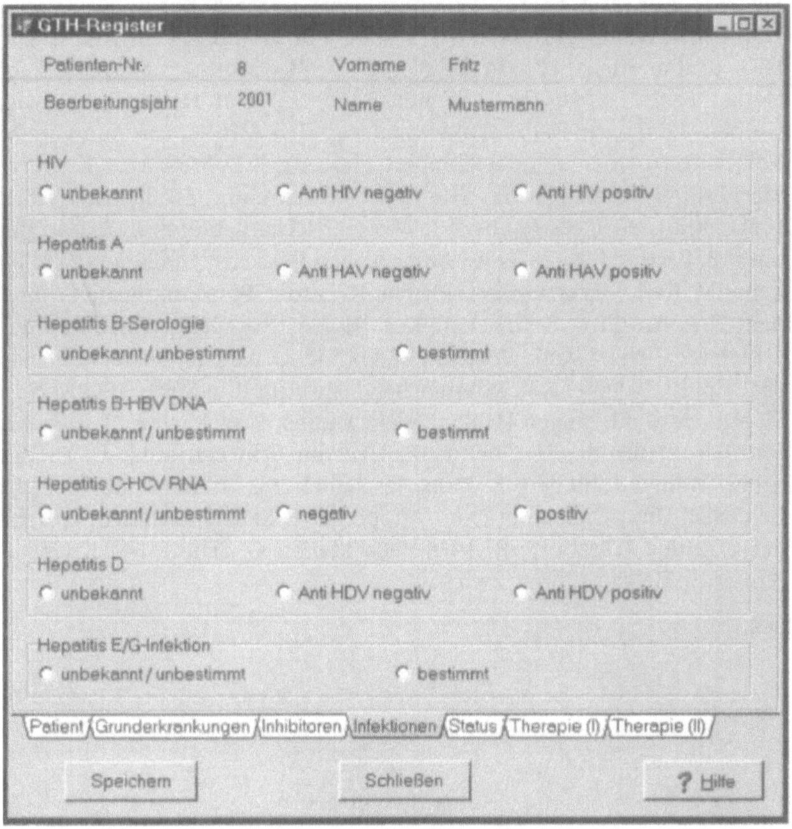

Fig. 11. Offline-Version of the GTH Hemophilia Registry

wald, Bremen; Holzhüter, Bremen; H. Leithäuser, Celle; F. Fiedler, Kerstin Wolf, Chemnitz; Klaus Hofmann, Chemnitz; J. Oppermann, Elisabeth Holfeld, Dagmar Möbius, Cottbus; Johann Böhmann, Claudia Niekrens, Delmenhorst; Joachim Mößeler, Dillingen; Wolfgang Kotte, Heiner Güldenring, Dresden; Jörg Wendisch, Dresden; Heiner Trobisch, Duisburg; U. Göbel, Lex, Düsseldorf; G. Vogel, Frau Winterstein, Erfurt; Jens Klinge, M. Girisch, Erlangen; R. Eckstein, Erlangen; Christian Klinkenstein, Frankfurt (Oder); Frau I. Scharrer, Frankfurt/Main; W. Kreuz, Klarmann, Frankfurt/Main; W. Mondorf, Frankfurt/M; Antje Nimtz, Frankfurt/Oder; A.H. Sutor, Barbara Ziegler, Freiburg; R. Mertelsmann, Karola Hasler, Freiburg; Pralle, PD Bettina Kemkes-Matthes, Gießen; G. Berger, Wilke (I Med), Doris Joachim, Görlitz; Rosemarie Schobeß, Halle-Wittenberg/S; Anatol Kurme, Bernhard Pauka, D.K. Hossfeld, Barbara Eifrig, Hamburg; Rolf Kuse, Wittkowsky, Hamburg; Schneppenheim, N. Muenchow, Hamburg; L. Balleisen, Hamm; A. Ganser, M. von Depka, Hannover; K. Welte, C. Wermes, Hannover; Rainer Zimmermann, Heidelberg; E. Wenzel, Pindur, Homburg /Saar; F.C. Sitzmann, Gerd

Dockter, Annegret Seider, Homburg/Saar; F. Zintl, Karim Kentouche, Jena; K. Höffken, K. Wollina, Fricke, Jena; Hirschmann, Frau B. Eggeling, Kassel; U.R. Fölsch, H.D. Bruhn, Kiel; Eckhard Lechler, Köln (Lindenthal); Mario Koksch, Leipzig; Harald Lenk, Leipzig; H. J. Siemens, Lübeck; Peter Hellstern, Ludwigshafen; R. Herbert, Lüneburg; D. Franke, Magdeburg; Uwe Mittler, von Aumann, Magdeburg; Volker Kretschmer, Monika Weippert, Marburg; K.U. Freiberger, K. Morgenschweis, Mechernich; Karin Kurnik, München; W. Schramm, München; H. Pollmann, Sr. Heike, Münster; C. G. Lipinski, J. Weisser, Neckargemünd; R. Arndt, Neubrandenburg; B. Berthold, Neubrandenburg; Jürgen Drescher, Oldenburg; Th. Wüst, Pforzheim; M. Karl, Maria Anstadt, Plauen; R. Pasold, Potsdam; Beate Schmeltzer, Potsdam-Drewitz; Prof Andreesen, Karl Huber, Regensburg; H. Konrad, Rostock; I. Richter; Ulrike Kyank, Rostock; M. Freund, O. Anders, Rostock; Bernhard Maak, Saalfeld; P.C. Clemens, R. Schumacher, Schwerin; Rita Subert, Schwerin; F.J. Göbel, Siegen; Osswald, Singen (Hohentwiel); Günter Syrbe, Schw. M. Stephan, Schw. H. Hädrich, Stadtroda; H. Edelmann, Heidrun Schwarz, Suhl; D. Niethammer, H. Scheel-Walter, Tübingen; L. Kanz, Jaschonek, M. Mohren, Tübingen; Debatin, W. Behnisch, Ulm; Dieter Böttcher, Wuppertal; F. Keller, U. Geisen, Würzburg; Speer, Petra Zeitler, Würzburg; Richter, Zella Mehlis; G. Schott, Ute Kreibich, Zwickau; Nentwich, Helga Gräbner, Zwickau

Hemophilia 2001 –
The Annual Survey of the Austrian Hemophilia Centers

U. Eidher, H.K. Hartl, U. Kunze, P. Arends, J. Falger, N.D. Jones,
M. Kronawetter, P. Kurnik, I. Pabinger, H. Ramschak, E. Reiter,
R. Schwarz, W. Streif, H. Türk, H. Wank, W. Zenz and K. Zwieauer

Patients and Methods

Each year the Institute of Social Medicine of Vienna (ISM) organizes the annual survey of the Austrian Hemophilia Centers where the anonymous questionnaires from all collaborating centers are collected and analyzed.

The patients data are collected by the co-authors of this report using specially designed questionnaires. To simplify the work for the survey, the centers receive their data report from the year before to compare and/or to complete their files.

The analysis 2001 shows the distribution of the patients within the Austrian counties in respect to the place where they live, the number of patients according to the severity of the disease and the distribution according to age. Further the type of the disease and the number of HIV-infections among Austria's hemophilia patients are analyzed.

For the first time we could receive data from centers in Vorarlberg this year. Unfortunately there is still a lack of data concerning adult patients in Tyrol and Upper Austria so that we still cannot show the complete epidemiological situation, but quite a representative overview on hemophilia in Austria in the year 2001.

Results

In total there are 508 patients with hemophilia registered. Their files are used for presentation of the following criteria:
– Hemophilia type and severity of the disease
– HIV-infection among the population
– Distribution within the Austrian counties
– Distribution according to age

Severity of the disease

We received data from 403 patients, 350 (68,9%) suffer from hemophilia A and 53 (10.4 %) from hemophilia B. There is a lack of information concerning the hemophilia type in 20.7 % of patients.

I. Scharrer/W. Schramm (Ed.)
32nd Hemophilia Symposium Hamburg 2001
© Springer-Verlag Berlin Heidelberg 2003

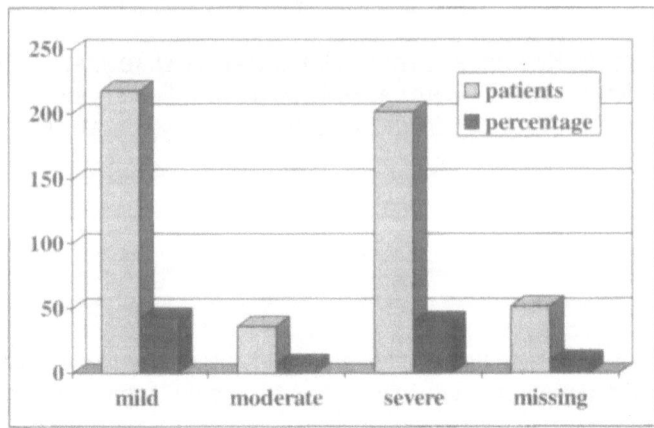

Fig. 1. Severity of the disease

The relation of patients with mild hemophilia to patients with the severe form in hemophilia A as well as in B, is similar, the relation of hemophilia A to hemophilia B is according to the literature.

Concerning the severity of the disease, 218 patients (42.9 %) show the mild form, 36 (7.1 %) the moderate and 202 (39.8 %) the severe form. Information is missing on 52 patients (10.2 %).

Distribution within Austria

The distribution of patients in the Austrian counties gives information on the registration as well as on the participation in the survey itself.

Counties like Lower Austria, Styria and Vienna, where most of the Austrian patients are registered, have reached a very high standard of documentation. But concerning for example average age there is a bias, because of still missing information from Tyrol and Upper Austria.

Table 1. Number of patients according to counties

County	Total	Percentage	Cumulative percent
Burgenland	19	3.7	3.7
Carinthia	34	6.7	10.4
Lower Austria	132	26.0	36.4
Upper Austria	31	6.1	42.5
Salzburg	20	3.9	46.5
Styria	109	21.5	67.9
Tyrol	13	2.6	70.5
Vorarlberg	5	1.0	71.5
Vienna	145	28.5	100.0
Total	508	100.0	

Age

The average age is 32.86 +/- 20.0 years. The oldest patient is 95, the youngest 2 years old. 96 patients are younger and 387 older than 15 years, information on age is missing in 25 patients.

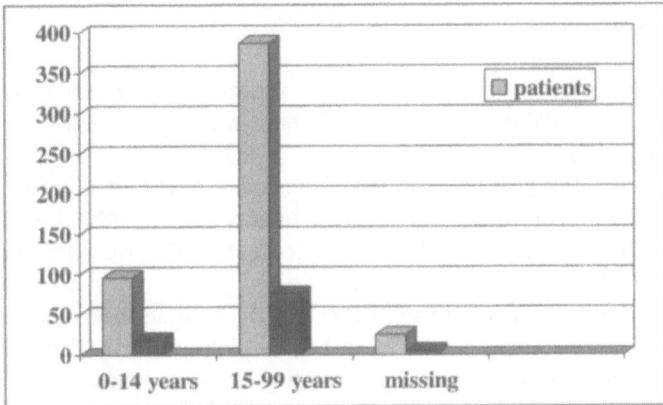

Fig. 2. Age

Table 2. Type of hemophilia according to counties

County		Hemotype		
		Hem. A	Hem. B	Total
Burgenland	number	13	3	16
	% of county	81.3%	18.8%	100.0%
Carinthia	number	20	1	21
	% of county	95.2%	4.8%	100.0%
Lower Austria	number	83	11	94
	% of county	88.3%	11.7%	100.0%
Upper Austria	number	27	1	28
	% of county	96.4	3.6%	100.0%
Salzburg	number	16	–	16
	% of county	100.0%	–	100.0%
Styria	number	79	25	104
	% of county	76.0%	24.0%	100.0%
Tyrol	number	13	–	13
	% of county	100.0%	–	100.0%
Vorarlberg	number	5	–	5
	% of county	100.0%	–	100.0%
Vienna	number	94	12	106
	% of county	88.7%	11.3%	100.0%
Total	number	350	53	403
	% of county	86.8%	13.2%	100.,0%

HIV infection

Unfortunately the data concerning HIV in our 2001 survey is less complete than in the year 2000 so that we used the 2000's survey's data in which 52 patients were HIV infected, 45 with hemophilia A and 7 with hemophilia B.

Discussion

The annual survey on hemophilia shows a representative overview on hemophilia in Austria though there is still data missing, especially on HIV infection and Hepatitis B.

For the year 2002 we have created a new and more simple to handle questionnaire, in which we also included questions on other bleeding disorders as there is for example von-Willebrand disease as well as questions concerning Hepatitis B and Hepatitis C.

Further we would of course like to include more and more hospitals in our survey to come closer to the real epidemiological situation. With the already collected data we now have the possibility of getting other important information, for example concerning home treatment, use of factor concentrates, frequency of treatment center visits, compliance, psycho-social and quality-of-life questions and other informations.

Finally we would like to thank all participants of the annual survey on hemophilia in Austria for their useful and successful cooperation.

Epidemiology of Hemophilia in Switzerland: A first Insight in the Data Base achieved by the Medical Committee of the Swiss Hemophilia Association

E. O. MEILI

Aim of the Swiss hemophilia data base

The medical committee of the Swiss hemophilia association decided in 1995 to set up a hemophilia data base. The aim was
1. to get an overview of hemophilia epidemiology in Switzerland.
2. to make the most important data of hemophilia patients available to treaters especially for situations patients ask for treatment in another than their original hemophilia centre.

Therefore the purpose was more a practical one than a scientific.

Data collection

Reporting of data from the 19 treatment centers began in 1996. The registry is managed by Serena Hartmann MD, a member of the medical committee, who developed software together with a computer specialist.

Patients suffering from the following coagulation disorders are registered: Hemophilia A and B with factor VIII/IX $\leq$ 30%[1]; von Willebrand disease with Ristocetin cofactor $\leq$ 30%, or > 30% with severe bleeding tendency (mainly type 2B); afibrinogenemia; clinically severe cases of homozygous or compound heterozygous factor XIII-, VII- and combined V/VIII-deficiency. At present there are no other clinically severe plasmatic factor deficiencies in Switzerland. Patients are identified by BGA code, date of birth and zip code. The coagulation disorder is defined by the missing coagulation factor, it's residual activity and the actual and earlier inhibitor status. Concerning treatment, the administered coagulation concentrate and the modality of administration (on demand, prophylactic) are registered. An update is once a year done. With the next update it is planned to extend the data base with the amount of used concentrates per year and the date of the last examination in the centre.

---

[1] According to the latest ISTH-definition for severity of hemophilia, patients with factor VIII/IX levels from <1 – <40% will be recorded in the data base with the next update (ThrombHaemost 2001;85:560)

I. Scharrer/W. Schramm (Ed.)
32nd Hemophilia Symposion Hamburg 2001
© Springer-Verlag Berlin Heidelberg 2003

Table 1. Data from the Swiss hemophilia data base (October 2001)

	Hemophilia A	Hemophilia B
Mean age	37.7 y	32.4 y
Severity		
severe <1%	148 (35%)	28 (28%)
moderate 1–5%	93 (22%)	42 (43%)
mild >5–30%	180 (42%)	25 (26%)
Inhibitors		
neg.	67%	82%
pos.	5%	1%
unknown	28%	17%
Treatment modality		
on demand	309 (73%)	76 (77%)
prophylaxis	75 (18%)	20 (21%)

Data

At the end of October 2001 complete data of 651 patients were collected: 421 patients with hemophilia A, 95 with hemophilia B, 85 with von Willebrand disease and 50 with other factor deficiencies.

The mean age of patients, severity of coagulation disorder, inhibitor status and treatment modality are shown in the table. From 1996 to 2001 21patients died at a mean age of 59 years (25–88); in non HIV-infected patients the mean age at death was 68 years (33–88), in six HIV-infected 46 years (25–55). The cause of death in two non HIV-infected patients was an intracranial hemorrhage (57 y, 88 y), in the remaining cardiovascular diseases, malignancies and one accident.

Overall Blood Supply Strategy with Regard to vCJD

R. Seitz

Introduction

While the »classical« Creutzfeldt-Jakob disease (CJD) has been transmitted in rare cases by therapeutic application of human brain-associated materials such as dura mater transplants or injection of pituitary hormones, there has been no documented transmission of CJD via human blood or blood products. The same is true also for the variant of CJD (vCJD). This rather new disease is thought to be a manifestation of BSE in humans, and both BSE and vCJD have been observed mainly in UK (Fig. 1). It is encouraging that in a neuropathological study of 33 UK deceased hemophilia patients, who had been treated for years with UK-sourced plasma products, no sign of vCJD was found [1]. However, the observation time has been too short yet to draw any conclusion on epidemiological grounds as to the transmissibility of vCJD by blood. In contrast to classical CJD, infectivity is found in lymphatic tissues of vCJD patients. Moreover, experimental data from several species point to the possibility that a low level of infectivity is present in their blood. Also the preliminary results of a transfusion experiment in sheep [2] raised such concerns. Taken together, the possibility of vCJD transmission by blood and blood products can so far neither be proven nor excluded.

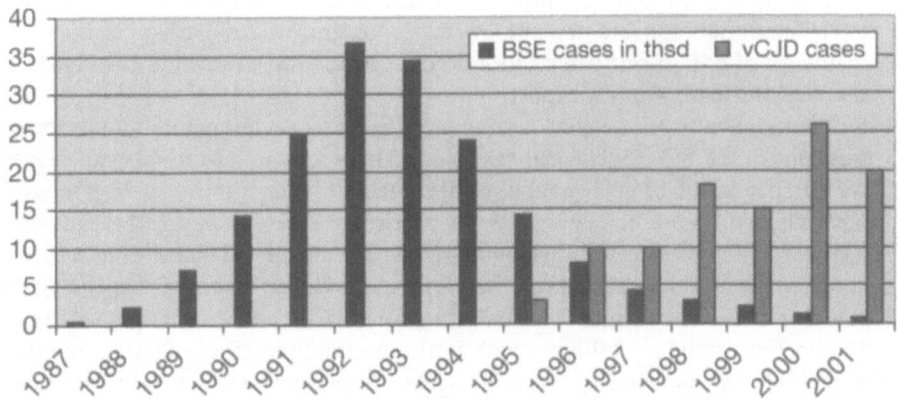

I. Scharrer/W. Schramm (Ed.)
32nd Hemophilia Symposion Hamburg 2001
© Springer-Verlag Berlin Heidelberg 2003

In such an unclear situation, to be on the safe side, it appears wise to treat such a hypothetical risk seriously and to consider any sensible precautionary measures. Following this line, the German Federal Minister of Health asked the president of the Paul-Ehrlich-Institut (PEI), Prof. Johannes Löwer (chairperson), and the chairman of the Arbeitskreis Blut, Prof. Reinhard Burger, to convene a group of experts in order to elaborate an overall blood supply strategy with regard to vCJD. This group met several times in order to review the existing statistical, epidemiological and experimental data in relation to the evolution, spread and future projection of BSE and vCJD as well as the risk of primary infection from the food chain and the possibility of secondary infection via human materials such as blood. This data base was used in order to elaborate an assessment of the vCJD risk in Germany and other European countries and to derive precautionary measures.

The comprehensive report of the group was published by the Federal Minister of Health, Mrs. Ulla Schmidt, on 16 October 2001 [3]. Besides the executive summary, the report contains a comprehensive compilation of scientific data and references to numerous official documents and assessments. In this short contribution, only some essential statements of the report shall be mentioned:

- The EU-wide ban on the processing of BSE risk materials, which has been in force since 1 October 2000, is aimed at preventing the transmission of BSE to humans. The rigorous observance of this ban is the essential precondition for ensuring that there is no further spread of vCJD as a result of foodstuffs contaminated with the BSE agent.
- By extrapolation of estimates in the UK [4], in »worst case« scenarios for France and Germany up to a total of 300 to 600 persons incubating vCJD after infection via foodstuffs would be expected. Overall, it is assumed that there will be no significant difference in the incidence of cases of vCJD in the various countries of West and Central Europe, with the exception of the United Kingdom. It is true that in some continental European countries (e.g. France) vCJD cases have already been observed. However, for estimating the number of individuals eventually incubating vCJD, and the evolution of vCJD in the upcoming years, the exposure to risk materials appears to be of crucial importance. A comparison of the peak incidence of BSE in cattle in relation to the population is shown in the Figure 2, reproducing Table 4 of the report.
- It is not known to what extent secondary infections, i.e. human to human transmissions of the vCJD agent, can take place. There are no indications whatsoever for a transmission of the agent by social contact. Investigations in animal models have yielded contradictory results; in particular cases, however, the causative agent of a spongiform encephalopathy can be detected in the blood, even if in low concentrations. As a precaution, therefore, it should be assumed that the agent can also be found in human blood in the case of vCJD, and in fact up to a titre of 10 infectious units per milliliter with intravenous administration (10 IU-iv/ml).
- A possible *transmission of the vCJD agent via* plasma products (e.g. immunoglobulins, albumin, *factor concentrates for hemophilia patients*) appears *very unlikely*, since the agent is already removed to a large extent during the manufacture of these blood products. Should the vCJD agent be transmissible via blood transfusions, this could however represent the only remaining route for its further

Table 4: BSE incidence at the peak of the BSE epidemic (reported cases of animals with clinical symptoms)

Country	Year (peak of the epidemic)	Number of cattle with clinical BSE	Cattle stock (age >2 years) in 1000 animals in specified year	Incidence (BSE cases per 1 million animals)	Human population (in millions)	Clinical BSE cases per 1 million inhabitants
UK	1992	36,682	6,196.1	5,920	58.015	632
Portugal	1999	170	715.8	237	10.03	17
Switzer-land	1995	68	810.3	84	7.166	6
Ireland	1999	91	3,853.9	24	3.753	24
France	2000	101	11,033.0	9	59.329	1.7
Belgium	1998	6	1,470.2	4	10.202	0.6

Fig. 2. Table 4 of the strategy paper [3]; right column shows relation between peak number of BSE cases and population for selected countries

spread (secondary infections) among the human population in addition to the theoretically conceivable transmission by surgical instruments.

- This secondary route of transmission could be prevented to a large extent if there were a suitable *detection test* that could be performed on each blood donation in order to screen the donation for the presence of the vCJD agent. *High priority should be given to the promotion of such projects.*
- In the meantime, other precautionary measures should be taken to prevent the theoretically conceivable transmission of vCJD by transfusion. Already in force are:
  - the exclusion of people as donors who spent more than 6 months in total in the United Kingdom between 1980 and 1996,
  - the separation of the white blood cells (leucodepletion) in the manufacture of red cell and platelet preparations, which would remove some of the vCJD agents, if they were present in the donated blood,
  - as another effective precautionary measure for reducing the potential risk of transmitting infectious agents, including vCJD, initiatives towards the critically indicated application of blood products (»optimal use«).
- Assuming that the route of infection via the food chain has been blocked in the mean time, a hypothetical way of »recycling« vCJD transmission might be supposed, via blood donated by people who have themselves received transfusions and thus been exposed to a theoretical risk of a vCJD infection. This hypothetical route could be prevented by excluding transfusion recipients from donating blood. Such a measure would affect around 4% of blood donors in Germany, a loss that according to the blood donation services would be difficult to overcome, in view of the prevailing blood shortage.

- Before the introduction of any exclusion of transfusion recipients from donating blood, sufficient measures would therefore have to be taken to guarantee the long-term stability of the blood supply in Germany. These measures would include making the most of potential savings (»optimal use of blood and blood products«) and the implementation of suitable advertising and motivational campaigns for the recruitment of donors.

The Ministry of health had mandated the group to analyze the situation and measures already in place and to explore possible future scenarios. The aim was to be prepared to take further precautions, if necessary, but equally important, to help to avoid unreflected overreactions under the impression of new situations. The paper was published to inform the public, and particularly patients and treating physicians about the situation and the thoughts of the authorities.

The group reinforced previous assessments and the measures already in place, and underlined the priority of developing suitable test methods. After revision of the current state of knowledge, the group could arrive at the statement that a transmission of vCJD by plasma derivatives, including hemophilia products, is highly improbable.

References

1. Lee, C.A., Ironside, J.W., Bell, J.E., Giangrande, P., Ludlam, C., Esiri, M.M., McLaughlin, J.E. Retrospective Neuropathological Review of Prion Disease in UK Hemophilic Patients. Thrombosis and Haemostasis, 80:909–911, 1998
2. Houston, F., Foster, J.D., Chong, A., Hunter, N., Bostock, C.J.:
   Transmission of BSE by blood transfusion in sheep.
   The Lancet, 356:999–1000, 2000
3. Report of the Working Group Overall Blood Supply Strategy with regard to vCJD. August 2001. Available on the PEI website under http://www.pei.de/pm/2001/14_2001.htm
4. Ghani, A. C., N. M. Ferguson, C. A. Donnelly, and R. M. Anderson. Predicted vCJD mortality in Great Britain. Nature 406:583–584, 2000

II. Genetic Diagnosis of Clotting Disorders

Chairmen:

E. O. MEILI (Zurich)
I. SCHARRER (Frankfurt/Main)

IIa. Human Genome Project

11 novel Mutations in the Factor VIII encoding Gene lead to severe or moderate Hemophilia A

C. Uen, N. Klopp, J. Oldenburg, H.-H. Brackmann, W. Schramm, R. Schwaab, and J. Graw

Summary

In Germany, approximately 5800 patients are suffering from hemophilia A. In a systematic large-scale analysis we will identify the genotype of all severe cases (approximately 3000 patients). A first screening for mutations causing hemophilia A analyzes the exons from genomic DNA by methods like DGGE, SSCP or dHPLC. Since this approach covers only approximately 97% of the mutations, the *FVIII* gene of the remaining patients has to be sequenced in total. Therefore, all exons including their flanking regions were amplified and subsequently sequenced. Here, we describe the results for a set of 35 patients. In 8 patients mutations have been identified, which have been described previously. Additionally, 11 novel mutations have been characterized during this study in 12 patients. The mutations are mainly base pair substitutions. The second group are deletions or insertions of 1 bp; only in one case, 4 nucleotides have been inserted. The mutations are predicted to cause amino acid exchanges or frameshifts leading to premature stop codons close to the mutation points. However, in 14 patients no mutation could be identified neither within the coding area nor in the promoter or the 3'-UTR of the *FVIII* gene. This indicates the need to consider also further noncoding regions of the *FVIII* gene to be causative for hemophilia A, like the intron-22 genes *F8A* and *F8B*.

Additionally, in 7 patients two known polymorphisms in exon 14 have been observed; however, only one of these leads to an amino acid exchange (D1241E). Moreover, in 8 of our patients a known polymorphic site in the 3'-UTR of exon 26 was identified. A further polymorphism was observed in the intron 7 in two patients. This polymorphic site was not reported in the HAMSTeRS database. It remains to be elaborated whether these polymorphisms have any influence on the stability of the FVIII mRNA (intron and 3'-UTR) or the processing of the protein (exon 14).

Introduction

Hemophilia A is caused by heterogeneous mutations in the gene coding for factor VIII (gene symbol: *FVIII*); it maps to Xq28 and consists of 26 exons. The genomic region covers approximately 186 kb and encodes for a mature protein of 2332 amino acids. The main cause (40–50%) for severe cases of hemophilia A is a homologous

I. Scharrer/W. Schramm (Ed.)
32nd Hemophilia Symposion Hamburg 2001
© Springer-Verlag Berlin Heidelberg 2003

recombination involving intron 22 and related sequences outside the *FVIII* gene (Naylor et al., 1993; Lakich et al., 1993).

For the detection of the other mutations affecting the *FVIII* gene, a number of mutation screening methods like the denaturing gradient gel electrophoresis (DGGE), single-strand conformation polymorphism (SSCP), conformational sensitive gel electrophoresis (CSGE) and chemical mismatch cleavage (CMC) have been applied. Most of these studies resulted in a mutation detection rate of 80–95% (Schwaab et al., 1997; for recent review see Oldenburg, 2001). Using these techniques, more than 600 mutations within the *FVIII* gene have been described in all coding as well as in some untranslated regions; for an overview refer to the hemophilia A mutation database *(http://europium.csc.mrc.ac.uk/usr/WWW/ WebPages/main.dir/main.htm)*. Despite the heterogeneity in *FVIII* mutations, carrier detection and prenatal diagnosis can be done by direct detection of selected mutations.

From a cohort of approximately 600 patients, the mutation could not be identified in 36 cases by the screening methods described above. Therefore, we established a direct sequencing protocol for the coding region including the promoter and the 3'-UTR of the *FVIII* gene. Among this subgroup of 36 patients, we could characterize the mutations in 20 cases, 11 of which have not yet been described in the HAMSTeRS database. Unexpectedly, 16 patients did not show a mutation neither in the coding region including the flanking intronic sequences, the promoter and the 3'-UTR thus suggesting further allelic or non-allelic regions to be causative for a Hemophilia A phenotype.

Material & Method

Patients were collected at the Hemophilia Center, University of Bonn, and written consent was received from all patients included into this study. DNA was prepared as described previously (Becker et al., 1996). 36 patients with hemophilia A were examined, which demonstrated no positive result in mutation screening methods (Southern-blot, CMC, DGGE, dHPLC; Becker et al., 1996; Oldenburg, 2001).

All 26 exons of the *FVIII* gene were amplified by PCR including flanking intron sequences. Most primer pairs and conditions were chosen according to the HAMSTeRS database; conditions for the promoters, for exons 3, 4 and 14 as well as for the 3'-UTR were optimized. Amplification of exons 21 and 22 were done as described by Vidal et al. (2001). Purified PCR products were sequenced; the data were managed by the program package Vector NTI (Suite 6.0; InforMax, Oxford, UK).

Results

We established a systematic high throughput sequencing in those hemophilia A patients, where no mutation was detected previously by CMC, DGGE or dHPLC screening methods (Oldenburg, 2001). Among 36 patients, we characterized 20 at the molecular level. The results are given according to the scheme in the HAMSTeRS database.

The mutations included 7 small insertions (4 of them in repeats), 1 deletion and 13 bp exchanges (two of them occurred in two patients). In 4 patients, the mutation leads immediately to a new stop codon; in 5 other cases, only a few new amino acids (between 2 and 26) were included followed by a premature stop codon. No mutations have been found in 16 patients.

Polymorphic sites

Moreover, during the systematic sequencing of the 36 patients, three known polymorphic sites were identified (Table 1): the first one occurs three times in this set of patients and could not be considered as causative for the phenotype. In the coding region, one of these additional polymorphic sites is located within codon 1241; the C→G exchange at the nucleotide level leads to a Asp→Glu exchange. This mutation effects one amino acid within the proteolytically removed B domain; therefore, it is concluded to be without effect on the FVIII activity. The causative mutations for two of the corresponding patients (#2 and 8) could not yet be identified; for patient #11 it is a stop codon further downstream in exon 14.

Additionally, the silent polymorphic site in exon 14 at codon 1269 (A→C, Ser→Ser) was observed in four patients and does not have any consequence for the amino acid composition. Moreover, the known polymorphic site in the 3'-UTR of exon 26 (position 8728 A→G) was confirmed in 6 patients (2, 8, 11, 15, 20, 28).

A novel polymorphism was identified in intron 7 in two patients (#8 and 11). While in patient 11 a causative nonsense mutation was found in exon 14, no mutation could be observed in patient 8 to be causative for the phenotype.

Table 1. Polymorphic Sites without Obvious Influences on the FVIII Activity

Region	Patients	Variation	Position	Consequence	HAMSTeRS
Promoter	24				
Intron 7	8;11	G→C	nt 32 (#271 according to M88635)	splicing?	novel
Exon 14	2; 8; 11	C→G	codon 1241	D→E	known
Exon 14	15; 20; 28; 42	A→C	codon 1269	S→S	known; Frequency 6% in Caucasians; 18% in oriental populations
Exon 26 (3'-UTR)	2, 8, 11, 15, 20, 28	A→G	position 8728	m-RNA-Stability?	known

Known mutations

Among the 36 patients tested, 9 mutations were identified, which are already described in the HAMSTeRS database (Table 2). One of them (C901T) was found twice (patients 25 and 29). In three patients, the mutations were observed in regions of high mutation frequency (R593C; R2159; R2116X; R2307Q). The 4 insertions observed in exon 14 occurred all in short polyA stretches.

Table 2. FVIII mutations described in the HAMASTeRS database

Exon	Patient	Mutation	nt cDNA	Codon	Amino Acid Exchange	Domain	Phenotype	HAMSTeRS (Frequency and Phenotype)	Antibody (HAMSTeRS)
7	29	C→T	901	282	R→C	A1	severe	1x mild	
7	25	C→T	901	282	R→C	A1	?		?
12	12	C→T	1834	593	R→C	A2	moderate	22x moderate/mild	yes
14	16	insA	3300–3301	1081	new 15aa, X	B	severe	1x severe	no
14	42	insA	3637–3638	1193	new 27aa, X	B	severe	3x severe	yes
14	18	insA	4379–4380	1441	N→K, X	B	severe	8x severe, 1x moderate	no
14	28	insA	4826–4827	1590	new 3aa, X	B	severe	3x severe	no
26	10	C→T	6537	2159	R→C	C1	mild	23x moderate/mild	no
26	41	G→A	6978	2307	R→Q	C2	moderate	13x moderate/mild	no

Novel mutations

11 novel mutations were identified in the coding region, which were not yet described (Table 3a, b). 6 of them create new stop codons and lead to truncations of the protein; three of them within the B domain. Most interestingly, the del7013 mutation leads to a loss of the last 14 amino acids and to a severe form of hemophilia A.

Moreover, also the mutations A440T, Val128Asp, A5834G, Met1925Val affect amino acids, which are important for the function of the protein. The exchange of an amino acid with a hydrophobic side chain (Val) by an acidic amino acid (Asp) caused a severe form of hemophilia A, while the exchange of one hydrophobic amino acid (Met) by another one (Val) leads to a rather moderate form of hemophilia A. Both missense mutations might be expected to be causative, as no polymorphisms are known in this region despite excessive analysis of more than 600/1000 patients (HAMSTeRS database). Moreover, other missense mutations in the very close neighbourhood (e.g. Asp126His; Asn1922Ser; Asn1922Asp; Gly1923Arg) have been reported in HAMSTeRS to be causative for hemophilia A.

Table 3. Novel Mutations in the FVIII Gene
a) Novel Mutations in the Coding Region

Exon	Patient	Mutation	nt cDNA	Codon	Amino Acid Exchange	Domain	Phenotype
4	24	A→T	440	128	V→D	A1	severe
14	11	T→G	2496	813	Y→X	B	severe
14	15	A→T	2893	946	K→X	B	severe
14	20	insT	3417–3418	1120	new 26aa, X	B	severe
17	13	insT	5696–5697	1880	new 3aa, X	A3	severe
18	27	A→G	5834	1926	M→V	A3	moderate
18	9	ins GGAG	5968–5972	1971	new 2aa, X	A3	severe
26	31	delC	7013	2319	L→X	C2	severe

b) Novel Mutations in Introns Leading most Likely to Splicing Defects

Intron	Patient	Mutation	Location	Effect on Splicing	Phenotype
22	35	T→A	2 nt	no splicing, new ORF?	severe
22	6	G→T	5 nt	no splicing, new ORF?	severe
22	39	G→T	5 nt	no splicing, new ORF?	moderate

Additionally, two novel mutations were observed in intron 22 (Table 3b). In patient 35, a T→A exchange was observed 2 bp downstream of the end of exon 22. This T at the intron position #2 is essential for correct splicing in all introns analyzed so far (Tarn and Steitz, 1997). Therefore, it is suggested that the altered splice site creates a novel ORF leading to a loss of FVIII activity. The other exchange affects the 5th bp downstream of the end of exon 22 (in patients 6 and 39) and is characterized as a G→T exchange. This particular position in the intron is not as conserved as the first two positions (Tarn and Steitz, 1997). Therefore, the consequence of this particular intron mutation on the FVIII protein remains to be elaborated. However, without the analysis of the mRNA no further suggestion can be made yet. In the HAMSTeRS database, no mutation affecting intron 22 is described so far.

No mutations

Unexpectedly, in 16 patients out of this subgroup of 36, no mutation could be identified in the *FVIII* coding region nor in the promoter or 3'-UTR region of the *FVIII* gene. It has to be recognized that this subgroup of 36 patients represents a pre-selected cohort from a total of 600 patients, which have been investigated before by rapid screening methods. Clinically, all these patients are suffering from a severe or moderate hemophilia A.

Discussion

Molecular characterization of hemophilia A is well established; more than 600 entries have been collected in the HAMSTeRS database. The most common mutation in the *FVIII* gene is the inversion affecting exon 22 and a homologous telomeric sequence leading to the inactivation of the *FVIII* gene. Additionally, also deletions of all sizes, insertions, and base-pair exchanges have been found and are mainly identified with screening methods like CMC or dHPLC. Therefore, for the remaining cases it was necessary to sequence the entire *FVIII* gene. Using this approach we could characterize mutations in 20 patients and identify 11 novel mutations, which have not been described before. They cover the A1, B, A3 and C2 domain, but also the splice sites in intron 22.

Most interestingly, in 16 patients no mutation could be detected in the entire coding region, the flanking intron sequences, the promoter nor the large 3'-UTR, which might be attributed to the phenotype. In patients #2 and 8, polymorphic alterations have been observed in intron 7, exon 14 and in the 3'-UTR. However, since they occur several times and also in patients with other mutations causative for the corresponding phenotype, they have to be considered not to contribute to the disease in these cases.

This observation is in line with the report by Vidal et al. (2001), who could not identify a mutation in one of his patients. Obviously, it is a rare but not a unique finding, which occurs in approximately 2% of the diagnosed hemophilia A patients (16 out of 600 as reported here or 1 out of 45 as reported by Vidal et al., 2001). In these cases further mutations loci have to be considered to be causative for the hemophilia A phenotype. These mutation loci might be located either within the *FVIII* gene (e.g. affecting regulatory elements upstream of the promoter region or the introns) or may be non-allelic and related to proteins, which interact with the FVIII protein during its synthesis or its function in the blood. Two such examples have been discovered recently: Mutations in the FVIII-binding region of *vWF* gene (encoding the von Willebrand factor) have been found to cause clinical features similar to hemophilia A (Mazurier et al., 1990; Gaucher et al., 1991). In our patients, mutations in this region have been excluded by direct sequencing of the respective exons 18–20 of the *vWF* gene (R. Schneppenheim, personal communication). Another form of a hemophilia A like phenotype combined with factor V deficiency is caused by a mutation in the *ERGIC53* gene coding for an endoplasmatic reticulum – Golgi intermediate compartment protein. The gene is hypothesized to have a chaperone function involved in the secretion process for both, FV and FVIII. The mutation, therefore, leads to a loss of activity of these factors and a hemophilia A like phenotype (Nichols et al., 1998). Therefore, it might be concluded that in approximately 2% of the diagnosed hemophilia A patients further investigations remain necessary to elaborate the underlying molecular lesion.

Acknowledgment. The expert technical assistance of Klara Fizi is gratefully acknowledged. Part of this work was supported by a grant from the German Human Genome Project (DHGP) to HHB, JG, JO, RS and WS (01KW9905). Part of the work was performed using the technical resources at the Genome Analysis Center (GAC) at the GSF-Research Center.

References

1. Becker J, Schwaab R, Möller-Taube A, et al. Characterization of the factor VIII defect in 147 patients with sporadic hemophilia A: Family studies indicate a mutation type dependent sex ratio of mutation frequencies. Am J Hum Genet 1996;58:657–670.
2. Gaucher C, Jorieux S, Mercier B, Oufkir D, Mazurier C. The »Normandy« variant of the von Willebrand disease: Characterization of a point mutation in the von Willebrand factor gene. Blood 1991;77:1937–1941
3. Lakich D, Kazazian HH jr, Antonarakis SE, Gitschier J. Inversions disrupting the factor VIII gene as a common cause of severe hemophilia A. Nat. Genet 1993;5:236–241
4. Mazurier C, Dieval, J., Jorieux S, Delobel, J, Goudemand M. A new von Willebrand factor (vWF) defect in a patient with factor VIII (FVIII) deficiency but with normal levels and multimeric patterns of both plasma and platelet vWF. Characterization of abnormal vWF/FVIII interaction. Blood 1990;75:20–26.
5. Naylor JA, Green PM, Pizza CR, Gianelli F. Analysis of factor VIII mRNA levels reveals defects in everyone of 28 haemophilia A patients. Hum. Mol. Genet. 1993;2:11–17
6. Nichols WC, Seligsohn U, Zivelin A, et al. Mutation in the ER-Golgi intermediate compartment protein ERGIC-53 cause combined deficiency of coagulation factors V and VIII. Cell 1998;93:61–70.
7. Oldenburg J. Mutation profiling in haemophilia A. Thromb Haemost 2001;85:577–9
8. Schwaab R, Oldenburg J, Lalloz MRA, Schwaab U, Pemberton S, Hanfland P, Brackmann H-H, Tuddenham EGD, Michaelides K. Factor VIII gene mutations found by a comparative study of SSCP, DGGE and CMC and their analysis on a molecular model of factor VIII protein. Hum Genet 1997;101:323–32.
9. Tarn W-Y, Steitz JA. Pre-mRNA splicing: the discovery of a new spliceosome doubles the challenge. Trends Biochem. 1997; 22:132–7.
10. Vidal F, Frassac E, Altisent C, Puig L, Gallardo D. Rapid hemophilia A molecular diagnosis by a simple DNA sequencing procedure: identification of 14 novel mutation. Thromb Haemost 2001; 85:580–3

IIb. Register and Genetic Diagnosis

Molecular Analysis of Hemophilia B: »Greifswald Registry FIX Deficiency (Hemophilia B)«

K. Wulff, W. Schröder, F.H. Herrmann and the study group*

Abstract

Hemophilia B (HB) is due to multiple defects in the factor IX gene. More than 90% of mutants are single substitutions, small additions (<30bp) or small deletions. In the »Greifswald registry FIX deficiency (hemophilia B)« the FIX mutations from 289 hemophilia B patients from 14 different countries were analyzed. These 289 FIX gene mutations include 257 point mutations: 193 (66.8%) missense mutations, 43 (14.9%) nonsense mutations, 13 (4.5%) splice site variations and 7 (2.4 %) point mutations in the promotor region. In 32 (11%) of all patients gene deletion, insertions or gene rearrangements were analyzed. These 298 FIX gene mutations represent 178 different FIX lesions. 123 of all are unique mutants which were found in only one family. 55 mutants were detected repeatedly, at least in two unrelated patients.

---

*Study group »GREIFSWALD REGISTRY OF FIX DEFICIENCY (HEMOPHILIA B)« Almagro, Cuba; Auerswald G., Bremen; Barthels M., Hannover; Becher, Frankfurt/Main; Bergmann F., Bremen; Blanco A., Buenos Aires (Argentina); Borjas L., Maracaibo (Venezuela); Brackmann Ch., Bonn; Bratanoff E., Erfurt; Bykowska X., Warsaw (Poland); De Bosch N., Caracas (Venezuela); Demuth, Erfurt; Eberl W., Braunschweig; Eifrig B., Hamburg; Escuriola-Ettingshausen C., Frankfurt; Franke D., Magdeburg; Ganser A., Hannover; Gazda H., Warsaw (Poland); Gencik, Frankfurt; Ghafer, A.-A., Singapore; Gilberg E., Neubrandenburg; Goebel U., Düsseldorf; Göhmann, Delmenhorst; Grimm T., Würzburg; Güldenring, Dresden; Haubold, Bielefeld; Heinrichs Ch., Berlin; Hempelmann L., Berlin; Hinkel G.-K., Dresden; Hulst, Berlin; Ivaskevicius V., Vilnkus (Lithuania); Kallas A., Tartu (Estonia); Klarmann D., Frankfurt/Main; Kley, Freiburg; Kluba U., Magdeburg; Kobelt R., Bern (Switzerland); Kretschmer V., Marburg; Kreuz W., Frankfurt/Main; Kurme A., Hamburg; Lenk H., Leipzig; Lopaciuk S., Warsaw (Poland); Mitulla B., Suhl; Nagy A., Pecs (Hungary); Nißle, Dresden; Nohe N., München; Oldenburg O., Bonn; Peter-Salonen K., Switzerland; Pindur G., Homburg; Pollmann H., Münster; Rauch, Erlangen; Roos, München; Rott, Erlangen; Ruiz-Saez A., Caracas (Venezuela); Salazar-Sanchez L., Costa Rica; Salazes N., Costa Rica; Scharrer I., Frankfurt; Scheel H., Leipzig; Schmeltzer B., Potsdam; Schobeß R., Halle; Schröder, Bremen; Schulte-Overberg U., Berlin, Serban M., Timisoara (Romania); Stuhe-Southeisser, Venkirche; Stuhrmann-Spangenberg, Hannover; Sutor A., Freiburg; Szergert, Hungary; Trobisch, Duisburg; Verma J.-C., India; Vogel G., Erfurt; Vorlova Z., Prague (Czechian); Weippert M., Rostock; Wending, Göttingen; Wendisch J., Dresden; Wenzel E., Homburg; Wolf H.-H., Halle; Wolf K., Chemnitz; Zeitler, Würzburg; Zimmermann R.-E., Münster.

I. Scharrer/W. Schramm (Ed.)
32nd Hemophilia Symposion Hamburg 2001
© Springer-Verlag Berlin Heidelberg 2003

Most mutations were detected in the codons Arg(-4), Arg180, Arg248 and Thr296. All these frequent lesions are located in a CpG island a hot spot for mutations. The same origin of these frequent mutations in all cases is not likely.

The results of this study emphasize the high molecular heterogeneity of hemophilia B.

Introduction

Hemophilia B is a recessive X-linked bleeding disorder caused by a deficiency of the clotting factor IX (F IX). The F IX gene is located on the long arm of X chromosome at Xq 27 and the genomic sequence was analyzed by Yoshitake et al. (1985).

The product of the F IX gene is a polypeptide of 415 amino acids (aa) preceded of a pre-pro signal peptide. The circulating F IX consists of a Gla domain and two epidermal growth factor-like (EGF) domains separated from the serine protease domain by an activation region (Yoshitake et al. 1985).

The available data (Database, FIX mutation, Green et al. 2000) clearly indicate that hemophilia B is highly heterogeneous at the molecular level. The spectrum of mutations which causes hemophilia B is different in the populations. Repeatedly observations in apparently unrelated individuals generally occur at either CpG dinucleotides or by founder effects (Peake et al. 1995, Tuddenham at al. 1994).

In the »Greifswald registry FIX deficiency (hemophilia B)« we analyzed the molecular basis of hemophilia B in unrelated patients from 14 different countries by analysis of the factor IX gene.

We have undertaken efforts to characterize the mutations of the F IX gene in 289 unrelated patients as a part of international wide approach to provide an efficient hemophilia B genetic counseling service. The results of the mutation study shall be summarized here.

Material and Methods

Patients

We have investigated more than 300 unrelated patients from different clinical centres from Germany and from Argentina, Czechia, Costa Rica, Cuba, Estonia, Hungary, India, Lithuania, Poland, Romania, Singapore, Switzerland and Venezuela (Table 1) with severe form of hemophilia B (F IX activity < 1 %), with moderate form (FIX activity 1% to 5%) and mild hemophilia B with FIX activities > 5% to 40% (White et al. 2001).

DNA studies

DNA was isolated from 10 ml EDTA blood, from white blood cells by standard methods (Miller et al. 1988).

PCR primer pairs for the FIX gene, derived from the F IX sequence (Yoshitake et al. 1985) and PCR conditions were described previously (Wulff et al. 1995, 1997c).

Table 1. »Greifswald study factor IX deficiency (hemophilia B)«: Origin of the hemophilia B patients

Countries	(symbols)	Number of unrelated patients
Germany	(G)	174
Poland	(P)	70
Argentina	(A)	11
India	(I)	7
Hungary	(H)	4
Lithuania	(Li)	4
Romania	(R)	3
Costa Rica	(CR)	3
Switzerland	(S)	3
Czechia	(C)	4
Cuba	(Cu)	2
Singapore	(Si)	2
Estonia	(E)	1
Venezuela	(Ve)	1

Southern blotting

The FIX gene was analyzed by Southern blot analysis after restriction of genomic DNA with endonuclease Eco RI or Taq I using a cDNA probe of the FIX gene (Herrmann et al. 1990).

Sequencing

The double-stranded PCR products were purified and concentrated in Microcon 100 concentrators (Amicon GmbH). The sequence analysis was performed as a cycle sequencing procedure using the Big Dye Terminator Cycle Sequencing Ready Reaction Kit Applied Biosystems and the automatic sequencer type 373 A from Applied Biosystems (Wulff et al. 1995).

Results and Discussion

In the »Greifswald registry FIX deficiency (hemophilia B)« in more than 300 HB patients all factor IX gene regions of likely functional significance were analyzed. In 289 unrelated HB patients a mutation in different parts of the FIX gene was detected (Table 2 and 3 and Fig. 1).

The 289 FIX lesions represent 178 different mutants. 123 mutants were unique molecular events.

Gross gene lesions (>30bp) were identified in 14 unrelated patients. 4 complete FXI gene deletions (Fig. 1) and 8 partial gene deletions were analyzed. 8 (67%) of these hemophilia B patients have developed factor IX antibodies (an inhibitor) after replacement therapy.

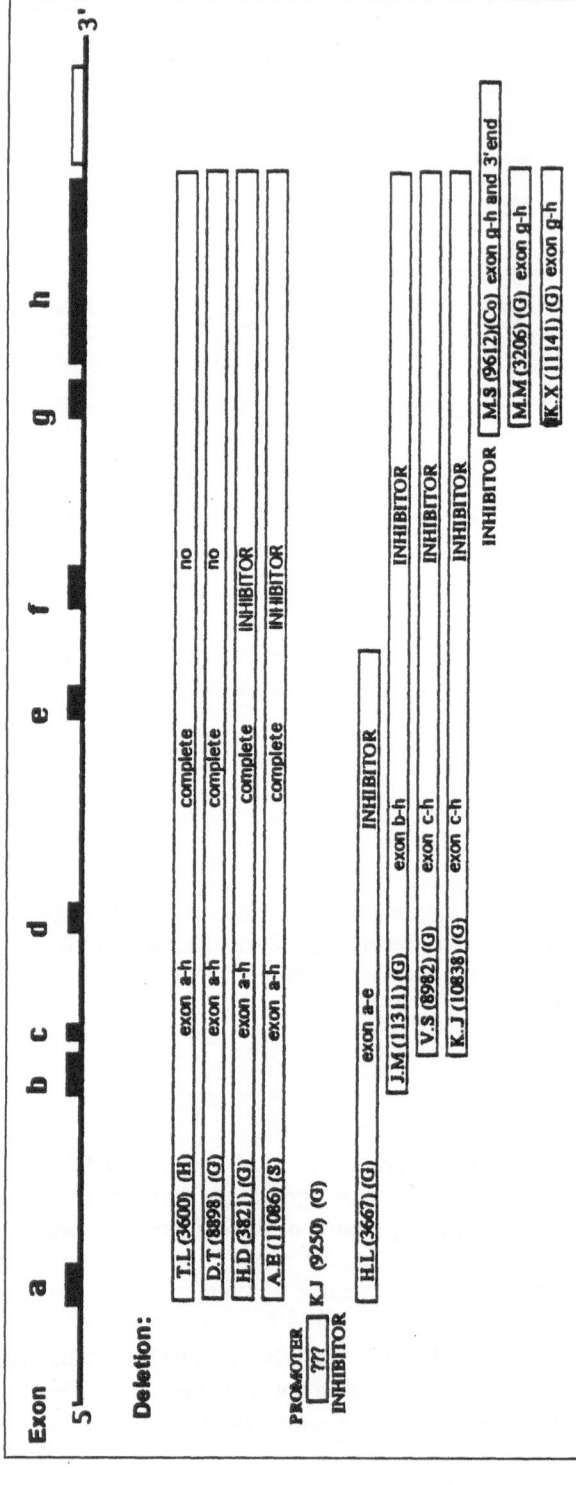

Fig. 1. Large factor IX gene deletions (<30bp) analyzed in the » Greifswald study FIX deficiency (hemophilia B)«

Table 2. Greifswald study factor IX deficiency (hemophilia B): Results of the mutation analysis in 289 unrelated patients

Type of Mutation	Number Mutants (%)	Number Repeated Mutants	Number Unique Mutants
Missense	193 (66.8%)	37	80
Nonsense	43 (14.9%)	9	10
Promoter	7 (2.4%)	–	7
Splice site	13 (4.5 %)	4	8
Donor splice site	10	1	8
Acceptor splice site	3	3	–
Deletions (<30bp)	17 (5.9%)	2	11
– in frame	5	1	2
– out frame	12	1	9
Branch site	1 (0.3%)	–	1
Insertions (<30bp)	1 (0.3%)	–	1
Summary	275 (95.2%)	52	118
Deletion >30bp	12 (4.2%)	3	3
– complete deletion	4	1	–
– partial deletion	8	2	3
Insertion >30 bp	1 (0.3%)	–	1
Chromosomal rearrangements	1 (0.3%)	–	1
Total	**289** (100%)	55	123

A large gene insertion, an addition of an Alu repeated element in exon e (Wulff et al. 2000) was analyzed in one patient. In a Polish hemophilia B patient was detected a chromosomal rearrangement (Schröder et al. 1998).

Gross deletions or insertion are easily detectable by standard methods. These lesions were found by Southern blot analysis of patient's DNA. The most lesions, point mutations, small nucleotide deletions or insertions could be defined by sequencing.

In 257 of the 289 (89%) examined patients with hemophilia B (Table 3) point mutations in a functional important region of the factor IX gene were identified (Herrmann et al. 1993, 1996, 1996a, 1997, 1997b, 1998, 1998a, 1999, Schröder et al. 1998, Wulff et al. 1994, 1994a, 1995, 1997, 1997a, 1999).

Single base mutations cause in 193 (66.8%) patients an amino acid substitution (missense mutations), in 43 (14.9%) patients a stop codon (nonsense mutations), in 13 (4.5%) cases a splice site variation. In 7 (2.4%) cases a promoter mutation and in one a branch site variation were found.

Small deletions of 1, 2, 3 or 6 base pairs were identified in 17 patients.

The 289 analyzed mutations represent 156 different types of single base substitutions in the promoter region, the exons or the splice sites of the factor IX gene (Table 2 and 3). FIX gene lesions were detected most frequently in the codons

Table 3. Point mutations and small deletions/ insertions (< 30 bp) in the FIX gene »Greifswald study factor IX deficiency (hemophilia B)«

Patient IDN	Pat. Origin	Clinical	Codon No.	Nucleotide Substitution	Exon No.
52	(P)	severe	Promoter	−26G>A	−
11459	(Ve)		Promoter	−24A>G	−
3792	(G)	moderate	Promoter	−20T>A	−
11228	(G)	severe	Promoter	−6G>A	
9845	(G)		Promoter	7T>C	−
9069	(I)		Promoter	9C>G	
3587	(G)		Promoter	13A>C	−
9189	(G)	mild	Ile(−40) Phe	48A>T	a
11294	(G)		Frame shift stop(−24)	81insCT	a
9169	(G)		Frameshift stop (−27)	del 84C	a
43	(P)	moderate	Cys(−19) Arg	111T>C	a
9280	(G)		Val(−17) Ile	117G>A	a
9857	(G)		IVSA+1G>A inhibitor	118G>A	IVSA
55	(P)	severe	IVSA+5G>A	122G>A	IVSA
37	(Si)		Donor splice delGTTT	del121−124	IVSA
3703	(G)	(female<15)	Asn(−11)Thr	6344A>C	b
8205	(R)		Arg(−4) Trp	6364C>T	b
1989	(G)	severe	Arg(−4) Trp	6364C>T	b
9232	(G)		Arg(−4) Trp	6364C>T	b
8478	(G)		Arg(−4) Trp	6364C>T	b
9171	(Li)		Arg(−4) Trp	6364C>T	b
10892	(I)		Arg(−4) Trp	6364C>T	b
10892	(I)		Arg(−4) Trp	6364C>T	b
31	(P)	severe	Arg(−4) Gln	6365G>A	b
48	(P)	severe	Arg(−4) Gln	6365G>A	b
3571	(P)	severe	Arg(−4) Gln	6365G>A	b
2252	(G)	severe	Arg(−4) Leu	6365G>T	b
2271	(G)	severe	Arg(−4) Leu	6365G>T	b
2272	(G)	severe	Arg(−4) Leu	6365G>T	b
8783	(G)	moderate	Arg(−4) Leu	6365G>T	b
11292	(G)	severe	Arg(−4) Leu	6365G>T	b
2269	(G)	severe	Lys(−2)delA frame shift	del 6370A	b
14	(P)	moderate	Arg(−1) Ser	6375G>T	b
3	(P)	severe	Glu7 Val	6395A>T	b
44	(P)	severe	Glu8 Asp	6399G>C	b
2705	(G)	severe	delArg15-Glu16	6420-25 del GAGAGA	b
3282	(G)	moderate	Cys18 Arg	6427T>C	b
9759	(G)	mild	Cys18 Arg	6427T>C	b
2232	(A)	moderate	Glu20 Val	6434A>T	b
9410	(G)	severe	Lys22delA frame shift	del 6440A	b
3408	(G)	severe	Cys23 Arg	6442T>C	b
9536	(G)		Cys23 Arg	6442T>C	b
3149	(A)	mild	Phe25 Ser	6449T>C	b
9503	(G)		Phe25 Ser	6449T>C	b
9172	(Li)		Glu26 Gln	6451G>C	b
2133	(H)		Arg29 stop	6460C>T	b
2225	(A)	severe	Arg29 stop	6460C>T	b
2230	(A)	severe	Arg29 stop	6460C>T	b

Table 3. Continued

Patient IDN	Pat. Origin	Clinical	Codon No.	Nucleotide Substitution	Exon No.
2237	(A)	moderate	Arg29 stop	6460C>T	b
3168	(G)	severe	Arg29 stop inhibitor	6460C>T	b
9048	(G)		Arg29 stop	6460C>T	b
65	(P)		Arg29 stop	6460C>T	b
2254	(G)	severe	Glu30 stop	6463G>T	b
2277	(G)	mild	Glu33 Asp	6474A>C	b
11466	(G)		IVSB branch site?	6653A>G	IVSB
2309	(Cu)		IVSB–1G>A acceptor splice	6677G>C	IVSB
2249	(G)	mild	Tyr45 Cys	6697A>G	c
1	(P)	severe	Asp47 Asn donor splice	6702G>A	d
1759	(P)	severe	IVSC+4A>G	6706A>G	IVSC
53	(P)	moderate	IVSC+5G>A	6707G>A	IVSC
9030	(G)		Gly48 Val	10395G>T	d
11154	(G)		Cys56 Ser	10418T>A	d
9174	(G)	(female)	Cys62 Tyr	10437G>A	d
2257	(G)	severe	Tyr69 Cys	10458A>G	d
2332	(S)	severe	Cys73 Phe	10470G>T	d
8135	(G)	moderate	Cys82 Tyr	10497G>A	d
2489	(G)	severe	IVSD-3T>C acceptor splice	17665T>C	IVSD
6	(P)	severe	Cys88 Arg	17677T>C	e
2798	(G)	(female)	Cys88 Tyr	17678G>A	e
2265	(G)	mild	Ile90 Thr	17684T>C	e
9182	(I)		Asn92 Asp	17689A>G	e
33	(P)	severe	Cys109 Phe	17741G>T	e
1760	(P)	severe	Ser110 Pro	17743T>C	e
62	(P)	severe	Ser110 Pro	17743T>C	e
8032	(G)	severe	Cys111 Arg	17746T>C	e
2243	(G)	moderate	Gly114 Glu	17756G>A	e
2268	(G)	mild	Gly114 Glu	17756G>A	e
2059	(G)	moderate	Gly114 Glu	17756G>A	e
11296	(G)		Gly114 Glu	17756G>A	e
9222	(G)		Gly114 Arg	17775G>A	e
3590	(G)	(female)	Tyr115 Cys	17759A>G	e
8650	(G)	moderate	Arg116 Arg	17761C>A	e
9274	(G)	moderate	Arg116 Arg	17761C>A	e
9556	(G)	severe	Arg116 stop	17761C>T	e
9371	(G)		Arg116 stop	17761C>T	e
2228	(A)	moderate	Gln121 His	17778G>T	e
2235	(A)	moderate	Gln121 His	17778G>T	e
2367	(A)		Gln121 His	17778G>T	e
11347	(G)	(female 14%)	Ser123 Ser	17784C>T	e
			Csy124 Phe double mutation	17786G>T	e
8070	(G)	severe	Ser123 Ser	17784C>T	e
			Csy124 Phe double mutation	17786G>T	e
8743	(G)	moderate	Ala127 Ala	17796A>G	e
9760	(G)	severe	Ala127 Ala	17796A>G	e

Table 3. Continued

Patient IDN	Pat. Origin	Clinical	Codon No.	Nucleotide Substitution	Exon No.
3647	(I)		IVSE+1G>A donor splice	17798G>A	IVSE
9509	(I)	(female)	IVSE+1G>A donor splice	17798G>A	IVSE
2276	(G)	severe	Cys132 Trp	20376T>G	f
8235	(G)	moderate	Arg145 Cys	20413C>T	f
8260	(G)		Arg145 Cys	20413C>T	f
8923	(G)		Arg145 Cys	20413C>T	f
8720	(G)	moderate	Arg145 Cys	20413C>T	f
11255	(G)	mild	Arg145 Cys	20413C>T	f
2253	(G)		Arg145 His	20414G>A	f
3997	(G)		Arg145 His	20414G>A	f
8987	(G)	moderate	Arg145 His	20414G>A	f
9426	(G)	moderate	Arg145 His	20414G>A	f
64	(P)	mild	Arg145 His	20414G>A	f
11098	(G)	moderate	Arg145 His	20414G>A	f
11233	(G)		Arg145 His	20414G>A	f
69	(P)		Arg145 Pro	20414G>C	f
9861	(G)		Ala146 del C frame shift	del 20417C	f
1763	(P)		Arg180 Trp	20518C>T	f
34	(P)	severe	Arg180 Trp	20518C>T	f
11580	(CR)		Arg180 Trp	20518C>T	f
11469	(G)	severe	Arg180 Trp	20518C>T	f
11380	(G)	severe	Arg180 Trp	20518C>T	f
2130	(H)		Arg180 Gln	20519G>A	f
2132	(C)		Arg180 Gln	20519G>A	f
1764	(P)	severe	Arg180 Gln	20519G>A	f
8469	(G)	moderate	Arg180 Gln	20519G>A	f
9170	(Li)		Arg180 Gln	20519G>A	f
68	(P)		Arg180 Gln	20519G>A	f
11150	(G)		Arg180 Gln	20519G>A	f
10566	(G)		Arg180 Pro	20519G>C	f
60	(P)	severe	Arg180 Pro	20519G>C	f
47	(P)	severe	Val181 Phe	20521G>T	f
2280	(S)		Val181 Asp	20522T>A	f
49	(P)	moderate	Pro193 Ser	20557C>T	f
8389	(G)	moderate	Trp194 stop	20561G>A	f
2352	(G)	severe	Gln195 Gln donor splice	20565G>A	f
58	(P)	severe	Gly207 Glu	30073G>A	g
2308	(Cu)		Gly207 Glu	30073G>A	g
10982	(G)		Gly207 Val	30073G>T	g
11151	(G)		Gly208 Asp	30076G>A	g
11140	(G)		Trp215 Leu	30097G>A	g
11305	(G)		Thr218 Ile	30106C>T	g
2274	(G)	mild	Ala219 Thr	30108G>A	g
9227	(G)	mild	Ala219 Thr	30108G>A	g
8711	(G)		Ala233 Thr	30150G>A	g
3906	(G)	severe	Gly234 Val splice site	30822G>T	h
8651	(G)	moderate	Gly234 Val splice site	30822G>T	h
57	(P)	severe	IVSG+1G>A splice site, inhibitor	30154G>A	IVSG
2128	(C)		Asn237 Asp	30830G>A	h

Table 3. Continued

Patient IDN	Pat. Origin	Clinical	Codon No.	Nucleotide Substitution	Exon No.
2244	(G)	severe	del Glu240 delGAG	30839-41	h
2259	(G)	severe	del Glu240 delGAG	30839-41	h
2260	(G)	severe	del Glu240 delGAG	30839-41	h
2267	(G)	severe	del Glu240 del GAG	30839-41	h
3814	(G)		Glu245 Lys	30854G>A	h
11312	(G)		Glu245 Lys	30854G>A	h
8504	(G)	mild	Glu245 Asp	30856G>T	h
952	(G)	severe	Arg248 Gly	30863C>G	h
17	(P)	severe	Arg248 stop	30863C>T	h
9409	(G)	severe	Arg248 stop	30863C>T	h
9141	(Si)		Arg248 stop	30863C>T	h
56	(P)	severe	Arg248 stop	30863C>T	h
11152	(G)	severe	Arg248 stop	30863C>T	h
2273	(G)	moderate	Arg248 Gln	30864G>A	h
3328	(G)	moderate	Arg248 Gln	30864G>A	h
9441	(G)	moderate	Arg248 Gln	30864G>A	h
9487	(G)	mild	Arg248 Gln	30864G>A	h
10989	(G)		Arg248 Gln	30864G>A	h
11112	(G)	severe	Arg248 Gln	30864G>A	h
11155	(G)		Arg248 Gln	30864G>A	h
19	(P)	severe	Arg248 Leu	30864G>T	h
3146	(G)	severe	Arg252 stop	30875C>T	h
8459	(G)		Arg252 stop	30875C>T	h
3867	(E)	moderate	Arg252 stop	30875C>T	h
9056	(G)		Arg252 stop	30875C>T	h
8948	(G)		Arg252 stop	30875C>T	h
54	(P)	severe	Arg252 stop	30875C>T	h
9365	(G)		Arg252 stop	30875C>T	h
8426	(G)	mild	Arg252 stop	30875C>T	h
2131	(H)		Frameshift stop 279	del 30892C	h
1986	(P)	severe	Tyr266 stop	30919C>A	h
51	(P)	severe	Tyr266 stop	30919C>A	h
10	(P)	severe	Asp269 Val	30927A>T	h
3969	(G)	severe	Ala271 Asp	30933C>A	h
11388	(G)	mild	Ala271 Val	30933C>T	h
3147	(G)	severe	Leu275 Gln	30945T>A	h
2266	(G)	severe	Frameshift stop 308	del 30968A	h
8839	(G)	severe	Frameshift stop 308	del 30968A	h
10995	(G)	severe	Frameshift stop 308	del 30968A	h
9589	(G)	mild	Ser283 Arg	30970G>C	h
9563	(G)	(female)	Tyr284 Tyr	30973C>T	h
2234	(A)	mild	Pro287 His	30981C>A	h
8832	(G)	(female)	Cys289 Arg	30986C>T	h
1757	(P)	severe	Tyr295 stop	31006C>G	h
40	(P)	severe	Tyr295 stop	31006C>G	h
8506	(G)	severe	Trp295 stop	31006C>A	h
2121	(C)	moderate	Frameshift stop 308	del 31007A	h
2722	(G)	mild	Thr296 Lys	31008C>A	h
1758	(P)	mild	Thr296 Met	31008C>T	h
2256	(G)	moderate	Thr296 Met	31008C>T	h

Table 3. Continued

Patient IDN	Pat. Origin	Clinical	Codon No.	Nucleotide Substitution	Exon No.
27	(P)	mild	Thr296 Met	31008C>T	h
9846	(G)	moderate	Thr296 Met	31008C>T	h
8643	(G)		Thr296 Met	31008C>T	h
8711	(G)		Thr296 Met	31008C>T	h
8796	(G)	moderate	Thr296 Met	31008C>T	h
8954	(G)		Thr296 Met	31008C>T	h
9113	(G)		Thr296 Met	31008C>T	h
9321	(G)	mild	Thr296 Met	31008C>T	h
9327	(G)		Thr296 Met	31008C>T	h
2507	(G)		Thr296 Met	31008C>T	h
11033	(G)		Gly303 Glu	31029G>A	h
11156	(G)		Gly305 Asp	31035G>A	h
1765	(P)	severe	Trp310 Arg	31049T>A	h
61	(P)	severe	Trp310 Arg	31049T>A	h
10568	(G)		Trp310 Arg	31049T>A	h
3913	(G)	mild	Trp310 Leu	31050G>T	h
9195	(G)		Trp310 Leu	31050G>T	h
2223	(A)	severe	Trp310 Cys	31051G>T	h
41	(P)	severe	Gly311 Arg	31052G>A	h
3371	(P)	severe	Gly311 Arg	31052G>A	h
5	(P)	severe	Gly311 Arg	31052G>A	h
50	(P)	severe	Gly311 stop	31052G>T	h
11454	(G)		Gly311 Val	31053G>T	h
8830	(G)	moderate	Lys316 Glu	31067A>G	h
1761	(G)	severe	Lys316 delA frame shift	del 31069A	h
4	(P)	severe	Gln324 Pro	31092A>C	h
9168	(Li)		Gln324 Pro	31092A>C	h
26	(P)	severe	Tyr325 stop	31096C>A	h
8471	(G)		Tyr325 stop	31096C>G	h
8095	(G)		Val328 Phe	31103G>T	h
1984	(P)	severe	Leu330/1 del TTG	31110–12	h
1766	(P)	severe	Arg333 stop	31118C>T	h
42	(P)	severe	Arg333 stop	31118C>T	h
3549	(P)	severe	Arg333 stop	31118C>T	h
9550	(CR)		Arg333 stop	31118C>T	h
8646	(G)	severe	Arg333 stop	31118C>T	h
10922	(G)		Arg333 stop	31118C>T	h
3294	(G)	moderate	Arg333 Gln	31119G>A	h
1756	(P)	severe	Arg333 Gln	31119G>A	h
9449	(I)		Arg333 Gln	31119G>A	h
70	(P)		Arg333 Gln	31119G>A	h
25	(P)	severe	Cys336 Arg	31127T>C	h
1990	(P)	severe	Arg338 stop	31133C>T	h
25	(P)	severe	Arg338 stop	31133C>T	h
16	(P)	severe	Arg338 stop	31133C>T	h
8472	(G)	moderate	Arg338 stop	31133C>T	h
37	(P)	moderate	Ser339 Pro	31136C>T	h
2245	(G)	moderate	lle344 Phe	31151A>T	h
2261	(G)	severe	lle344 Phe	31151A>T	h
2120	(G)		Tyr345 stop	31156T>A	h

Table 3. Continued

Patient IDN	Pat. Origin	Clinical	Codon No.	Nucleotide Substitution	Exon No.
8433	(G)	mild	Phe349 Tyr	31167T>A	h
45	(P)	severe	Cys350 Arg	31169T>C	h
965	(G)	severe	Cys350 Ser	31170G>C	h
9684	(I)		Cys350 Tyr	31170G>A	h
41	(P)	severe	Gly352 Asp	31176G>A	h
11580	(G)		Gly352 Asp	31176G>A	h
9629	(G)	moderate	Gly356 Arg	31187G>A	h
8511	(G)	severe	Asp359 del GA frame shift	del 31196–97	h
2248	(G)	severe	Cys361Ser	31202T>A	h
9	(P)	severe	Cys361Gly	31202T>G	h
1780	(P)	severe	Ser365 Asn	31215G>A	h
3918	(G)	mild	Gly366 Trp	31217G>T	h
9429	(G)	moderate	Pro368 Ser	31223C>T	h
35	(P)	severe	Pro368 His	31224C>A	h
1762	(P)	severe	Pro368 His	31224C>A	h
3299	(G)	severe	Glu374stop	31241G>T	h
8712	(G)		Leu379 stop	31257T>G	h
3254	(G)	moderate	Gly381 Arg	31262G>A	h
59	(P)	moderate	Ser384 Cys	31271A>T	h
9403	(G)		Ser384 Asn	31272G>A	h
3591	(H)		Ser384 Arg	31273C>G	h
2227	(A)	moderate	Trp385 Arg	31274T>A	h
66	(P)		Trp385 Cys	31276G>T	h
2251	(G)	severe	Gly386 Ser	31277G>A	h
3633	(G)		Gly386 Ala	31278G>C	h
8787	(G)	moderate	Gly386 Ala	31278G>C	h
8200	(R)		Gly386 Asp	31278G>A	h
36	(P)	moderate	Glu387 Lys	31280G>A	h
10505	(G)		Glu387 Lys	31280G>A	h
63	(P)	severe	Glu387 Lys	31280G>A	h
9559	(G)		Glu387 Lys	31280G>A	h
3625	(G)		Glu387 Ala	31281A>C	h
3625	(G)		Glu387 Ala	31281A>C	h
8200	(R)	moderate	Glu387 Ala	31281A>C	h
39	(P)	severe	Cys389 Tyr	31287G>A	h
1987	(P)	severe	Cys389 Tyr	31287G>A	h
3550	(G)		Gly396 Val	31308G>T	h
2229	(G)	mild	Arg403 Trp	31328C>T	h
22	(P)	severe	Trp407 stop	31342G>A	h
28	(P)	severe	Trp407 stop	31342G>A	h
8027	(G)	mild	Trp407 Cys	31342G>C	h

Origin of patients: Argentina (A), Czechia (C), Costa Rica (CR), Cuba (Cu), Estonia (E), Germany (G), Hungary (H), India (I), Lithuania (Li), Poland (P), Romania (R), Singapore (Si), Switzerland (S), Venezuela (Ve)

Arg(-4) (CGG), Arg180 (CGG), Arg248 (CGA) and Thr296 (ACG). The lesions Arg(-4) Trp (6364C>T), Arg(-4) Asn (6365G>A) or Arg(-4) Leu (6365G>T) were detected in 6, 3 or 4 patients respectively from Romania, Germany, Lithuania, India or Poland (Table 2).

In 13 patients from Germany, Poland, Hungary, Lithuania and Costa Rica the codon Arg180 were mutated by the lesions: transition 20518C>T with substitution Arg180 Trp (5 cases), transition 20519G>A with substitution Arg180 Gln (6 cases) or transversion 29519G>C with substitution Arg180 Pro (two cases).

The codon Arg248 in exon h was substituted in 14 unrelated patients from Germany (10 cases), Poland (3 cases) and Singapore (one case). The amino acid substitutions Arg248 Gly (30863C>G) in one case, Arg248 stop (30863C>T) in 5 cases, Arg248 Gln (30864G>A) in 7 cases and Arg248 Leu (30864G>T) in one patient were analyzed.

The most frequent lesion of the »Greifswald study factor IX deficiency (hemophilia B)« is the lesion Thr296 Met which has been analyzed in 10 cases from Germany and two patients from Poland..

All of these frequent FIX gene lesions are located in a CpG dinucleotides. The same origin of all cases is not likely. The C>T transversion in CpG islands is now recognized to be the most frequent DNA change in the human genome, arising from apparent spontaneous desamination of methylated cytosine residues. It is becoming clear that the high number of repeated observations of identical F IX mutations at same CpG doublets, particularly those which caused mild disease [e.g. 93 examples at Thr296 Met (HGMD Database FIX, 2000)] are caused by the CpG island and, at least in a part, by founder effect.

The mutations could influence the F IX function in different ways. The promotor mutation could have an influence of the transcription of the factor IX. The position (–26) in the promotor is located in the liver-enriched transcription factor HNF4 and caused severe hemophilia B (Peak et al. 1995, HGMD Database FIX, 2000).

Point mutations in promotor position –23 to 13 could lead to the hemophilia B type Leyden. This factor IX variant is characterized by severe childhood hemophilia which is ameliorated at puberty. In the »Greifswald study FIX deficiency (hemophilia B)« a point mutation in the »Leyden« region was identified in five patients in positions –20, –6, 7, 9 and 13.

Splice site mutations are analyzed in 14 unrelated patients. In a study in Polish hemophilia B patients we could show that in all cases the splice mutation lead to severe disease, with phenotype CMR- (Triplett et al. 1985), with a reduction of FIX activity (FIX:C), with similarly reduced antigen level (FIX:Ag), with the absence of dysfunctional F IX molecules in the plasma (Wulff et al. 1999).

Most of the lesions in the FIX gene, 196 (67%) of all 289 mutants are missense mutations, the substitution of one amino acid by another. Missense mutations cause hemophilia B varying from severe to mild phenotype. In two patients were detected two point mutations (double mutations) in exon e of the FIX allele, the silent mutation Ser123 Ser and the missense mutation Cys124 Phe .

Hemophilia B is caused by a large number of different mutations in the region of the factor XI gene. Hemophilia B is mostly due to small changes in the F IX gene affecting either the transcription, the mRNA maturation, the mRNA translation or the fine structure of the factor IX. To date, over 689 unique molecular mutations have been analyzed from 1,918 unrelated patients (HGMD Database FIX 2000). Only 2–3% of the patients showed gross deletions (>30bp) or rearrangements. Repeated observations in apparently unrelated individuals generally applied at either CpG dinucleotides or founder effects (Peak et al. 1995).

Direct sequencing of individually PCR – amplified factor IX exon sequences – has emerged as a relatively rapid and accurate method of diagnostic analysis in hemophilia B families (Herrmann et al. 1990, 1993, 1994, 1995, 1996, 1997, 1997a, 1998). The practical application to genetic analysis of the factor IX genes are accurate carrier detection and prenatal diagnosis. Counseling of potential carriers and their relatives is an extremely important part of the procedure.

Acknowledgements. The authors would like to acknowledge the technical assistance Ingeborg Keller and Eva-Maria Denecke for performance of the sequence analysis and DNA isolation.

References

1. Green P.M., Giannelli F., Sommer S., Poon M.-C., Ludwig M., Schwaab R., Reitsma P.H., Goossens M., Yoshioka A., Figueiredo M.S., Brownlee G.G. (2000) Hemophilia B: Database of point mutations and short additions and deletions. 9th Edn. http://www.uwcm.ac.uk/molgen/haemBdatabase.htm
2. Herrmann FH, Wulff K, Schröder W, Machill G, Wehnert M (1993) Molecular genetics and genomic diagnosis of X-linked disorders in the man. Genet Live Sci Adv. 12: 43–53
3. Herrman FH, Schröder W, Wehnert M, Wulff K (1994) Zur genomischen Diagnostik von Hämophilie A und B in den fünf neuen Bundesländern. In: A. Kurme, Klose HJ, Beer H-J (Eds) Psychosoziale Aspekte bei Hämophilie und HIV. Georg Thieme Verlag Stuttgart-New York 222–231.
4. Herrmann FH, Scharrer I (1995) Humangenetische Beratung bei Hämophilie A und B. In: Deutsche Hämophiliegesellschaft, Hamburg (Hrsg.) Mitteilungen der Deutschen Hämophiliegesellschaft zur Bekämpfung von Blutungskrankheiten e.V. Hamburg 3–30 (Sonderdruck 2/95)
5. Herrmann FH, Wulff K, Schröder W, Wehnert M, Machill G, Ebener U (1995a) Molekulargenetik und genomische Diagnostik bei Hämophilie A und B. Med. Genetik 7: 376–381
6. Herrmann FH, Schröder W, Wulff K, Wehnert M (1996) Neue Ergebnisse zur Mutationscharakterisierung bei Hämophilie A und B In: I. Scharrer, W. Schramm (eds.) 25. Hämophilie-Symposion Springer Verlag Berlin Heidelberg New York, S. 235–246
7. Herrmann FH Genomische Diagnostik bei Hämophilie B (1) (1996a) mta 11; 12: 958–963
8. Herrmann FH, Schröder W, Wulff K, Bendix M, Wehnert M, Anders O, Aumann V, Bratanoff E, Ebener U, Franke D, Güldenring A, Heinrichs Ch, Lenk H, Mitulla B, Pindur G, Seyfert UT, Thiele G, Vogel G, Weippert M, Wendisch J, Wenzel E (1997) Genomische Diagnostik bei Hämophilie A und B : Ergebnisse einer multizentrischen zehnjährigen Zusammenarbeit. In: I. Scharrer, W. Schramm (eds.) 26. Hämophilie-Symposion Springer Verlag Berlin Heidelberg New York S. 261–267
9. Herrmann FH (1997a) Genomische Diagnostik bei Hämophilie B (2). mta 12; 1: 15–18
10. Herrmann FH (1997b) Genomische (DNA) Diagnostik bei Hämophilie A und B - DNA-Analyse zur Konduktorinnendiagnostik. Hautnah Pädiatrie. 9, 479–487.
11. Herrmann FH, Vogel G (1998) Molekulargenetik hereditärer Hämostasedefekte In: Ganten, D, Ruckpaul, K: Handbuch der molekularen Medizin, Band 3. Kreislauf-Erkrankungen. Springer-Verlag Berlin Heidelberg New York, S. 223–287

12. Herrmann F.H., Wulff K. (1998a) Molekulare Genanalyse und Gendiagnostik bei Hämophilie B und Faktor VII Mangel. Hämostaseologie. 3: 129- 139.
13. Herrmann FH, Scharrer I (1999) Humangenetische Beratung bei Hämophilie A und B. In: Deutsche Hämophiliegesellschaft, Hamburg (Hrsg.) Mitteilungen der Deutschen Hämophiliegesellschaft zur Bekämpfung von Blutungskrankheiten e.V. Hamburg 3–33 (Sonderdruck 1/99), 2. Auflage
14. Miller M., Dykes D.D., Polesky H.F (1988) A simple salting out procedure for extracting DNA from human nucleated cells. Nucleic Acids Res.16: 121
15. Peake I. (1995) Molecular Genetics and Counseling in Hemophilia. Thromb.Haemost. 74: 40–44.
16. Schröder W, Wulff K, Wollina K, Herrmann FH (1997) Hemophilia B in female twins caused by a point mutation in one Factor IX gene and nonrandom inactivation patterns of the X-chromosomes. Thromb Haemost 78: 1347–51
17. Schröder W, Wollina K, Wulff K, Herrmann FH (1998) Unbalancierte X Chromosomen-Inaktivierung in weiblichen Zwillingen mit Hämophilie B. In: I. Scharrer, W. Schramm (ed.) 27. Hämophilie-Symposion Hamburg 1996 Springer Verlag Berlin Heidelberg New York, S. 306–313
18. Schröder W, Poetsch M, Gazda H, Werner W, Reichelt T, Knoll W, Robicka-Milewska R, Zieleniewka B (1998a) A de novo translocation 46,X(X15) causing hemophilia B in a girl: a case report. Brit J Haematol 100: 750–757
19. Triplett DA, Brandt JT, McGann, Batard MA, Schaeffer Dixon JL, Fair DS (1985) Hereditary factor VII deficiency: Heterogeneity defined combined functional and immunochemical analysis. Blood 66:1284–1287.
20. Tuddenham EGD,Cooper DN (1994) The molecular genetics of haemostasis and its inherited disorders. pp. 78–110, Oxford University Press, New York Tokyo.
21. White GC, Rosendaal F, Aledort LM, Lusher JM, Rothschild C, Ingerslev J: Definition behalf of the Factor VIII and Factor IX Subcommittee (2001) Definitions in Hemophilia. Thromb Haemost. 85:560
22. Wulff K, Schröder W, Blanco A, Wehnert M, Herrmann FH (1994) Factor IX structural gene mutations in hemophilia B patients from Argentina. Rev Iberoamer Tromb Hemostasia 7: 256–258
23. Wulff K, Wehnert M, Schröder W, Herrmann FH (1994a) Mutationen im Strukturgen des Faktor IX In: I. Scharrer, W. Schramm (eds.) 24. Hämophilie-Symposion Springer Verlag Berlin Heidelberg New York, S. 130–134
24. Wulff K., Schröder W., Wehnert M., Herrmann F.H. (1995) Twenty-five novel mutations of the factor IX gene in haemophilia B. Hum Mutat. 6, 346 –348.
25. Wulff K, Gazda H, Schröder W, Robicka-Milewska R, Herrmann FH (1997) Mutationsanalyse bei 27 Hämophilie B-Patienten aus Polen. In: Scharrer I, Schramm W. 28. Hämophilie-Symposion Hamburg 1997. Springer Verlag Berlin Heidelberg New York, S 157–162
26. Wulff K, Schröder W, Herrmann FH (1997a) Molekulare Defekte bei 116 Hämophilie B (Faktor IX Mangel) Patienten und bei Patienten mit Faktor VII Mangel. In: Herrmann F.H. (Hrsg) Molekulargenetik hereditärer Hämostasedefekte. Pabst-Verlag, pp.157–162
27. Wulff K, Bykowska K, Lopaciuk S, Herrmann FH (1999) Molecular analysis of hemophilia B in Poland: 12 novel mutations of the factor IX gene. Acta Biochimica Polonica. 46: 721–726
28. Wulff K, Gazda H, Schröder W, Robicka-Milewska R, Herrmann FH (2000) Identification of an novel F9 gene mutation-an insertion of an Alu repeated element in exon e of the factor IX gene. Hum Mutat. 2000 web/109
29. Yoshitake S, Schach BG, Foster DC, Davie EW, Kurachi K (1985) Nucleotide sequence of the gene of human factor IX (hemophilia factor B). Biochemistry 24: 3736–3750.

Gly222Asp and Ser379Lys – Novel Factor X Gene Mutations in severe FX Deficiency – Greifswald Registry of Factor X congenital Deficiency

F. H. HERRMANN, K. WULFF, S. LOPACIUK, and H. POLLMANN

Introduction

Factor X (FX) is a vitamin K-dependent plasma protein which plays a central role in blood coagulation. It is activated into the serine protease factor Xa (FXa) either by the intrinsic tenase complex (factor IXa/factor VIIIa) or by the tissue factor (extrinsic) pathway. FXa, in complex with its cofactor factor Va, forms the prothrombinase complex and is the important physiological activator of prothrombin. In the liver the 488-amino acid FX precursor is synthesized. Before secretion, the precursor undergoes several post-translational modifications. These steps include removal of the 40-amino acid pre-pro leader sequence (–40 to –1), γ-carboxylation of the first 11 glutamin acid residues, β-hydroxylation of Asp63, and excision of the Arg 140-Lys-Arg tripeptide. The resulting two chain zymogen consists of a 139-amino acid light-chain linked to a 306-amino acid heavy-chain by a single disulphide bond between Cys132 and Cys302. The light-chain includes the amino-terminal γ-carboxy-glutamic acid (Gla) domain that contains the 11 Gla residues. A short helical stack is present downstream of the Gla domain, followed by two consecutive epidermal growth factor like domains (EGF1 and EGF2). The amino terminus of the heavy-chain includes a 52-amino acid activation peptide, followed by the protease domain which contains the active site triade of His236, Asp282, and Ser379 typical of serine proteases [1].

The gene encoding FX is located on chromosome 13q34. The FX gene lies 2,8 kb downstream of the factor VII gene. The FX gene is more than 27 kb in length and is organized in 8 exons: exon 1 encodes the signal peptide, exons 2 encodes the propeptide and Gla domain, exon 3 encodes the aromatic amino acid stack domain, exons 4 and 5 each code for the EGF-like regions, exon 6 encodes the activation domain, and exons 7 and 8 encode the catalytic domain.

Factor X deficiency is a very rare hemostatic disorder. The first case was described in the Prower [13] and Stuart [6} pedigrees . Both cases are characterized by a prolonged prothrombin time (PT). Other factor X variants have been reported which are associated with prolonged PT and activated partial thromboplastin times (aPTT), which were correctable by addition of normal serum but not of absorbed plasma.

FX deficiency is normally transmitted as an autosomal recessive trait [3,9] and is frequently associated with consanguinity.

The variable severity manifested by individuals with FX deficiency correlates poorly with laboratory phenotype. In the classical deficiency state exemplified by

I. Scharrer/W. Schramm (Ed.)
32nd Hemophilia Symposion Hamburg 2001
© Springer-Verlag Berlin Heidelberg 2003

Stuart, both activity and antigen are severely decreased (CRM-), in the case of Prower, only factor X activity is reduced (CRM+). Factor X [Red] is characterized by reduced activity and antigen but with antigen markedly higher than activity (CRM[R]).

In 1998 the »**Greifswald Registry of FX congenital deficiency**« was started by Herrmann FH and Wulff, K. The aims of this registry are:
a) to characterize the molecular defects (mutations, polymorphisms) of the FX gene,
b) to analyze the genotype-phenotype correlation of the clinical symptoms as well as
c) to describe the epidemiology of FX deficiency.

Until now more than 24 centers (Table 1) are involved in this study. More than 30 patients/families are under investigation. Here the results of the molecular genetic and clinical characterization are reported of two patients with severe factor X deficiency caused by two novel mutations.

Table 1. Greifswald registry of factor X congenital deficiencies

Study group			
F.H. Herrmann	Greifswald	K. Kurnik	Munich
K. Wulff	Greifswald	S. Lopaciuk	Warsaw (Poland)
M. Arlt	Stuttgart	B. Maak	Saalfeld
G. Auerswald	Bremen	G. Marx	Hamburg
N. de Bosch	Caracas (Venezuela)	B. Mitulla	Suhl
A Batorova	Bratislava (Slovakia)	G. Pfanner	Feldkirch
F. Bergmann	Hamburg	H. Pollmann	Muenster
U. Budde	Hamburg	A. Ruiz-Saez	Caracas (Venezuela)
R. Eisert	Hamburg	I. Scharrer	Frankfurt/Main
B. Eifrig	Hanover	G. Syrbe	Stadtroda
S. Halimeh	Muenster	M. v. Depka Prondzinski	Hanover
K. Kentouche	Jena	J. Wendisch	Dresden
U. Kluba	Magdeburg	K. Wolf	Chemnitz

Material and Methods

The identification of the patients with FX deficiency and the analysis of the hemostaseological parameters were carried in the home hospital of the members of the study group (Table 1).

DNA Isolation

EDTA-blood was collected of patients with FX deficiency. DNA was extracted of white blood cells by NaCl extraction method [10]

Sequencing

The molecular basis of inherited factor X deficiency was analyzed by sequencing of the FX gene (all coding regions and the 5'flanking region containing the promoter) in probands with reduced FX level.

The double stranded PCR products were purified and concentrated in Microcon 100 concentrators (Amicon GmbH). The sequence reaction was performed as a cycle sequencing procedure using Taq Dye Deoxy-terminator Cycle sequencing Kit (Applied Biosystems) [15]. All sequences were analyzed at least twice.

Haplotype analysis

The haplotype of FX alleles were determined by the following polymorphisms (Table 2): Hexanucleotide (TTGTGA) deletion in nt-343 to nt-348, the base changes in the promoter region –222C>T and –220C>A [7,11] as well as the exon 7 polymorphism Thr224 Thr (817T>C).

The polymorphisms were identified by sequencing or in cause of deletion TTGTGA by heteroduplex analysis [14]. The FX haplotypes were detected by family studies or/and analysis of homozygosity of the mutation.

Table 2. Analyzed polymorphisms of FX gene

Gene region	Polymorphisms	Genotype	Symbols
Promoter region	Deletion TTGTGA nt –348 to –343	WT/WT WT/del del/del	A1/A1 A1/A2 A2/A2
Promoter region	–222C>T	C/C C/T T/T	B1/B1 B1/B2 B2/B2
Promoter region	–220C>A	C/C C/A A/A	C1/C1 C1/C2 C2/C2
Exon 7	817T>C Thr224 Thr	T/T T/C C/C	D1/D1 D1/D2 D2/D2

Results and discussion

Analysis of mutations in FX deficiency - Mutation spectrum

In the »Greifswald Registry of FX congenital deficiency« more than 30 patients/families with FX deficiency are under investigation. Until now 21 different mutations are detected in different genetic conditions. 15 of these are novel mutati-

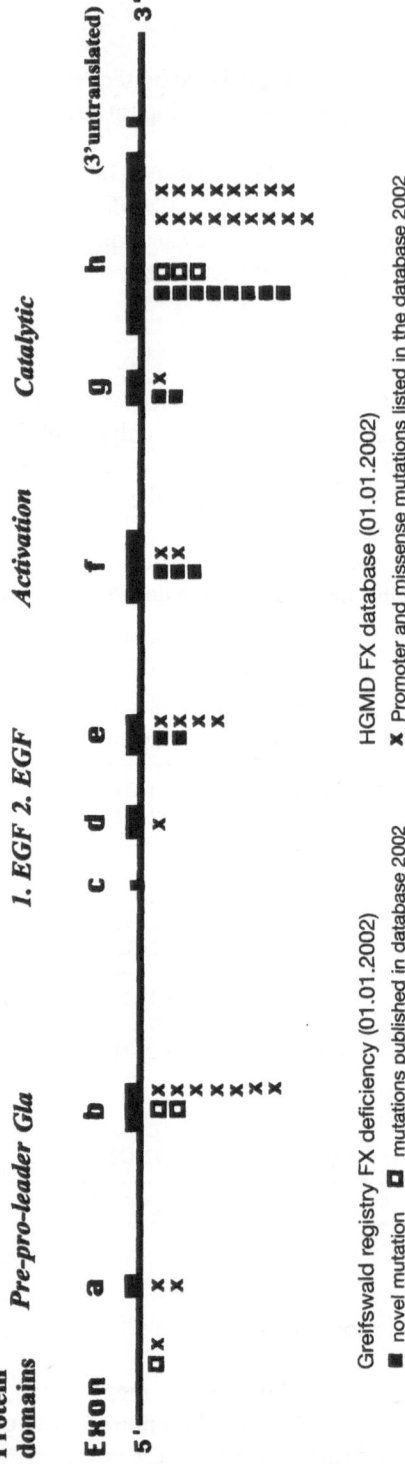

Fig. 1. Localization of 21 different mutations in the factor X gene analyzed in the »Greifswald Registry of FX congenital deficiency«

ons, previously unreported (HGMD database FX, 2002 [5]). Figure 1 shows the distribution of the different FX lesions along the FX gene. Most of the mutations are detected in exon h encoded for the catalytic domain.

All detected mutations are caused by single nucleotide-substitutions. One mutation is located in the promoter region, 20 lesions were missense mutations.

Genomic diagnosis of two families with FX deficiency

Family KS

Patient KS has a FX activity < 1% and FX:Ag <1% (CRM⁻, Type 1 deficiency). He is homozygous for the novel mutation Gly222 Asp. The symptomatic is characterized by epistaxis, gumbleeding, GI bleeding. Family study has shown that the mother and the sister are heterozygous for the same mutation and both are asymptomatic (Table 3). On the basis of the homozygosity for this mutation the haplotype A1,B1,C1,D1 was detected (Fig. 2) for the Gly222 Asp substitution.

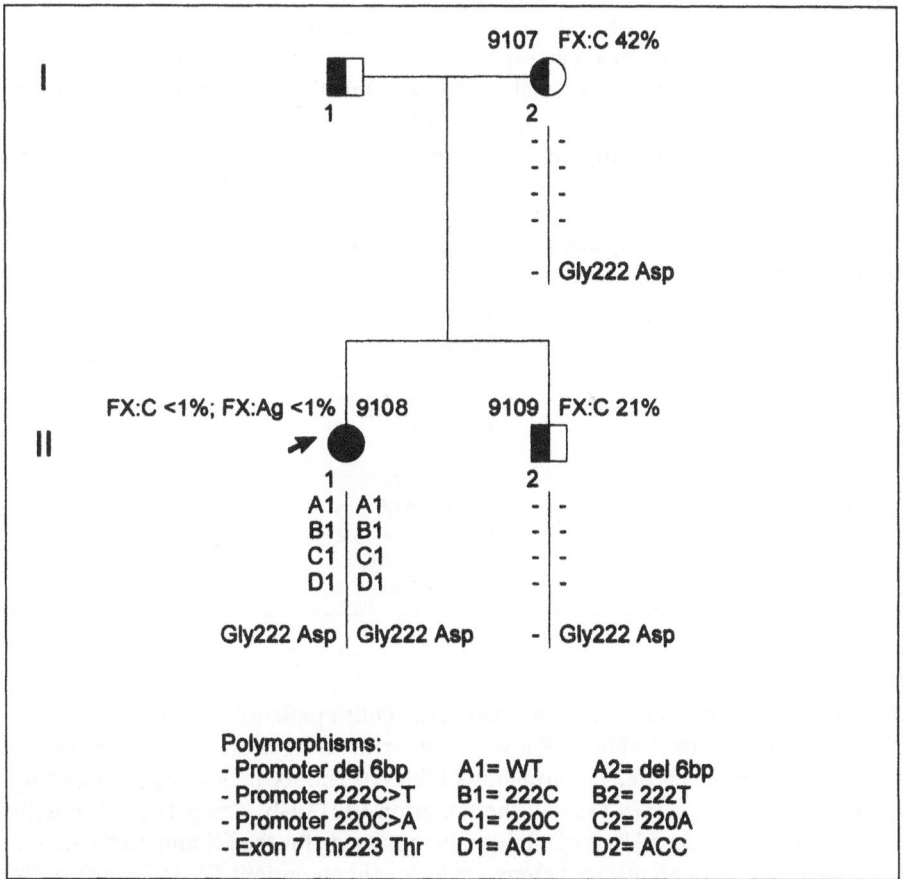

Fig. 2. Pedigree of family KS

Table 3. Factor X deficiency in proband KS and family members

Family Member (PIN)	FX:C (FX:Ag)	Mutation and Genet. Condition	Clinical Phenotype
Proband KS (9108)	<1% (<1%)	Gly222 Asp homozygous	Epistaxis, gumbleeding, Gl bleeding, prophylactic treatment
Brother (9109)	21%	Gly222 Asp heterozygous	Asymptomatic
Mother (9107)	42%	Gly222 Asp heterozygous	Asymptomatic

The substitution of Gly222 by the negative charged Asp222 lies adjacent of Cys221 and may interfere with the ability of Cys221 to disulphide link to Cys237 in the catalytic domain. Thereby the function of the catalytic site His236 might be influenced and the stability of the molecule is decreased.

The Gly222 Asp substitution occur in a residue which is strictly conserved in factor X, IX and VII. The lesion is responsible for severe type 1 deficiency, consistent with findings reported for several analogous substitutions [3,16] in factor IX (Table 4). An analogous substitution in factor VII is Gly179 Arg, which was described recently (2) in two compound heterozygous patients with Ala244 Val (FVII:C 3%, FVII:Ag 10%) and IVS1a+5 (FX:C 2%, FX:Ag 62%), respectively.

Table 4. FX variant Gly222 Asp and substitutions in analogous residue in factors VII and IX, causing severe deficiency

FX Gly 222	FVII Gly 179	FIX Gly207
Gly 222 Asp	Gly 179Arg	Gly 207 Glu
		Gly 207 Glu
FX:C <1%		Gly 207 Glu
		Gly 207 Arg
		Gly 207 Arg
		Gly 207 stop
		All severe HB
		FIX:C <1%

Family MB

Severe clinical symptoms were described in the Polish patient MB showing bleeding diathesis like moderate hemophilia with hemarthrosis, epistaxis, muscle hematomas, CNS bleeding, chronic arthropathy (Table 5). The FX deficiency is caused by the novel mutation Ser379 Lys and the mutation Glu14 Gly. The patients MB with FX :C < 2% and FX:Ag 57 % is compound heterozygote for the FX mutations Ser379 Lys/ Glu14 Gly. His parents are heterozygous for the mutations Glu14Gly or Ser379 Lys, respectively (Fig. 3), and they are asymptomatic.

Table 5. Factor X deficiency in proband MB and family members

Family Member	FX:C (FX:Ag)	Mutation and Genet. Condition	Clinical Phenotype
Proband MB (10370)	2% (57%)	Glu14 Gly / Ser379 Lys compound heterozygote	Bleeding diathesis like moderate hemophilia, epistaxis, CNS bleeding, hematomas (both knees, both elbows), chronic arthropathy
Father (10372)	60% (97%)	Ser379 Lys heterozygous	asymptomatic
Mother (10371)	52% (55%)	Glu14 Gly heterozygous	asymptomatic

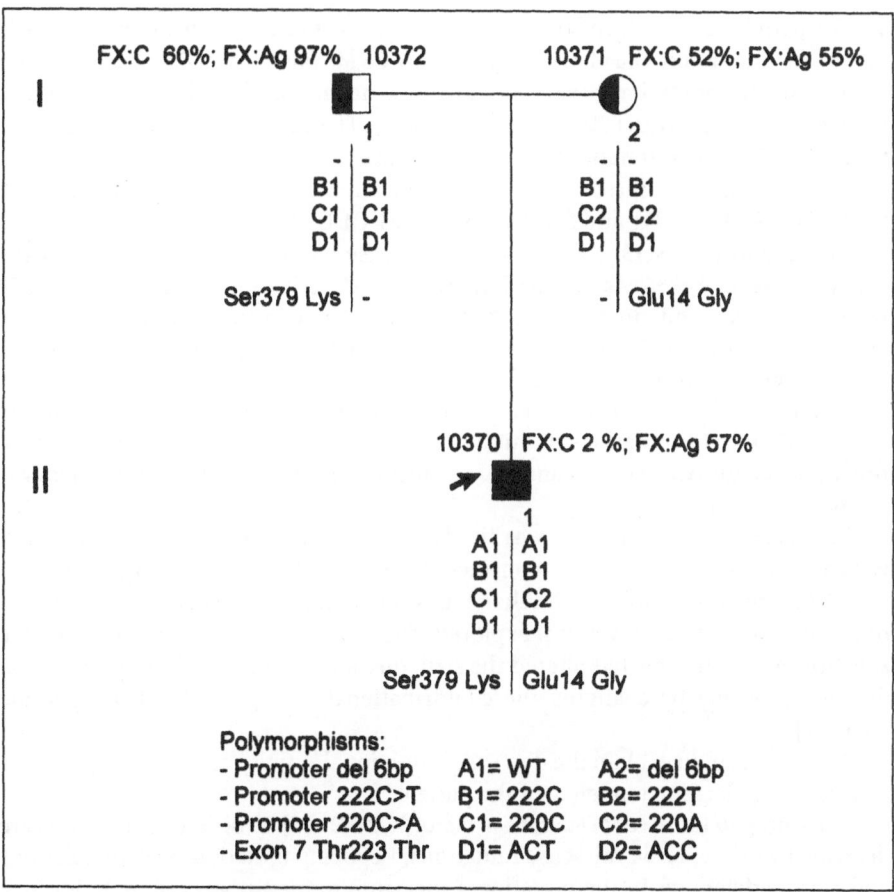

Fig. 3. Pedigree of Family MB

Table 6. FX variant Ser379 Lys, and substitutions in the analogous active site in factor IX, causing severe deficiency

FX Ser379	FIX Ser365
Ser379 Lys	Ser365 Gly CRM⁺
	Ser365 Gly n.d.
	Ser365Asn n.d.
	Ser365Asn n.d.
	Ser365 Ile n.d.
	Ser365Arg CRM⁺
	Ser365Arg CRM⁺
	All severe HB
	FIX:C <1%
	FIX:Ag 90–100

The FX activity and antigen level of near 50% in the heterozygous mother (Table 5, Fig. 3) for the lesion Glu14 Gly indicates an CRM⁻ phenotype. The heterozygous father with the mutation Ser379 Lys shows a normal antigen level (97%) and a reduced FX activity with 60% of the normal level. The substitution Ser379 Lys seems to result a CRM⁺ (dysfunctional) protein variant.

On the basis of pedigree studies (Fig. 3) the following haplotypes were detected: Glu14 Gly -A2 B1 C2 D1 and Ser379 Lys - A1 B1 C1 D1.

The amino acid Ser379 in the serine protease factor FX is one residue of the catalytic triade His236, Asp282 and Ser379. The described novel mutation Ser379 Lys of factor X results in a severe FX deficiency. The equivalent mutations in FIX gene Ser365 Asn, Ser365 Gly, Ser365 Ile and Ser 365 Arg [3] caused in all patients severe forms of hemophilia B (Table 6).

The antigen level of the heterozygote father of index patient MB was normal. As shown, FX and FIX mutations in this active site are obviously characterized as dysfunctional factor (CRM+). An analogous substitution (Ser344) in FVII deficiency is unknown until now.

The Glu14 Gly substitution was firstly described by Kim et al. [8] as factor X variant Ketchikan. The authors considered the patient to be homozygous for the defect, but the possibility of a simultaneous occurrence of an undetected deletion in one of the factor X genes was not explored. The low activation time implies that the substituting Gly residue has altered the structure and hence the function of the Gla domain, probably by changing the conformational entropy of local polypeptide chain [1].

The defect could explain the decreased functional activity of circulating factor X and the mild bleeding tendency of the patient.

According to the »HGMD database factor X, 2002« [5] 41 different mutations are described worldwide: 34 missense mutations, 1 splicing mutation, 3 small deletions and 3 gross deletions. In the mutational spectrum never a nonsense mutation was observed.

The started registry gives the unique possibility to characterize the causative mutations of FX deficiency and to study the genotype-phenotype correlation by genomic diagnosis and clinical evaluation. The »Study Group FX deficiency« invites for collaboration on this multicenter study in order to characterize the molecular defects of FX deficiency, to complete epidemiological data and offers on the basis of the genomic diagnosis genetic counseling for patients and families.

References

1. Cooper DN, Millar DS, Wacey A, Pemberton S, Tuddenham EGD. Inherited factor X deficiency: Molecular genetics and pathophysiology Thromb Haemost 1997; 78:161–172
2. Giansily-Blaizot M, Aguilar-Martinez P, Biron-Andreani C, Jeanjean P, Igual H, Schved JF. Analysis of the genotypes and phenotypes of 37 unrelated patients with inherited factor VII deficiency. Eur J Hum Genet 2001;9 :105–112
3. Green PM, Giannelli F, Sommer SS, Poon M-C, Ludwig M, Schwaab R, Reitsma PH, Goossens M, Yoshioka A, Figueiredo MS and Brownlee GG. Haemophilia B: database of point mutations and short additions and deletions – v9.0. 2001, http://umds.ac.uk/molgen/haemBdatabase.html
4. Herrmann FH, Wulff K, Lopaciuk S, Pollmann H. Two novel factor X mutations in severe factor X deficiency . Thromb Haemost 2001;Suppl:P1126
5. HGMD Database Factor X, 2002, http://uwcm.ac.uk/uwcm/mg/hgmd0.html
6. Hougie C, Barrow HM, Graham JB: Stuart clotting defect. Segregation of a hereditary hemorrhagic state from the heterozygous heretofore called »stable factor« (SPCA, proconverting factor VII deficiency). J Clin Invest 1957; 36: 485–493
7. Huang, MN, Hung HL, Stanfield-Oakley SA, High KA. Characterization of the human blood coagulation factor X promotor. J Biol Chem 1992; 267: 15440–15446
8. Kim DJ, Thompson AR, James HL. Factor X (Ketchikan): a variant molecule in which gly replaces a gla residue at position 14 in the light chain. Hum. Genet 1995; 95: 212–214
9. Millar DS, Elliston L,Deex P,Krawczak M, Wacey AI, Reanaud J, Nieuwenhuis HK, Bolton-Maggs P, Mannucci PM, Reverter JC, Cachia P, Pasi KJ, Layton DM, Cooper DN. Molecular analysis of the genotype-phenotype relationship in factor X deficiency. Hum Genet 2000; 106:249–257
10. Miller M, Dykes DD, Polesky HF. A simple salting out procedure for extracting DNA from human nucleated cells. Nucleic Acid Res 1988;16:121
11. Miao Ch, Leytus SP, Chung DW, Davie EW. Liver-specific expression of the gene coding for human factor X, a blood coagulation factor. J BiolChem 1992; 267: 7395–7401
12. MRC FVII Mutation Database 2001, http://europium.csc.mrc.ac.uk/
13. Telfer TP, Denson KW, Wright DR . A »new« coagulation defect. Brt J Haematol 1956; 2: 308–316
14. Wulff K, Ebener U, Wehnert, Ch-S, Ward, PA, Reuner U, Hiebsch W, Herrmann FH, Wehnert M. Direct molecular genetic diagnosis and heterozygote identification in X-linked Emery-Dreifuss Muscular Dystrophy by heteroduplex analysis. Disease Markers 1997; 13: 77–86
15. Wulff K, Herrmann FH. Twenty two novel mutations of the factor VII gene in factor VII deficiency. Hum Mutat 2000; 15:489–496
16. Wulff K, Schröder W, Wehnert M, Herrmann FH. Twenty-five novel mutations of the factor IX gene in haemophilia B. Hum. Mutat 1995;6: 346–348

IIc.   Gene Therapy

Hematopoietic Stem Cells as Targets for Gene Therapy of Hemophilia A

T. Tonn, S. Becker, C. Herder, M. Grez, and E. Seifried

Abstract

Considering the plasticity of hematopoietic stem cells (HSC), they would be ideal targets for gene therapy of hemophilia A by virtue of their progeny providing immediate access to the blood stream. However, several attempts to show expression of recombinant factor VIII (rFVIII) by primary hematopoietic cells and cell lines have failed, which was attributed to the inability of HSC to secrete rFVIII. Here we describe the generation of stable, FVIII-secreting hematopoietic cell lines representing different blood-cell types using a bicistronic lentiviral vector encoding for a B-domain deleted FVIII (FVIIIΔB) and enhanced green fluorescence protein (EGFP). Transduced cell lines with erythroid and/or megakaryocytic background, (K562-F8 and TF-1-F8), secrete high levels of FVIII in the order of 76.4 and 41.6 ng FVIII:C/ml, while moderate and low levels are observed in B-lymphoblastoid Raji-F8 cells and the T leukemia line Jurkat-F8 which secrete 6.73 and 1.83 ng FVIII:C/ml, respectively. The capacity to secrete rFVIII appeared to depend on factors related to the cell lineage, rather than on the transduction efficacy. The established cell lines should be helpful in further elucidating mechanisms which are able to improve FVIII secretion in hematopoietic cells on a post-translational level and suggest reanalysis of hematopoietic cells as target for gene therapy of the hemophiliacs.

Introduction

Hemophilia A is a monogenetic X-linked inherited bleeding disorder caused by a deficiency in blood coagulation factor VIII (FVIII). Current treatment options consist of prophylactic and therapeutic infusions of either plasma-derived or recombinant FVIII [1–3]. Recently alternative approaches to FVIII therapy have been proposed using somatic gene therapy [4–6]. Hemophilia A is particularly suitable for gene therapy since even low amounts of plasma FVIII can significantly reduce the severity of the disease and since the expression of FVIII does not require precise regulation [6].

While under physiological conditions FVIII synthesis mainly occurs in hepatocytes [7,8] and liver sinusoidal endothelial cells (LSECs) [9,10], a variety of different cell types, such as fibroblasts [11,12], skin [13], endothelial cells [9,14,15],

I. Scharrer/W. Schramm (Ed.)
32nd Hemophilia Symposion Hamburg 2001
© Springer-Verlag Berlin Heidelberg 2003

muscle [12], hepatocytes [16,17] and bone marrow stromal cells [18,19] have been tested for their usefulness in gene therapeutic approaches. Recently, the implantation of genetically altered fibroblasts that produce factor VIII, was shown to be well tolerated and lead to increased FVIII plasma levels in patients with severe hemophilia A [20].

As a further appealing target for gene therapy of hemophilia A, hematopoietic stem cells have been suggested since they promise long term transgene expression with immediate access to the blood stream by virtue of their progeny representing all blood-cell types [21,22]. Moreover, hematopoietic stem cells have been shown to be able to transdifferentiate into non-hematopoietic tissue, such as endothelial [23] cells and hepatocytes [24], which holds the option of site directed gene therapy with ex vivo transduced hematopoietic stem cells [25]. However, attempts to express recombinant FVIII in hematopoietic cells and cell lines have failed thus far – a fact which has been attributed to the inability of these cells to secrete detectable amounts of FVIII [21,22,26].

In mammalian cells expression of recombinant FVIII is 5–10 fold less than that of most other proteins, irrespective of the host cell or vector system used. The diminished yield of recombinant FVIII is apparently mediated by a combination of different factors, that include inhibitory sequences within the FVIII coding region [27–29] and lead to 100–1000 times lower yields in retroviral vector titers and transcribed RNA [27, 28, 30, 31], inefficient intracellular transport, inefficient FVIII secretion and the susceptibility of FVIII to proteolytic degradation [4, 32, 33].

While these observations were mainly obtained in FVIII-transduced Chinese hamster ovarian (CHO) and fibroblast cells, the mechanisms accounting for the lack of FVIII secretion by hematopoietic cells have not been addressed. We therefore transduced human hematopoietic cell lines representing different leukocyte subsets with a bicistronic lentiviral vector encoding the B-domain deleted FVIII (FVIIIΔ) cDNA and the enhanced green fluorescence protein (EGFP) as marker gene to reanalyze the capacity of hematopoietic cells to express recombinant FVIII. Lentiviral vectors are best suited for stable transduction of quiescent hematopoietic and adult stem cells and are able to promote long-term transgene expression after transplantation of ex vivo transduced cells [34, 35]. Using this vector system and cells highly enriched for transgene expression, we were able to show high amounts of FVIII secretion by individual hematopoietic cell lines. Moreover, these hematopoietic cells could be established as stable FVIII-secreting lines which are suitable for the further analysis of the subcellular characteristics of blood cells with regard to FVIII translation and secretion.

Materials and Methods

Cloning of a B-domain deleted FVIII

The full length FVIII-cDNA [36] (accession number K01740) was obtained from ATCC (American Tissue Culture Collection, Rockville, USA) and deleted of a large portion of the B-domain (nucleotides 2,428–5,067) by overlapping PCR. Briefly, a polymerase chain reaction (PCR) fragment starting 5´of the Bgl lI restriction site at nucleotide 1,830 and overspanning nucleotide 2,427, as well as a PCR fragment starting at nucleotide 5,068 and spanning 3´of the PflM I site at nucleotide 5,870 were designed to overlap for 17 bp, while sparing out the B-domain between the nucleotides indicated. The complementary single strands were used for a second PCR step to obtain a product that combines both fragments. The PCR fragment was cloned into the pCR2.1 vector (Invitrogen, Groningen, NL) and excised with Bgl II and PflM I. This Bgl II-Pflm I fragment was then cloned into the Bgl II-Pflm I dige- sted full-length cDNA. The resulting FVIIIΔB cDNA was excised with Sal I and clo- ned into a pcDNA3 vector. The lack of mutations due to the PCR amplification and cloning was confirmed by sequencing.

Vector construction

To generate the lentiviral vector C(FVIIIΔB)IGWS, two cloning steps were required. First, the HIV-1-based, monocistronic self-inactivating vector pRRL-CMV-GFP-WPRE-SIN (CGWS, derivative of the vectors pRRL-PGK-GFP-SIN-18 and pHR'-CMV-LacZ-SIN-18 kindly provided by D. Trono, Geneva, Switzerland) encoding the EGFP gene (enhanced green fluorescence protein) as a marker gene flanked 5' by an internal CMV promoter and 3' by the woodchuck hepatitis virus posttranscriptio-nal regulatory element (WPRE) was modified by insertion of a multiple cloning site (MCS) and the internal ribosome entry site (IRES) of the encephalomyocarditis virus (ECMV; MCS and IRES from pIRES2-EGFP, Clontech, Heidelberg, Germany).

Then the FVIIIΔB fragment was excised from the pcDNA3 vector and cloned into the Sal I site of the MCS between CMV promoter and IRES to yield a bicistronic lentiviral vector. Due to the deletion in the U3 region of the 3' LTR, the transcription of the integrated provirus is regulated only by the CMV promoter upstream of the FVIIIdelB-IRES-EGFP expression cassette.

Cell lines and culture conditions

Hematopoietic cell lines representing different lymphoid and myeloid subsets were obtained from ATCC or the DSMZ (Deutsche Sammlung für Mikroorganismen und Zellkulturen GmbH, Braunschweig, D). The cell lines K562 (chronic myeloid leuke-mia), TF-1 (erythroleukemia), Raji (Burkitt B cell lymphoma), Jurkat (acute T cell leukemia), PLB-985 (acute myeloid leukemia), and KG-1 (acute myeloid leukemia) were cultured in RPMI (plus 5 ng/ml rhIL-3 for TF-1) or IMDM (for KG-1) supple-mented with 10% heat inactivated fetal calf serum (HI-FCS), 4mM L-glutamine, 100 U/ml penicillin G sodium, and 100 µg/ml streptomycin sulfate. 293T cells were maintained in DMEM/10%HI-FCS with 4mM L-glutamine, 100 U/ml penicillin G sodium, and 100 µg/ml streptomycin sulfate and grown in tissue culture flasks or plates precoated with 0,1% gelatin.

Vector supernatant production

To generate lentiviral particles C(FVIIIΔB)IGWS vector DNA was transiently introduced into 293T cells by triple cotransfection with the packaging construct
pCMVΔ8.93 encoding gag, pol and rev [37] and the pseudotyping construct pMD.G
[38] coding for the vesicular stomatitis virus glycoprotein (VSV-G). Transfection of
plasmid DNA was performed via calcium phosphate coprecipitation. 16 hrs after
transfection, the cell culture medium was replaced by medium containing 10 mM
sodium butyrate (Upstate, Lake Placid, NY) for 11 hrs. Then this medium was
removed, the cells were washed with PBS and virus was collected twice after incubation periods of 12 hrs in X-Vivo10 supplemented with 1% human serum albumin
(HSA; BSD Hessen), 2 mM L-glutamine, 100 U/ml penicillin G sodium, and 100
µg/ml streptomycin. The VSV-G pseudotyped lentiviral particles were concentrated
tenfold by ultrafiltration (Vivaspin, Greiner, D) and used for transduction of target
cell lines at titers of 1–2x10^6 TU/ml (TU, 293T-transducing units).

Transduction of different cell types and sorting of highly transduced cells

The transductions of hematopoietic cell lines and 293T cells were performed in 24-
well plates. For the transduction of hematopoietic cell lines, 10^5 cells were transduced in each well with 500–1000 µl concentrated virus in the presence of 4 µg/ml pro-
tamine sulfate (and 5 ng/ml rhIL-3 for TF-1). 293T cells were seeded at a density of
5x10^4 cells per well and transduced with 500 µl concentrated virus in the presence
of 4µg/ml polybrene. After spinoculation (1250 g, 90 mins, 32°C), the cells were
incubated for further 16 hrs with the virus. Cells were then washed and cultured in
vitro until FACS analysis and sorting. In order to obtain efficiently transduced cell
populations, the cells were sorted using EGFP gene expression as marker for transduction efficiency by means of a MoFlo high-speed cell sorter (Cytomation, USA).
The cells with the brightest EGFP fluorescence (about 1% of each mixed population) were then cultured and used for analysis of FVIII expression.

FVIII quantification

To assess the amount of secreted FVIII protein, transduced EGFP-sorted hematopoietic cell lines and 293T cells as well as untransduced controls were seeded at a
concentration of 5x10^5 cells/ml in a 24 well plate. After 48 hrs the supernatants were
harvested and stored at –20°C until analysis. FVIII activity (FVIII:C) was quantified
by measuring the FVIII-dependent generation of factor Xa from factor X using a
chromogenic assay (Immuno GmbH, Heidelberg, D).

FVIII antigen (FVIII:Ag) was determined according to the manufacturer's
instruction using a commercially available sandwich ELISA (Immuno GmbH,
Heidelberg, D). Results are represented as mean of at least four (FVIII:C) or six
experiments (FVIII:Ag). Human plasma of known FVIII activity (1IU = 200ng/ml)
was used as standard. In all experiments, supernatants of non-transduced cell lines

were run as negative controls. Activity and antigen concentration in these controls was always <1ng/ml FVIII:C and FVIII:Ag, respectively. In addition, media containing heat-treated FCS did not yield any detectable FVIII activity or antigen.

Results

Transduction efficiency of hematopoietic cell lines

To generate stable FVIII-expressing cell lines, hematopoietic cells representing different leukocyte subsets were transduced with VSV-G pseudotyped lentiviral particles derived from the vector C(FVIIIΔB)IGWS (Fig. 1) encoding FVIIIΔB and enhanced green fluorescence protein (EGFP). The vector titers, were about tenfold decreased for the FVIIIΔB-containing construct C(FVIIIΔB)IGWS, when compared to the corresponding control vector CGWS. The transduction efficiency as determined by the number of EGFP-positive cells varied considerably between the different cell lines and ranged between 4% and 64%, being highest in cell lines K-562 and TF-1 (55%, 64%) and lowest in lines KG-1 and Raji (4%, 5%), respectively (data not shown). To further enrich for transduced cells, cells with high EGFP fluorescence intensity were sorted using a high-speed fluorescence activated cell sorter. With this technique, we were able to establish populations of transduced cells which contained at least 72% EGFP-positive cells (Table 1). There was no correlation between EGFP expression and FVIII secretion.

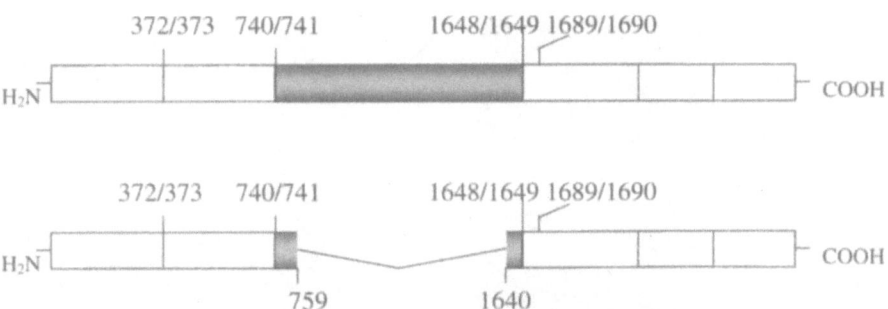

Fig. 1. Schematic representation of FVIIIΔB. The B-domain deleted FVIIIc DNA used in our experiments is represented was obtrained by multiple cloning steps. The deletion of nucleotides 2428 to 5067 of the FVIII full length cDNA leads to a protein with a deletion from amino acids 760 to 1639

Comparison of FVIII expression in lentivirally transduced cell lines

RT-PCR with FVIIIΔB specific primers confirmed the transcription of the integrated FVIII cDNA in all hematopoietic cell lines (data not shown). Analysis of the supernatants of transduced cells for FVIII secretion gave highest amounts of FVIII

Table 1. Characteristics of lentivirally transduced hematopoietic cell lines. Control plasma with 100% FVIII activity (200 ng/ml served as a reference. Detection limit (1 ng/ml)

Transduced cell line	Origin	EGFP-expression after sorting (%)	rFVIII expression FVIII:C	FVIII:Ag
K562	Chronic myeloid leukemia	74.2	76.4	74.8
TF1	Erythroleukemia	93.3	41.6	49.1
Raji	Burkitt B cell lymphoma	87.6	6.73	6.88
Jurkat	Acute T cell leukemia	72.3	1.83	1.95
PLB	Acute myeoloid leukemia	91.5	<1	<1
KG-1	Acute myeloid leukemia	74.4	<1	<1

secretion by the erythrocytic/megakaryocytic leukemia cell lines K-562-F8 and TF-1-F8, which secrete 74.8 and 49.1 ng FVIII:Ag per $5x10^5$ cells in 48 hrs, respectively. The Burkitt B cell lymphoma line Raji exhibits moderate FVIII levels with 6,88 ng FVIII:Ag, whereas the acute T cell leukemia derived cell line Jurkat does produce low levels of transgene FVIII protein (1.95 ng FVIII) (Fig. 2). However, despite the high transduction efficacy and the detection of transcribed FVIII mRNA, no FVIII protein could be detected in the supernatants of the acute myelogenous leukemia cell lines KG-1-F8 and PLB-985-F8 (Table 1).

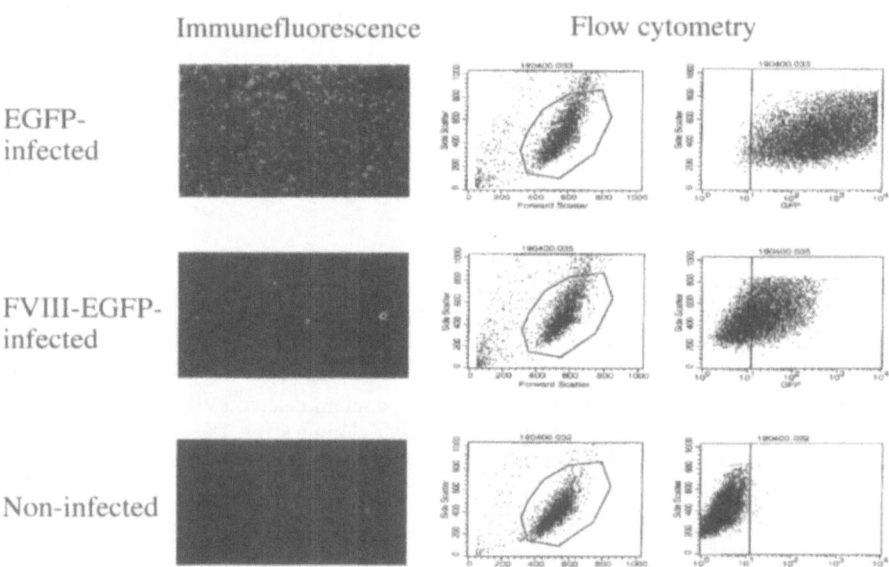

Immunefluorescence   Flow cytometry

EGFP-infected

FVIII-EGFP-infected

Non-infected

Fig. 2. Immunefluorescence and FACS analysis of EGFP expression in K562 cells. K562 cells were either transfected with a lentiviral vector encoding for EGFP (top line), or for FVIII and EGFP. Untransduced cells served as control (bottom line). EGFP expression and transduction efficiency in K562 cells that were transduced with the lentiviral construct encoding for both, FVIIIΔB and EGFP, was markedly reduced when compared to EGFP-transduced cells

To prove the functionality of the recombinant FVIIIΔB-protein, the coagulation activity of the secreted FVIII was assessed using a chromogenic assay. In all cell lines, the FVIII clotting activity (FVIII:C) corresponded well with the amounts of FVIII:Ag (Table 1). The human embryonal kidney cell line 293T which was transduced with the same vector C(FVIIIΔB)IGWS to give rise to 293T-F8, served as a reference cell line for FVIII expression throughout the experiments. While these cells were not sorted for transduced cells and exhibited up to 400ng FVIII activity per 5x10^5 cells in 48 hrs shortly after transduction (data not shown), the amount of FVIII protein secreted declined over time to remain stable at approximately 86 ng/ml. In EGFP-sorted hematopoietic cell lines, FVIII secretion remained stable over the observation period of now 6 months. Supernatants of non-transduced cells were always run as controls and did never exhibit FVIII:C or FVIII:Ag activity.

Discussion

The capacity of hematopoietic stem cells (HSC) to differentiate into a large number of blood cells and as recently reported to trans-differentiate into non-hematopoietic tissue such as liver and endothelial cells [23,24], makes them attractive targets for ex vivo gene therapeutic approaches of the hemophilias. Small numbers of genetically engineered hematopoietic stem cells could potentially provide a patient with stable populations of FVIII-secreting cells of all blood-cell types as well as liver and endothelial cells, providing long-term expression of the transgene and immediate access to the blood stream [25].

However, several attempts have failed to show recombinant FVIII expression after transduction of primary hematopoietic cells or hematopoietic cell lines. Hoeben et al. have successfully transferred the B-domain deleted FVIII cDNA into progenitor cells but despite the proof of transcribed FVIII-mRNA in hematopoietic colonies, they failed to detect secretion of recombinant FVIII protein by these cells [21]. Since this was accompanied by successful integration of the FVIII cDNA into the genome of hematopoietic cells, the lack of FVIII secretion was mainly ascribed to the inability of hematopoietic cells to synthesize and secrete FVIII [21]. Using an improved FVIII retroviral splicing vector Chuah et al. have demonstrated high FVIII expression (10–60 ng of FVIII/10^6 cells/24hrs) in cell lines derived from human medullary thyroid carcinoma, skin primary fibroblasts as well as human umbilical vein endothelial cells. This study however failed to show functional FVIII protein expression in transduced human T-lymphoma cells (SupT1) and the human Burkitt B-lymphoblastoma cells (Raji) [22]. With the same vector system Evans and Morgan were able to induce tolerance to transgene FVIII in hemophilia mice through transplantation of transduced hematopoietic progenitor cells. However, while the induction of tolerance in these experiments suggests the secretion of FVIII protein or fragments thereof in the context of tolerogenic compartments of the immune system through antigen presenting cells (APC), the transplanted mice failed to show detectable FVIII plasma levels [26].

Using a new generation bicistronic lentiviral construct encoding FVIIIΔB and EGFP which allows stable transduction and enrichment of hematopoietic cells, our present work aimed to reanalyze the capacity of hematopoietic cells to express recombinant FVIII protein. Using this combined approach of stable transduction and enrichment of transduced cells, we were able to establish stable FVIII-secreting hematopoietic cell lines representing different blood-cell subtypes.

Among the cell lines analyzed, K562-F8 and TF-1-F8 cells were shown to secrete high levels of FVIII:Ag, 74.8 ng/ml and 49.1 ng/ml/5x10^5/48 hrs, respectively, while moderate FVIII secretion was observed in the B lymphoblastoid cell line Raji (6.8 ng/ml) and low levels of FVIII in the T cell leukemia line Jurkat (1.9 ng/ml). The monocytic cell lines KG-1 and PLB did not show any detectable FVIII protein.

The differences in FVIII secretion between transduced hematopoietic cell lines seem not to be related to the transduction efficacy, since we did not observe any correlation between the mean copy number of integrated FVIII genes and the amount of secreted FVIII protein. Despite stable integration of 20 and 5 copies per cells and transcription of FVIII cDNA's, PLB-F8 and KG-1-F8 did not secrete detectable amounts of FVIII protein. Using flow cytometry, we were not able to detect intracellular FVIII in these cells, which would have suggested that the lack of FVIII in the supernatants of transduced PLB-F8 and KG-1-F8 cells is due to the inability of these cells to secrete FVIII (data not shown). However, flow cytometry might not be sensitive enough to exclude low levels of intracellular FVIII protein and we therefore feel that further analysis on the subcellular level using e.g. confocal laser scanning microscopy should be necessary to answer this question. Of note is that in the present study we were able to achieve stable expression of FVIII at moderate levels in B lymphoblastoid Raji cells and the T cell line Jurkat. Previous studies have failed to show recombinant FVIII secretion in Raji cells and the human T cell line SupT1 using moloney-based retroviral vectors and enrichment of transduced cells by G418-selection [18]. Interestingly, cell lines that proved to be most effective in secreting recombinant FVIII protein, i.e. the proerythroblastic leukemia line K562 and the megakaryoblastic line TF-1, are both described to be able to differentiate into the megakaryocytic lineage [44,45], and it is conceivable that compared to other blood cells, megakaryocytes are especially suited to express and secrete recombinant FVIII. Besides endothelial cells, megakaryocytes are the natural site of von Willebrand factor (vWF) production [46,47]. vWF serves as an important carrier for FVIII protein, and binding of FVIII to vWF leads to stabilization of the FVIII protein and reduced proteolytic cleavage. In cell lines, coexpression of vWF- and FVIII-cDNA leads to increased FVIII expression as well as secretion [32]. In endothelial cells vWF alters the intracellular trafficking of FVIII from a constitutive to a regulated secretory pathway, thus creating a releasable storage pool of colocalized FVIII and vWF in Weibel-Palade bodies [14].

In conclusion, our experiments show for the first time stable FVIII secretion by individual hematopoietic cell lines, which suggests reanalysis of HSC as targets for gene therapy of hemophilia A. Moreover, the established cell lines should be a valuable tool to further elucidate factors that might be able to increase efficacy of FVIII secretion in hematopoietic cells at the post-translational level.

Acknowledgments. T.T. is recipient of a research fellowship through the »Stiftung Hämotherapie-Forschung«. This work was supported in part by research funding from the »Gesellschaft für Thrombose- und Hämostaseforschung e.V. (GTH)« to T.T and the »Hermann J. Abs Program of the Deutsche Bank AG«. The Georg-Speyer-Haus is supported by the »Bundesministerium für Gesundheit« and the »Hessische Ministerium für Wissenschaft und Kunst«.

References ·

1. Furie B, SA Limentaniand, CG Rosenfield. (1994). A practical guide to the evaluation and treatment of hemophilia. Blood 84: 3–9.
2. Hoyer LW. (1994). Hemophilia A. N Engl J Med 330: 38–47.
3. Ginsburg D. (1997). Hemophilias and other disorders of hemostasis. In: Principle and Practice of Medical Genetics. DL Rimoin, JM Connor, RE Pyeritz, eds. (New York: Churchill Livingstone) Vol 3. pp. 1651–1674.
4. Kaufman, RJ (1999). Advances toward gene therapy for hemophilia at the millennium. Hum Gene Ther 10: 2091–2107.
5. Thompson, AR (2000). Gene therapy for the haemophilias. Haemophilia 6 (Suppl): 115–119.
6. High, KA (2001). Gene transfer as an approach to treating hemophilia. Circ Res 88: 137–144.
7. Wion KL, D Kelly, JA Summerfield, EGD Tuddenham and RM Lawn. (1985). Distribution of factor VIII mRNA and antigen in human liver and other tissues. Nature 317: 726–729.
8. Zelechowska MG, JA van Mourik and T Brodniewicz-Proba. (1985). Ultrastructural localization of factor VIII procoagulant antigen in human liver hepatocytes. Nature 317: 729–730.
9. Do H, JF Healey, EK Waller and P Lollar. (1999). Expression of Factor VIII by murine sinusoidal endothelial cells. J Biol Chem 28: 19587–19592.
10. Hollestelle MJ, T Thinnes, K Crain, A Stiko, JK Kruijt, TJ van Berkel, DJ Loskutoff and JA van Mourik. (2001). Tissue distribution of factor VIII gene expression in vivo – a closer look. Thromb Haemost 86(3):855–861.
11. Zatloukal K, M Cotton, M Berger, W Schmidt, E Wagner and ML Birnstiel. (1994). In vivo production of human factor VIII in mice after intrasplenic implantation of primary fibroblasts transfected by receptor-mediated, adenovirus-augmented gene delivery. Proc. Natl. Acad. Sci. (USA) 91: 5148–5152.
12. Dwarki VJ, P Belloni, T Nijjar, J Smith, L Couto, M Rabier, S Clift, A Berns and LK Cohen. (1995). Gene therapy for hemophilia A: Production of therapeutic levels of human factor VIII in vivo in mice. Proc Natl Acad Sci (USA) 92: 1023–1027.
13. Fakharzadeh SS, Y Zhang, R Sarkr and HH Kazazian. (2000). Correction of the coagulation defect in hemophilia A mice through factor VIII expression in skin. Blood 95: 2799–2805.
14. Rosenberg JB, JS Greengard and RR Montgomery. (2000). Genetic induction of a releasable pool of factor VIII in human endothelial cells. Arterioscler Thromb Vasc Biol 20: 2689–2695.
15. Lin Y, L Chang, A Solovey, JF Healey, P Lollar and RP Hebbel. (2002). Use of blood outgrowth endothelial cells for gene therapy for hemophilia A. Blood 99:457–462.
16. Conelly S, JM Gardner, RM Lyons, A McClelland and M Kaleko. (1996). Sustained expression of therapeutic levels of human factor VIII in mice. Blood 87: 4671–4677.
17. Park F, K Ohashi and MA Kay. (2000). Therapeutic levels of human factor VIII and IX using HIV-1-based lentiviral vectors in mouse liver. Blood 96: 1173–1176.
18. Chuah MKL, H Brems, V Vanslembrouck, D Collen and T VandenDriessche. (1998). Bone marrow stromal cells as targets for gene therapy of hemophilia A. Hum Gene Ther 9: 353–365.

19. VandenDriessche T, V Vasslembrouck, I Goovaerts, H Zwinnen, ML Vanderhaeghen, D Collen and MKL Chuah. (1999). Long-term expression of human coagulation factor VIII and correction of hemophilia A after in vivo retroviral gene transfer in factor VIII-deficient mice. Proc Natl. Acad. Sci. (USA) 96: 10379–10384.

20. Roth DA, NE Tawa, JM O'Brien, DA Treco, Rf Selden and the factor VIII transkaryotic therapy study group. (2001). Nonviral transfer of the gene encoding coagulation factor VIII in patients with severe hemophilia A. N Engl J Med 344: 1735–1742.

21. Hoeben RC, MP Einerhard, E Briet, H Van Ormondt, D Valerio and AJ Van Der Eb. (1992). Toward gene therapy for hemophilia A: retrovirus-mediated transfer of a FVIII gene into murine haematopoietic progenitor cells. Thromb. Haemost 67: 341–345.

22. Chuah MKL, T VandenDriessche and RA Morgan. (1995). Development and analysis of retroviral vectors expressing human factor VIII as a potential gene therapy for hemophilia A. Hum Gene Ther 6: 1363–1377.

23. Gehling UM, S Ergun, U Schumacher, C Wagener, K Pantel, M Otte, G Schuch, P Schafhausen, T Mende, N Kilic, K Kluge, B Schafer, DK Hossfeld and W Fiedler. (2000). In vitro differentiation of endothelial cells from AC133-positive progenitor cells. Blood 95: 3106–3112.

24. Lagasse E, H Connors, M Al-Dhalimy, M Reitsma, M Dohse, L Osborne, X Wang, M Finegold, IL Weissman and M Grompe. (2000). Purified hematopoietic stem cells can differentiate into hepatocytes in vivo. Nat. Med 11: 1229–1234.

25. Brenner MK (1996). Gene transfer to hematopoietic cells. N Engl J Med 335: 37–339.

26. Evans GL and RA Morgan. (1998). Genetic induction of immune tolerance to human clotting factor VIII in a mouse model for hemophilia A. Proc Natl Acad Sci (USA) 95: 5734–5739.

27. Lynch CM, DI Israel, RJ Kaufman and AD Miller. (1993). Sequences in the coding region of clotting factor VIII act as dominant inhibitors of RNA accumulation and protein production. Human Gene Ther 4: 259–272.

28. Koeberl DD, CL Halbert, A Krumm and AD Miller. (1995). Sequences within the coding regions of clotting factor VIII and CFTR block transcriptional elongation. Hum Gene Ther 6: 469–479.

29. Fallaux FJ, Hoeben RC, Cramer SJ, DJM van den Wollenberg, E Briet, H van Ormondt and AJ van der Eb. (1996). The human clotting factor VIII cDNA contains an autonomously replicating sequence consensus- and matrix attachment region-like sequence that binds a nuclear factor, represses heterologous gene expression, and mediates the transcriptional effects of sodium butyrate. Mol Cell Biol 16: 4264–4272.

30. Hoeben RC, RC van der Jagt, F Schoute, NH van Tilburg, MP Verbeet, E Briet, H van Ormondt and AJ van der Eb. (1990). Expression of functional factor VIII in primary human skin fibroblasts after retrovirus-mediated gene transfer. J Biol Chem 265: 7318–7323.

31. Hoeben RC, FJ Fallaux, SJ Cramer, DJ van den Wollenberg, H van Ormondt, E Briet and AJ van der Eb. (1995). Expression of the blood-clotting factor VIII cDNA is repressed by a transcriptional silencer located in its coding region. Blood 85: 2447–2454.

32. Kaufman RJ, LC Wasley, MV Davies, RJ Wise and DI Israel. (1989). The effect of von Willebrand factor coexpression on the synthesis and secretion of factor VIII in Chinese hamster ovarian cells. Mol Cell Biol 9: 1233–1242.

33. Tagliavacca L, Q Wang and RJ Kaufman (2000). ATP-dependent dissociation of non-disulfide-linked aggregates of coagulation factor VIII is a rate-limiting step for secretion. Biochem 39: 1973–1981.

34. Case SS, MA Price, CT Jordan, XJ Yu, L Wang, G Bauer, DL Haas, KD Xu, R Stripecke, L Naldini, DB Kohn and GM Crooks. (1999). Stable transduction of quiescent CD34+CD38- human hematopoietic cells by HIV-1-based lentiviral vectors. Proc Natl Acad Sci (USA) 96: 2988–2993.

35. Miyoshi H, KA Smith, DE Mosier, IM Verma and BE Torbett. (1999). Transduction of human CD34+ cells that mediate long-term engraftment of NOD/SCID mice by HIV vectors. Science 283: 682–686.

36. Toole JJ, JL Knopf, JM Wozney, LA Sultzman, JL Buecker, DD Pittman, RJ Kaufman, E Brown, C Shoemaker, EC Orr, GW Amphlett, WB Foster, ML Coe, GJ Knutson, DN, Fass and NF Hewick. (1984). Molecular cloning of a cDNA encoding human antihaemophilic factor. Nature 312: 342–347.
37. Dull T, R Zufferey, M Kelly, RJ Mandel, M Nguyen, D Trono and L Naldini. (1998). A third-generation lentivirus vector with a conditional packaging system. J Virol 72: 8463–8471.
38. Ory DS, BA Neugeboren and RC Mulligan. (1996). A stable human-derived packaging cell line for production of high titer retrovirus/vesicular stomatitis virus G pseudotypes. Proc Natl Acad Sci (USA) 93: 11400–11406.
39. Zanetta L, SG Marcus, J Vasile, M Dobryansky, H Cohen, K Eng, P Shamamian and P Mignatti. (2000). Expression of von-Willebrand-Factor, an endothelial cell marker, is unregulated by angiogenesis factors: a potential method for objective assessment of tumor angiogenesis. Int J Cancer 85: 281–288.
40. Denis CV, K Kwack, S Saffaripour, S Maganti, P Andre, RG Schaub and DD Wagner. (2001). Interleukin 11 significantly increases plasma von Willebrand factor and factor VIII in wild type and von Willebrand disease mouse models. Blood 97: 465–472.
41. Stirling D, WA Hannant and CA Ludlam. (1998). Transcriptional activation of the factor VIII gene in liver cell lines by interleukin-6. Thromb Haemost 79: 74–78.
42. Cardier JE, DC Foster, S Lok, SE Jacobsen and MJ Murphy. (1996). Megakaryocytopoiesis in vitro: from the stem cells' perspective. Stem Cells 14(suppl):163–172.
43. Drayer AL, CT SIbinga, NR Blom, JT De Wolf and E Vellenga. (2000). The in vitro effects of cytokines on expansion and migration of megakaryocyte progenitors. Br J Haematol 109: 776–784.
44. Tetteroo PA, F Massaro, A Mulder, R Schreuder-van Gelder and AE von dem Borne. (1984). Megakaryoblastic differentiation of proerythroblastic K562 cell-line cells. Leuk Res 8: 197–206.
45. Testa U, F Grignani, HJ Hassan, D Rogaia, R Masciulli, V Gelmetti, R Guerriero, G Macioce, C Liberatore, T Barberi, G Mariani, PG Pelicci and C Peschle. (1998). Terminal megakaryocytic differentiation of TF-1 cells is induced by phorbol esters and thrombopoietin and is blocked by expression of PML/RARalpha fusion protein. Leukemia 12: 563–570.
46. Nachman R, R Levine and EA Jaffe. (1977). Synthesis of factor VIII antigen by cultured guinea pig megakaryocytes. J Clin Invest 60: 914–921.
47. Greenberg SM and C Chandrasekhar. (1991). Hematopoietic factor-induced synthesis of von Willebrand factor by the Dami human megakaryoblastic cell line and by normal human megakaryocytes. Exp Hematol 19: 53–58.

Adenovirus-mediated regulatable Expression of human Factor IX *in vitro* and *in vivo*

M.A. Srour, H. Fechner, X. Wang, U. Siemetzki, T. Albert,
J. Oldenburg, P. Hanfland, W. Poller, H.-H. Brackmann,
and R. Schwaab

Abstract

The ability to modulate transgene expression *in vivo* not only will mimic the expression of endogenous genes but is also important for therapeutic and safety reasons in gene therapy protocols. Regulated gene expression systems should be able to induce long-term expression and allow for exogenous control of expression. For this aim, the high gene transfer capacity of adenoviral vectors (Ad) and the high inducibility of the tetracycline-regulatable systems were combined in this study to develop a tetracycline-regulatable Ad vector for expression of human factor IX (hFIX). *In vitro* studies showed a dose dependent and high induction potential of the hFIX expression system resulting in 65-fold increase in hFIX expression after induction with doxycycline. The use of a liver-specific promoter has been shown to induce a relatively high expression of hFIX compared to CMV promoter in HepG2. In contrast to this, the liver specific promoter showed no hFIX expression when tested in three other non-hepatic human cell lines. The expression of hFIX can either be maintained by continuous induction of doxycycline or up- and down-regulated by mutual presence and absence of doxycycline. When mice were injected with Ad vector for hFIX and induced by doxycycline they showed a therapeutic level of circulating hFIX for one week. These results report on the development of a regulated Ad vectors for the expression of hFIX and demonstrate that FIX gene expression is regulatable *in vitro* and *in vivo*. These vectors should be useful not only for gene therapy protocols in haemophilia B but also for diverse applications in gene therapy studies.

Introduction

In vivo, endogenous genes are expressed in specific cells at specific levels. Therefore, for gene therapy pharmacological control over the level of expression is necessary. One of the most used regulatable expression systems is the Tet-system of which transcriptional regulation can be driven by the antibiotic tetracycline or its derivatives [1,11]. This system has been used for gene therapy purposes with adenovirus vectors (AdV) [6,18,29], retroviral [3,4,33] or adeno-associated viral vectors [5].

Recombinant AdVs are one of the attractive vectors' group for gene transfer into mammalian cells. In experimental animals, following intravenous administration of the AdVs, the vector tends to accumulate preferentially in the liver [9,12,19]. More-

I. Scharrer/W. Schramm (Ed.)
32nd Hemophilia Symposion Hamburg 2001
© Springer-Verlag Berlin Heidelberg 2003

over, the development of a new helper-dependent AdV has dramatically reduced the immunogenecity of AdV and resulted in a long-term expression of the transgene [22,28].

One of the most attractive models for gene therapy is the hemophilia B disease. Reasons for this are the existence of hemophilic animals, the good monitoring of the factor IX (FIX) protein after transferring of the transgene and the long life expectancy of haemophiliacs [24,38,40]. Until now, the expression of FIX *in vitro* and *in vivo* from AdVs [8,19,24,31,35,37], adeno-associated vectors [14,16,17,30,38], retroviral vectors [21,25,39,41] and naked plasmids [26,27] have been described. Moreover, based on species-specific results four clinical trials are either completed or currently underway: two for hemophilia B [20,40] and two for hemophilia A [32,40].

Recently, it has been shown that expression of high levels of FIX (above 129U/dl) increase the risk of venous thrombosis in normal individuals about 2- to 3-folds [36]. Therefore, it must be our intention to develop gene therapy protocols with a controlled expression of the FIX gene.

In this study, we have developed Tet-On regulatable AdVs for the expression of human FIX *in vitro* and *in vivo*, whereas the regulator AdV was driven by the CMV promoter/enhancer or alternatively, the liver-specific hAAT promoter (human alpha1-antitrypsin).

Materials and Methods

Development of recombinant adenoviral vectors (AdV)

Ad5 vectors (Fig. 1) were constructed by *in vitro* ligation of the *XbaI*-restricted shuttle plasmid to the *XbaI* long fragment of Ad5-*dl309* (3.3 –36 kb), followed by rescue of the Ad5 vectors in HEK 293 cells [31].

Cell cultures
Cell culture studies were performed using standard cell culture techniques in: EAhy926 cells (stable hybrids resulting from fusion of primary human umbilical vein endothelial cells (HUVEC) with the human epithelial cell line A549), HepG2 cells (liver carcinoma cells), KYSE140 cells (esophageal epithelial squamous carcinoma cells) and Colo320 cells (human colorectal Adenocarcinoma cells).

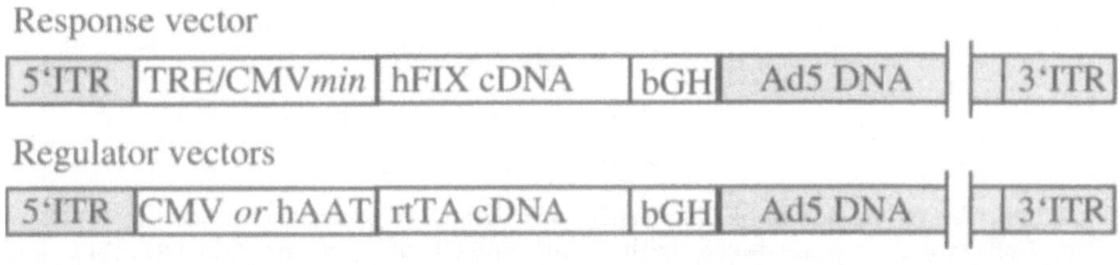

Fig. 1. Structure of AdVs. »Ad5 DNA« represents the long *XbaI* fragment of Ad5-*dl309* after restriction with *XbaI*. TRE: tetracycline responsive element; rtTA reverse tetracycline transactivator.

Animal experiments

Female C57BL/6 mice (8-10 weeks old; Charles River Sulzfeld, Germany) were injected intravenously via the tail vein with 4×10^{10} virus partiale (vp) per mouse, containing 2×10^{10} vp of regulator vector and 2×10^{10} vp of response vector (ratio 1:1). For induction of transgene expression, mice received a subcutaneous injection of Dox once a day starting two days before vector injection. For hFIX assay blood was collected by retro-orbital bleeding and mixed with 3.2% sodium citrate (9:1). After centrifugation of blood at 2000 xg at 4°C for 15 min, plasma was collected and stored at –80°C until determination of FIX:C and FIX:Ag.

Results

Inducible expression of hFIX in HepG2 cells with CMV promoter (in Ad5.CMV.rtTA) *in vitro*

The level of hFIX increased with Dox concentration, and maximum induction of hFIX was 64.9 in induced cells vs. 0.0 ng/10^6 cell/24 hours in un-induced cells at 200 ng/ml Dox (Fig. 2). Higher concentrations of Dox did not increase the hFIX expression.

Expression of hFIX by CMV promoter (Ad5.CMV.rtTA) and hAAT promoter Ad5.hAAT.rtTA) in four different cell lines

When HepG2 cells had been transduced with the response AdV (Ad5.TRE.hFIX) and the regulator AdV vector (either Ad5.CMV.rtTA or Ad5.hAAT.rtTA), the level of

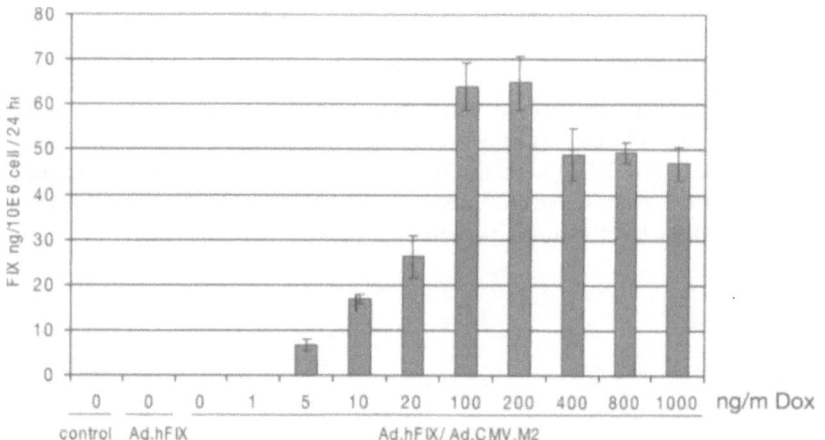

Fig. 2. Inducible expression of hFIX in HepG2 cells with CMV promoter (in Ad5.CMV.rtTA) *in vitro*. Cells were co-transduced with 2x10³ vp/cell of each of Ad5.TRE.hFIX and Ad5.CMV.rtTA, respectively, at 37°C for 20 min and then induced with different Dox concentration for 24 hours. hFIX concentration was determined in the medium supernatant by ELISA (Asserchrom IX:Ag ELISA kit (Roche)). Data are means ± SD

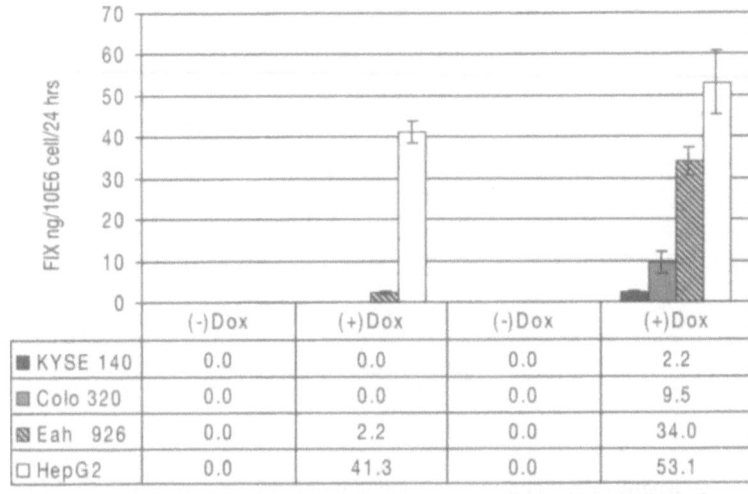

	(-)Dox	(+)Dox	(-)Dox	(+)Dox
■ KYSE 140	0.0	0.0	0.0	2.2
▨ Colo 320	0.0	0.0	0.0	9.5
▨ Eah 926	0.0	2.2	0.0	34.0
□ HepG2	0.0	41.3	0.0	53.1
	Ad.hFIX/ Ad.hAAT.rTA		Ad.hFIX/ Ad.CMV.rTA	

Fig. 3. Expression of hFIX by CMV promoter (Ad5.CMV.rtTA) and hAAT promoter Ad5.hAAT.rtTA) in four different cell lines. All cells were co-transduced with 2×10^3 vp/cell of each of the regulator and response AdV (Ad5.TRE.hFIX/Ad5.hAA.rtTA or Ad5.TRE.hFIX/Ad5.CMV.rtTA), respectively, and then incubated with 200 ng/ml Dox (+) or without Dox (-) for 24 hours. hFIX was determined in the medium supernatant by ELISA. The value »0.0« shown in the above table means that no detectable levels of hFIX was found in these samples. Data are means ± SD.

hFIX expression promoted by hAAT promoter was about 80% of that observed with CMV promoter (Fig. 3). When Ad5.TRE.hFIX plus Ad5.CMV.rtTA were used to co-transduce three non-hepatic cell lines, variable levels of hFIX have been observed with CMV promoter: 34.0, 9.5 and 2.2 ng/10^6 cell/24 hours for EAhy926, Colo320 and KYSE140 cells, respectively. In contrast, with hAAT promoter in the regulator AdV, very low levels of hFIX could only be detected in EAhy926 cells (2.2 ng/10^6 cell/24 hours), while in Colo320 and KYSE140 cells the level of hFIX was not detectable by ELISA.

Repetitive and continuous induction of hFIX in EAhy926 cells

To examine whether Dox-induced expression of hFIX can be up- and down-regulated by adding or removing Dox from the medium or maintained under continuous induction, EAhy926 cells were co-transduced with Ad5.TRE.hFIX/Ad5.CMV.rtTA (Fig. 4). For the first aim, cells were induced with 100 ng/ml Dox (R) for 24 hours, then Dox was removed and cells were kept for six days without Dox. On the seventh day, cells were re-induced using the same Dox dose for another 24 hours. For the second aim, EAhy926 cells were kept under continuous induction by three different Dox concentrations ((C) 20, 100, 200 ng/ml) for eight days. As shown in Figure 4, the level of hFIX after one-day induction with Dox reached 41 ng/10^6 cell/24 hours.

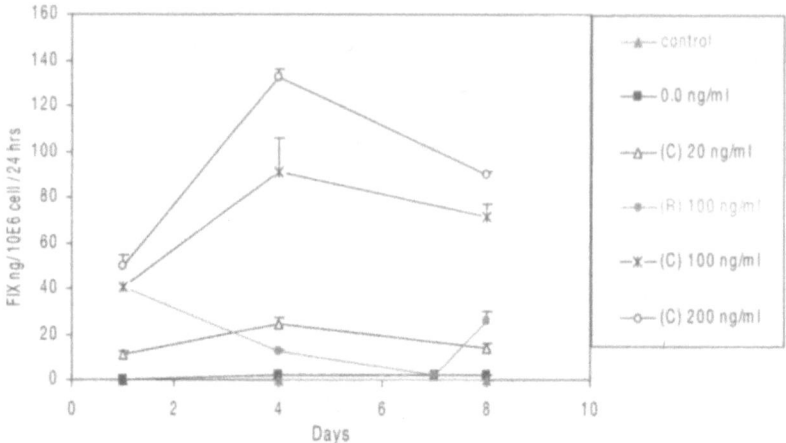

Fig. 4. Repetitive and continuous induction of hFIX expression in EAhy926 cells. Cells in 12-well plate were co-transduced with 2x10³ vp/cell of each of Ad5.TRE.hFIX and Ad5.CMV.rtTA and then incubated for 8 days with or without Dox (0.0 to 200 ng/ml). Control cells received neither vectors nor Dox (control) or only vectors (0.0 ng/ml Dox). The medium was collected every 24 hours for hFIX assay, and the cells were re-fed with fresh medium +/- Dox. Cells referred to with (R) were induced with 100 ng/ml Dox for 24 hours, then Dox was removed for six days, and re-induced with the same Dox dose again on the seventh day for another 24 hours. Cells referred to with (C) were induced with Dox (20, 100, 200 ng/ml) during the whole experiment (eight days). Data are means ± SD.

Upon removal of the inducer the expression declined about 3-folds after three days, and then almost returned to the basal level (2 ng/10⁶ cell/24 hours) at day seven. Re-induction with the same Dox dose on the seventh day has shown an increase in hFIX expression (26 ng/10⁶ cell/24 hours) on the eighth day. Additionally, Figure 4 shows that cells maintained under continuous induction with Dox express hFIX continuously and in amounts which are dependent on the Dox concentration during the experiment time (eight days).

Induction of FIX transgene expression *in vivo*

Based on preliminary results with luciferase expression, mice injected with Ad5.TRE.hFIX/Ad5.CMV.rtTA were treated with 250 μg Dox/mouse. The hFIX antigen level was determined in plasma at 2, 4, and 7 days post-infection. Figure 5 shows different expression within mice, however all hFIX values were above those of the control mice. Summarizing the results of all four mice induced with Dox, the average expression level for hFIX after 2, 4 and 7 days were 117, 131 and 13 ng/ml, respectively (corresponding to 2%, 2.5% and 0.2% of hFIX plasma antigen level, respectively). The hFIX has reached a maximum by the fourth day followed by about 10-fold reduction of the expression level on the seventh day.

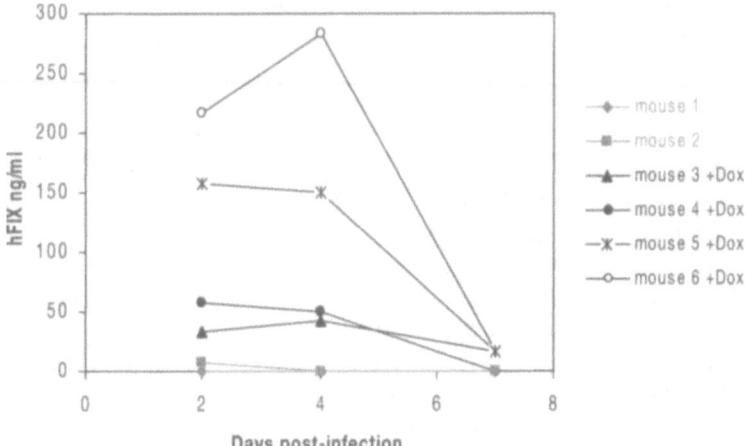

Fig. 5. Induction of hFIX expression in immunocompetent C57BL/6 mice. Mice were injected with $2x10^{10}$ vp per mouse of the response AdV (Ad5.TRE.hFIX) and the regulator AdV (Ad5.CMV.rtTA). Transgene expression was induced by subcutaneous injection of Dox once a day. Levels of hFIX in plasma are shown at 2, 4 and 7 days post-infection from mice induced with 250 µg Dox per mouse (mice 3-6) or those that received no Dox (mice 1-2). Each line represents an individual mouse. The level of hFIX in control mice (no vectors, no Dox) was not detectable by ELISA.

Discussion

Several adenoviral expression vectors in animals have been described [8,10,19,24,31,37]. In these studies, the level of FIX expression was extremely variable ranging from 100–1000 ng/ml (2–20%) [8] to several folds above normal FIX levels [24,31]. Moreover, it has been shown recently that increased levels of hFIX above normal levels (above 129U/dl) increase the risk for deep vein thrombosis by 2 to 3-folds [36]. Therefore, it should be desirable within gene therapy protocols, if hFIX level can be either up or down-regulated to maintain it within the therapeutic range for both therapeutic and safety reasons.

In this study the high gene transfer capacity of AdVs and the high inducibility of the Tet-system [1,11] have been combined to construct a tetracycline-regulatable AdVs for expression of hFIX. *In vitro* investigations have shown a high induction level of about 65-fold with hFIX (Ad5.TRE.hFIX/Ad5.CMV.rtTA) in HepG2 cells (Fig. 2). The Dox-induced expression in HepG2 cells was highly sensitive to the Dox concentration until 200-400 ng Dox/ ml. Similar results reported by other groups, using Tet-regulated vectors for Interleukin-12 [29] or erythropoietin [3], have also shown several fold increase in transgene expression *in vitro*.

For gene therapy, a liver-specific expression of hFIX is very important, since hFIX undergoes extensive post-translation modifications [2,7] in its natural site of synthesis. In order to achieve a liver specific expression of hFIX, the CMV promoter of Ad5.CMV.rtTA was replaced by the strong liver-specific hAAT promoter [13,26] and then Ad5.TRE.hFIX/Ad5.hAAT.rtTA constructs were used to co-transduce four different human cell lines representing four different organs *in vitro*. The only high expression rate of hFIX has been observed in HepG2 cells, where hFIX antigen level was about 80% of that observed with CMV promoter. In the three non-hepatic cell lines, hFIX expression was either extremely low in EAhy926 cells or undetectable in Colo320 and KYSE140 cells (Fig. 3). This is consistent with the *in vivo* distribution of hAAT gene expression, which is predominantly expressed in the liver and to a much lesser extent (<5% of the liver) in other organs such as kidney and stomach [34]. Using the CMV promoter, hFIX was expressed at different levels in all four cell lines, but as expected [23]. Thus, this assay could demonstrate, that a high and tissue-specific expression of hFIX can be achieved using hAAT promoter combined with an AdV/Tet-regulated expression system.

To demonstrate a successful Tet-regulated expression of hFIX, it should be possible to either maintain or up- and down-regulate transgene expression by manipulating Dox concentration. EAhy926 cells which had been co-transduced with Ad5.TRE.hFIX and Ad5.CMV.rtTA, and which had been continuously induced with Dox showed a high increase in hFIX expression for at least eight days. In a parallel experiment, when Dox was removed after one day, hFIX expression was reduced by more than 3-folds after three days and it further declined to basal level within six days (Fig. 4). Upon re-induction of the cells with the same Dox dose six days after removing Dox, hFIX expression increased again. These results indicate that hFIX expression levels can indeed be regulated over time by Dox in cultured cells transduced with Tet-regulated Ad5.TRE.hFIX. Similar results for repetitive induction of erythropoietin in primary myoblasts transduced with retroviral vectors by Dox *in vitro* have been reported by Bohl *et al.* [4].

When C57BL/6 mice were injected with Ad5.TRE.hFIX/Ad5.CMV.rtTA, they have shown an increase in hFIX expression (Fig. 5) with an average of 117, 131 and 13 ng/ml at 2, 4, and 7 days post-infection, respectively. Additionally, determination of hFIX activity in plasma from mice injected with Ad5.TRE.hFIX/Ad5.CMV.rtTA has shown that hFIX was also functional (data not shown). However, the rapid decline in hFIX antigen level after the fourth day is probably due to the loss of the AdV genome caused by the immune response of the mice, which seems to be directed against the vector proteins and/or against the cells harboring these vectors [10,15]. Using similar Tet-regulated Ad vectors for expression of interleukin-12, Nakagawa *et al.* [29] have observed that interleukin-12 level in mice peaked after 24 hours following infection, however was not detectable any more at day six.

In conclusion, the Tet-regulated AdVs for hFIX have been shown to be inducible, to achieve a dose-dependent expression of hFIX, and to allow a tissue-specific and repetitive induction of hFIX *in vitro*. This system also produced an inducible and therapeutic level of functional hFIX for about one week (end of experiment) in mice. At least this or other regulative expression systems should not only be useful for hemophilia, but also for other gene therapy applications, particularly if the vector persistence *in vivo* has been improved.

Acknowledgment. This study was supported by a research grant from Aventis, Germany. Additionally, MAS was supported by a scholarship from the German Academic Exchange Service.

References

1. Gossan M, Bujard H. Tight control of gene expression in mammalian cells by tetracycline-responsive promoters. Proc Natl Acad Sci USA. 1992;89:5547-5551
2. Arruda VR, Hagstrom JN, Deitch J, *et al*. Posttranslational modifications of recombinant myotube-synthesised human factor IX. Blood. 2001;97:130-138
3. Bohl D, Heard JM. Modulation of erythropoietin delivery from engineered muscles in mice. Hum Gene Ther. 1997;8:195-204
4. Bohl D, Naffakh N, Heard JM. Long-term control of erythropoietin secretion by doxycycline in mice transplanted with engineered primary myoblasts. Nature Med. 1997;3:299-305
5. Bohl D, Salvetti A, Moullier P, Heard JM. Control of erythropoietin delivery in mice after intramuscular injection of adeno-associated vector. Blood. 1998;92:1512-1517
6. Corti O, Sabate O, Horellou P, *et al*. A single adenovirus vector mediates doxycycline controlled expression of tyrosine hydroxylase in brain grafts of human neural progenitors. Nat Biotechnol. 1999;17:349-354
7. Dahlbäck B. Blood coagulation. Lancet. 2000;355:1627-1632
8. Dai Y, Schwarz EM, Gu D, Zhang WW, Sarvetnick N, Verma IM. Cellular and humoral immune response to adenoviral vectors containing factor IX gene: tolerization of factor IX and vector antigens allows for long-term expression. Proc Natl Acad Sci USA. 1995;92:1401-1405
9. Fechner H, Haack A, Wang H, *et al*. Expression of coxsackie adenovirus receptor and alpha,-integrin does not correlate with adenovector targeting *in vivo* indicating anatomical vector barrier. Gene Ther. 1999;6:1520-535
10. Fields PA, Armstrong E, Hagstrom JN, *et al*. Intravenous administration of an E1/E3-deleted adenoviral vector induces tolerance to factor IX in C57BL/6 mice. Gene Ther. 2001;8:354-361
11. Gossan M, Freundlieb S, Bender G, Muller G, Hillen W, Bujard H. Transcriptional activation by tetracycline in mammalian cells. Science. 1995;268:1766-1769
12. Guo ZS, Wang L-H, Eisensmith RC, Woo SLC. Evaluation of promoter strength for hepatic gene expression *in vivo* following adenovirus-mediated gene transfer. Gene Ther. 1996;3:802-810
13. Hafenrichter DG, Wu X, Rettinger SD, Kennedy SC, Flye MW, Ponder KP. Evaluation of liver-specific promoters from retroviral vectors after *in vivo* transduction of hepatocytes. Blood. 1994;84:3394-3404
14. Hagstrom JN, Couto LB, Scallan C, *et al*. Improved muscle-derived expression of human coagulation factor IX from a skeletal actin/CMV hybrid enhancer/promoter. Blood. 2000;95:2536-2542
15. Harvey E-G, Hacket NR, El-Sawy T, *et al*. Variability of human systemic humoral immune responses to adenovirus gene transfer vectors administered to different organs. J Virol. 1999;73:6729-6742
16. Herzog RW, Hagstrom JM, Kung S-H, *et al*. Stable gene transfer and expression of human blood coagulation factor IX after intramuscular injection of recombinant adeno-associated virus. Proc Natl Acad Sci USA. 1997;94:5804-5809
17. Herzog RW, Yang EY, Couto LB, *et al*. Long-term correction of canine hemophilia B by gene transfer of blood coagulation factor IX mediated by adeno-associated viral vector. Nature Med. 1999;5:56-63
18. Hu SX, Ji W, Zhou Y, Logothetis C, Xu HJ. Development of an adenovirus vector with tetracycline rgulatable human tumor necrosis factor alpha gene expression. Cancer Res. 1997;57:3339-3343
19. Kay MA, Landen CN, Rothenberg SR, *et al*. *In vivo* hepatic gene therapy: complete albeit transient correction of factor IX deficiency in hemophilia B dogs. Proc Natl Acad Sci USA. 1994;91:2353-2357
20. Kay MA, Manno CS, Ragni MV, *et al*. Evidence for gene transfer and expression of factor IX in haemophilia B patients treated with an AAV vector. Nature Genet. 2000;24:257-261.

21. Kay MA, Rothenberg S, Landen CN, *et al.. In vivo* gene therapy of hemophilia B: sustained partial correction in factor IX-deficient dogs. Science. 1993;262:117-119
22. Kochanek S. Development of high-capacity adenoviral vectors for gene therapy. Hum Gene Ther. 1999;10:2451-2459
23. Kriegler M. Gene transfer and expression: a laboratory manual. New York: W.H. Freeman and Company; 1991
24. Kung S-H, Hagstrom JN, Cass D, *et al.* Human factor IX corrects the bleeding diathesis of mice with hemophilia B. Blood. 1998;91:784-790
25. Louis DS, Verma IM. An alternative approach to somatic cell gene therapy. Proc Natl Acad Sci USA. 1988;85:3150-3154
26. Miao CH, Oashi K, Patijn GA, *et al.* Inclusion of the hepatic locus control region, an intron and untranslated region increases and stabilizes hepatic factor IX gene expression *in vivo* but not *in vitro.* Mol Ther. 2000;1:522-532
27. Miao CH, Thompson AR, Loeb K, Ye X. Long-term and therapeutic-level hepatic gene expression of human factor IX after naked plasmid transfer in vivo. Mol Ther. 2001;3:947-957
28. Morsy MA, Gu M, Motzel S, *et al.* An adenoviral vector deleted for all viral coding sequences results in enhanced safety and extended expression of a leptin transgene. Proc Natl Acad Sci USA. 1998;95:7866-7871
29. Nakagawa S, Massie B, Hawley RG. Tetracycline regulatable adenovirus vectors: pharmacologic properties and clinical potential. Europ J Pharm Sci. 2001;13:53-60
30. Nakai H, Herzog RW, Hagstrom JN, *et al.* Adeno-associated viral vector-mediated gene transfer of human blood coagulation factor IX into mouse liver. Blood. 1998;91:4600-4607
31. Poller W, Schneider-Rasp S, Lieber U, *et al.* Stabilization of transgene expression by incorporation of E3 region genes in an adenoviral factor IX vector and treatment by transient anti-CD4 treatment of the host. Gene Ther. 1996;3:521-532
32. Roth DA, Tawa NE, O'Brien JM, Treco DA, Selden RF. Non-viral transfer of the gene encoding coagulation factor VIII in patients with severe hemophilia A. N Engl J Med. 2001;344:1735-1742
33. Serguera C, Bohl D, Rolland E, Prevost P, Heard M. Control of erythropoietin by doxycycline or mifepristone in mice bearing polymer-encapsulated engineered cells. Hum Gene Ther. 1999;10:375-383
34. Shen R-F, Clift SM, DeMayo JL, Sifers RN, Finegold MJ, Woo SLC. Tissue-specific regulation of human alpha1-antitrypsin gene expression in transgenic mice. DNA. 1989;8:101-108
35. Smith TAG, Mehaffey MG, Kayda DB, *et al.* Adenovirus mediated expression of therapeutic plasma levels of human factor IX in mice. Nature Genet. 1993;5:397-402
36. Van Hylckama Vlieg A, van der Linden IM, Bertina RM, Rosendaal FR. High levels of factor IX increase the risk of venous thrombosis. Blood. 2000;95:3678-3682
37. Walter J, You Q, Hagstrom JN, Sands M, High KA. Successful expression of human factor IX following repeat administration of an adenoviral vector in mice. Proc Natl Acad Sci USA. 1996;93:3056-3061
38. Wang L, Takabe K, Bidlingmaier SM, Ill CR, Verma IM. Sustained correction of bleeding disorder in hemophilia B mice by gene therapy. Proc Natl Acad Sci USA. 1999;96:3906-3910
39. Wang Y, Xu J, Pierson T, O'Malley BW, Tsai SY. Positive and negative regulation of gene expression in eukaryotic cells with an inducible transcriptional regulator. Gene Ther. 1997;4:432-441
40. White GC. Gene therapy in hemophilia: clinical trials update. Thromb Haemost. 2001;86:172-177
41. Yao S-H, Wilson JM, Nabel EG, Kurachi S, Hachiya HL, Kurachi K. Expression of human factor IX in rat capillary endothelial cells: toward somatic gene therapy for hemophilia B. Proc Natl Acad Sci USA. 1991;88:8101-8105

III. Hemophilia

Chairmen:

H.-H. BRACKMANN (Bonn)
W. KREUZ (Frankfurt/Main)

IIIa. Orthopedics

Experiences with MRI Examination of the Joints of hemophilic Children

K. Kurnik, N. Nohe, K. Stehr, M. Praun, A. Lieb, and Th. Pfluger

Introduction

Magnetic resonance imaging (MRI) enables exact evaluation of synovial and carti-laginous structures of the joints. In contrast, conventional radiology describes changes in bony structures, cartilage is not visualized. Bony defects, however, repre-sent irreversible, long-term damage due to recurrent bleeding into hemophilic joints. MRI thus is the method of choice for early diagnosis of beginning joint damage with the opportunity to start therapeutical interventions in time.

Patiens and Methods

In 32 hemophilic children MRI examinations (T1 and T2-sequences with and with-out contrast medium) of different joints were performed. Children were aged 7 to 17 years, 12 children had an age of 7 to 10 years, 20 children an age of 10 to 17 years. Half of the children were under our treatment since school age. 26 patients suffered from hemophilia A, 6 children from hemophilia B of the severe form, mainly 82% were on prophylaxis; in more than the half prophylaxis was started after the 4th year of life. 6 patients were on demand treatment.

A total of 69 joints (49 ankles, 8 elbows, 5 knees and 7 hips) were examined. 49/69 (71%) joints were the affected index joints, 20/69 (29%) joints (19 ankles, 1 hip) the clinically healthy joints on the contrary side. Here the evaluation of both joints was possible in a single MRI session.

Indications for the MRI examination were orthopedic abnormalities in 29/49 (59%) and isolated pain with normal orthopedic examination in 20/49 (41%) joints. In 39/49 (80%) index joints at least 10 bleeding episodes, in 10/49 (20%) index joints less than 5 bleeding episodes had occurred. The time interval between MRI and last joint bleed was 4 weeks at least.

Aim of this study was to evaluate the need for a change in our therapeutical con-cept: do we have to increase the substitution dose or even, do we have to consider operative interventions?

For the analysis of the radiologic results 4 MRI grades were defined: grade 0 for no pathological changes, grade I for effusion and/or bone marrow edema, grade II for synovial hypertrophy and/or mild cartilaginous defects and grade III for severe cartilaginous defects, bony defects and/or diminishing of joint cavity.

I. Scharrer/W. Schramm (Ed.)
32nd Hemophilia Symposion Hamburg 2001
© Springer-Verlag Berlin Heidelberg 2003

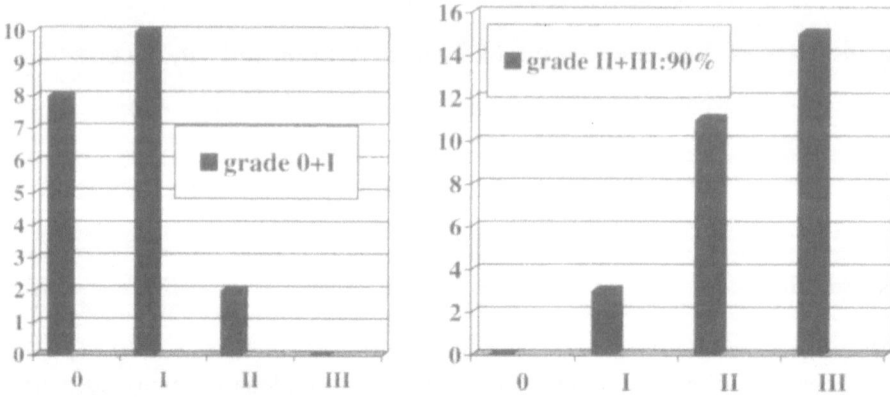

Fig. 1. Subjective pain and orthopedic abnormalities

Table 1. Score of the examined joints

Grade	0	I	II	III
hip (n = 7)	6	1	–	–
knee (n = 5)	2	3	–	–
elbow (n = 8)	–	1	4	3
ankle (n = 49)	2	19	16	12

Results

In the over-all analysis 10/69 (14%) joints were classified grade 0, 24/69 (35%) joints grade I, 20/69 (29%) grade II and 15/69 (22%) grade III. 90% of the joints with isolated subjective pain had no or grade I changes, 90% of the joints with abnormalities in the orthopedic examination on the other hand, were related to grade II or III (Fig. 1). These results exactly correspond to the clinical symptoms.

Table 1 summarizes the MRI scores of all joints examined. Knees and hips were the joints with the lowest bleeding frequency (<5 bleeding episodes) and the mildest MRI changes (grade 0 and I). With one exception, the indication for MRI in this group was subjective pain only. These results again are in clear concordance with the clinical examination. On the other hand, indications for MRI of the elbows were severe orthopedic abnormalities, represented by MRI scores of III or IV.

In the group of the ankle joints (target joints as well as clinically healthy joints of the contrary side) scores ranged from I to III in 47/49 (96%) joints, only 2/49 (4%) joints were normal (grade 0). The results of the 30 target ankles are shown in Figure 2. All ankles had experienced more than 10 bleeding episodes. In 2/3 of the patients prophylaxis was started after the 4th year of life. In more than half of the patients MRI was performed at an age of 10 to 17 years. 75% of the target joints were assigned to grade II or III, with increasing age the MRI score worsened. The remaining 25% target ankles joints despite a high bleeding rate had a MRI score of

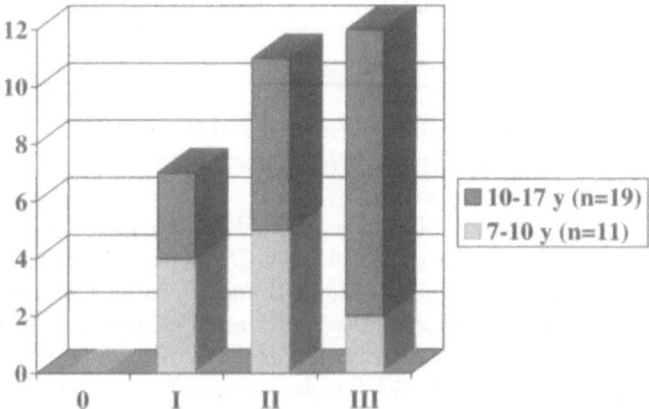

Fig. 2. Index ankles

I with a comparable distribution between both age groups. None of the ankle joints fulfilled the criteria for score 0.

The results of the 19 contralateral ankle joints with a normal orthopedic examination and 0 to 5 intraarticular bleedings are represented in Figure 3. Surprisingly, only 2/19 (11%) ankle joints of this group had normal MRI results. 12/19 (65%) ankles – independent of the patients age – were graded into score I. 5/19 (26%) ankles were graded into score II with a positive correlation between patients age and MRI score. No ankle joint fulfilled the criteria for score III.

According to these radiological results therapeutic consequences have to be discussed. In our patients we did not change the substitution regimen. 4 ankles and 2 elbows with MRI scores of III had a synovectomy with or without an arthrolysis. With regard to pain, range of motion and bleeding frequency all patients had a benefit from the operation. In 3 children aged 7 to 15 years with MRI scores of II the discussion about the indication for an early synovectomy at the ankle or knee joint is still ongoing.

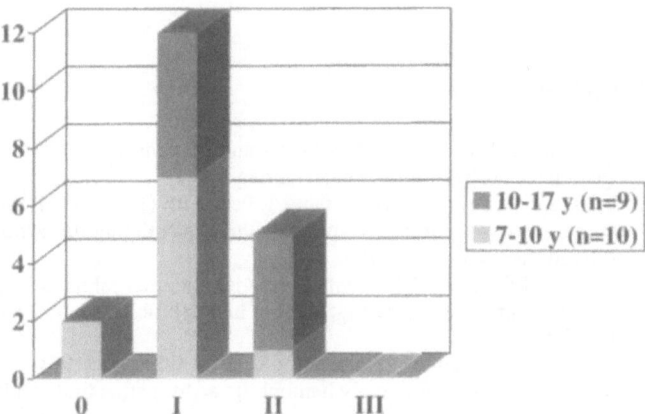

Fig. 3. Contralateral ankles

Discussion and Summary

The clinical symptoms correlated well with the MRI results: joints with subjective pain and normal orthopedic examination were assigned to score 0 and I, joints with orthopedic abnormalities to score II and III.

Joint damage was more pronounced in the age group 10 to 17 years than in the age group 7 to 10 years.

Joints with a low bleeding rate had discrete joint damage. The radiological outcome in joints with a high bleeding frequency varied. As expected, most of them were assigned to the MRI scores II and III. 25% of the index joints, however, had only mild radiological changes with an MRI score I. This observation can not be explained by the age distribution, as the number of patients aged 7 to 10 years and of patients aged 10 to 17 years was comparable. It can be speculated that the group with an MRI score I might have experienced milder bleeding episodes with just small amounts of intraarticular blood or might have had an earlier substitution of factor concentrate compared to the group with MRI scores II and III. These observations correspond to the few reports published in literature.

In summary, MRI was found to be a simple method for evaluation of joint damage. Even early changes in synovial and cartilaginous structures that usually are missed by routine clinical examinations can be diagnosed.

Our results give reason to discuss the following points:

In hemophilic children MRI should be performed routinely with the aim to diagnose early changes in synovia or cartilage. After the 5th bleeding episode into the same joint a first MRI followed by annually controls should be recommended.

The results of the MRI examinations should be the basis for further therapeutical interventions.

The importance of an early prophylaxis in childhood and adolescence is undisputed.

According to the MRI findings dose or frequency of substitution might have to be increased. On the other hand early synovectomy at the onset of joint damage might come to the fore.

These consequences together might be the key for reduction of irreversible joint damage in adolescence.

References

1. Erlemann R, Wörtler K (1999) Bildgebende Diagnostik der hämophilen Osteoarthropathie. Orthopäde 28: 329–340. Springer-Verlag
2. Erlemann R, Pollmann H, Vestring T, Peters PE (1992) MR Tomographie der hämophilen Osteoarthropathie unter besonderer Berücksichtigung der synovialen und chondrogenen Alterationen. RöFo 156: 270–276
3. Nuss R, Kilcoyne RF, Geraghty S, Wiedel J, Manco-Johnson M (1993) Utility of magnetic resonance imaging for management of hemophilic. Osteoarthropathie in children. J Pediatr 123: 388–392
4. Wörtler K, Pollmann H, Winkelmann B, Linnenbecker S (1998) MR imaging of synovial alterations in children with early hemophilic arthropathy: first results. Radiology 209: 480

Rhenium-186 Hydroxyethylidenediphosphonate (^{186}Re HEDP) – A novel Treatment for hemophilic Arthropathies?

T.A. Wallny, L. Hess, H.-H. Brackmann, A. Seuser, H. Palmedo, and C. Kraft

Patients diagnosed with hemophilia before the era of home infusion frequently suffer from severe hemarthropathies. Treatment usually relies on physiotherapy for muscular atrophy and to improve, or at least maintain, the limited range of motion of the afflicted joints. For acute pain non-steroidal anti rheumatical drugs (NSAR) are typically given, though in cases of marked arthritis and hepatobiliary contraindications, efficacy is questionable and the long-term value of this therapy can be disputed. This seems reason enough to contemplate alternative strategies for pain-treatment of hemophilic arthropathies. In this context local therapy with Rhenium 186 may be a feasible option.

Rhenium-186 (^{186}Re) is a radioisotope with therapeutically exploitable beta emission (92.2%) and a physical half-life of 3-7 days. The maximal distance of the emitted energy into surrounding soft tissue is 3.7 mm, with an average of 1.2 mm. Furthermore ^{186}Re also has gamma emission which can be utilized as a diagnostic tool, in that it allows whole-body imaging, with a standard gamma camera, and dose estimations. Hydroxyethylidenediphosphonate (HEDP) is an osteotropic diphosphonate which, in combination with technetium 99m (^{99m}Tc), has been used for many decades for bone scanning. ^{186}Re-HEDP is a combination of these two components. While the radiopharmaceutical adheres to the hydroxyapatite crystal mediated by the metabolic activity of osteoblastic cells by means of HEDP, the therapeutic effect is achieved by beta emission from ^{186}Re. Hypermetabolic regions of the bone and joints receive a significantly higher radiation dose than regions that have normal metabolism. ^{186}Re-HEDP is available from the producer (Mallinckrodt Medical b.v., Westerduinweg 3, 175 LE Petten, Holland) as a ready-to-use solution.

Materials and methods

12 hemophilic patients over the age of 45 with at least 3 painful joints were included in this prospective study. All patients were informed about the character of the study and possible side effects and provided written consent. Patients had persistent joint pain and either showed little or no improvement despite the use of NSAR or did not tolerate NSAR because of side effects. Symptoms were resistant to further conservative treatment. Approval for this study was obtained from the ethical committee of the University of Bonn.

I. Scharrer/W. Schramm (Ed.)
32nd Hemophilia Symposion Hamburg 2001
© Springer-Verlag Berlin Heidelberg 2003

Exclusion criteria:

a) patients with only slight subjective or objective loss of quality of life; clinical evidence or a history of one of the following diseases: malignoma, renal dysfunction, gastrointestinal ulcera

b) pathological results in one of the following tests: erythrocyte, retikulocyte, leukocyte and platelet count; marked deficiencies in red and white blood-cell count or serum iron-level, serum-creatinine and serum electrolyte-levels.

Before begin of therapy a sequential bone scintigraphy was performed, on the one hand to verify the diagnosis of polyarthritic manifestation and evaluate the degree of bony manifestation, on the other to obtain dose estimations of the afflicted joints. The radiopharmaceutical was intravenously applied. Each patient received a dose of 15mCi. Owing to local radiation protection laws, the patient remained in the isolation ward for 48h. 12h after injection of ^{186}Re-HEDP whole-body scintigraphy was again performed to document the periarticular accumulation of the tracer.

Prior to and 12 weeks after ^{186}Re-HEDP-therapy patients answered a questionnaire using a visual analogous scale (VAS), which ranges from 0-10, 0 being completely pain-free and 10 being the worst pain the patient can imagine. The patients general pain status, specific regions of joint-pain (when resting, standing and walking), the 3 most painful joints and the range of movement were assessed. Questions concerning activities of daily life and the patients quality of life were also asked.

Results

According to patients, 19 of 36 of the most painful joints (3 most painful joints per patient) improved after ^{186}Re-HEDP-therapy, whereby improvement was only documented if the VAS decreased by at least 2 points (Fig. 1).

On average, 2 joints per patient improved (range: 1-5). The general pain status was 1.75 VAS-points lower than before therapy. Initially patients claimed to have 6 painful joints prior to therapy, which then improved to an average of 5 painful joints (median) after application of the radiopharmaceutical. This only moderate success can be explained by the fact that patients were specifically questioned with regards to pain of all large joints, even those that were subjectively inconspicuous prior to therapy. It was therefore possible that 12 weeks after ^{186}Re-HEDP-therapy patients then claimed to have pain in joints that were initially clinically unremarkable. The overall number of painful joints therefore remained unchanged in 6 patients, increased in one patient and was found to be reduced in the remaining 5. An increase of mobility after therapy was not found. The quality of life increased for 4 patients, remained unaltered for a further 4 and the remaining 4 patients claimed that quality of life had in fact decreased since the therapy.

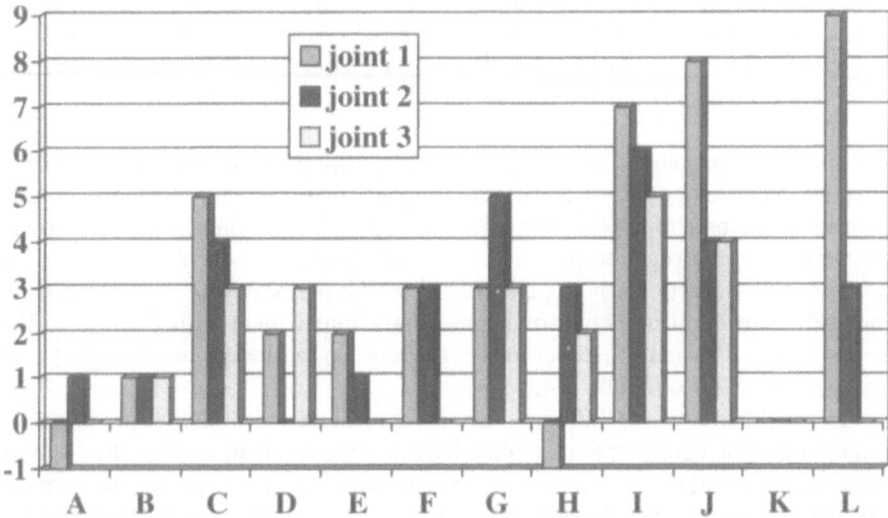

Fig. 1. Change of pain of the three most painful joints / patient before to after ^{186}Re-HEDP-therapy. On the y-axis the change of visual analogous scale (VAS) is shown: a positive value indicates an improvement of the subjective pain status, while negative values show deterioration.

Side effects

The radiopharmaceutical was tolerated well by all patients. Pre- and post-therapeutical (1day, 1 week, 4 weeks and 12 weeks) red and white blood cell-counts, as well as creatinine-values remained inconspicious, indicating good tolerance by the hematological and renal system.

Discussion

Hemophilic patients, growing up before the era of early prophylaxis, usually have multiple joints damaged through recurrent bleeding episodes. These polyarticularly afflicted patients are chronic pain-plagued patients (Wallny et al. 2001). Adequate orthopedic management of these patients is typically compounded by a number of problems:

1. Conservative methods such as physiotherapy, electrotherapy and orthopedic shoe wear frequently cannot alleviate pain sufficiently (Wallny et al. 2001)
2. Selective therapeutical measures such as intraarticular injections (e.g. hyaluronic acid, cortisone) make factor-substitution necessary (Wallny et al. 2000)
3. Non-steroidal anti rheumatical drugs (NSAR) show gastrointestinal, renal and, particularly in patients with an accompanying viral hepatitis, marked hepatological side-effects. Despite the fact that these drugs are effective and can be well steered, the limitations lie in the fact that the underlying cause of pain is not

adequately treated. This frequently leads to excessive and/or long-term use of the pharmaceutical and inadvertently to an unjustifiable increase of side-effects.

4. Patients suffering from HIV-infection usually need numerous tablets and are therefore frequently particularly critical towards further oral medication.

For the pain management of hemophilic arthropathy there is an abundant array of effective drugs. Yet no matter how successful these may be, all have in common that their use remains symptomatically oriented. As the disease typically takes a chronic course, long-term drug therapy is necessary and subsequent adverse side-effects are not uncommon. Particularly in patients with a high premorbidity or existing drug-induced gastrointestinal, renal or hepatobiliary impairment with damage to the hematopoetical system, the decisions regarding begin, dosage or change of oral analgesics remains difficult.

On the other hand local therapy such as surgical treatment modalities or radio-synovectomy of single impaired joint have shown excellent results (Rodriguez-Merchan et al. 2001). In this context it seems important to point out that this type of isolated intervention has the advantage of firstly being a very circumscribed measure, secondly a long-term solution and lastly shows virtually no cross-reaction with regards to side-effects of commonly subscribed drugs. Yet despite the documented success, the use of these measures in patients with multifocal arthritis seems questionable, due to the very localized character of the interventional therapy.

Systemic application of [186]Re-HEDP in hemophilic arthropathy has the advantage, that numerous joints can simultaneously be targeted. In a study with 77 joints with patients suffering either from chronic polyarthritis or psoriasis arthritis, Palmedo et al. (2001) could show a decrease of pain and disease activity over an observation period of 9 months after [186]Re-HEDP-therapy. Though the basic pathology as well as the symptoms found are similar, and one may hypothesize that the effect of HEDP-Rhenium is comparable, above mentioned good results cannot simply be transferred to the treatment of hemophiliacs.

Due to the benign nature of the disease, the maximum radiation doses in our study were purposely chosen moderately low. Levels of activity administered were significantly lower than values estimated for the palliative pain-treatment of bone metastases (Maxon et al. 1991), where extensive experience in regards to induction of side-effects has already been gained. With levels of activity of 1295 MBq (35 mCi), De Clerk et al. (1994) did not detect induction of permanent hematological damage. Reversible bone-marrow suppression, which receded 4-6 weeks after [186]Re-HEDP-therapy, was found in patients particularly after chemo- or radiation-therapy. A Dutch doses-escalation study (De Klerk et al. 1994) demonstrated that intolerable hematological side-effects did not occur up to doses of 2960 MBq (80 mCi). Calculated dose estimates for the red bone marrow after administration of a standard therapy of 1295 MBq amounted to 0.87 Gy (Maxon et al. 1988). From this prior experience with [186]Re-HEDP one can conclude that the maximal applied activity dose of 740 MBq, as used in this study, is well below those doses which are already known to be well tolerated.

By performing systemic therapy with [186]Re-HEDP for pain palliation of osseous metastases, Maxon et al. (1988) found that radiation doses of 10-100 Gy can be achieved in bone metastases. In our study we administered half these levels of activity, and we calculated dose estimates to achieve doses of a minimum of 5 Gy per joint.

When a dose of ^{186}Re HEDP between 496 and 688 MBq was administered systemically, the effective dose was about 200 MSv. This value was not much higher than the values of 80-155 mSv for whole-body radiation doses after radiosynovectomy, even if the treated joint was immobilized for 48 hours (Gratz et al. 1999). Further conservative treatment options were not available for the patients in this study, who were all older than 45 years, because their arthropathies did not respond to treatment with medication or they experienced severe side effects of medication. We did not see substantial changes in blood cell counts with a bone marrow dose of 0.4 Gy for each injection of ^{186}Re HEDP.

Conclusion

^{186}Re-HEDP accumulates in hypermetabolic bone and joint regions. Following the criteria as set forth by evidence-based medicine, the study design does as yet not allow the conclusion that ^{186}Re-HEDP-therapy induces a definite decrease of joint pain in hemophilic arthropathies over the observation period. A placebo-controlled, randomized study as well as a longer observation period to evaluate long-term results is necessary.

References

1. De Klerk JM, Zonnenberg BA, van het Schip AD, van Dijk A, Han SH, Quirijnen JM, Blijham GH, van Rijk PP. Dose escalation study of rhenium-186 hydroxyethylidene diphosphonat in patients wich metastatic prostate cancer. Eur J Nucl Med 1994; 21: 1114-1120.
2. Maxon HR, Schroder LE, Hertzberg VS, Thomas SR, Englaro EE, Samaratunga R, Smith H, Moulton JS, Williams CC, Ehrhardt GJ. Rhenium-186 (Sn) HEDP for treatment of painful osseous metastases: Results of a doubleblind crossover comparison with placebo. J Nucl Med 1991; 32: 1877-1881.
3. Maxon HR, Deutsch EA, Thomas, SR, Libson K, Lukes SJ, Williams CC, Ali S. Re-186 (Sn) HEDP for treatment of multiple metastatic foci in bone: Human biodistribution and dosimetric studies. Radiology 1988; 166: 501-507.
4. De Klerk JM, van het Schip AD, Zonnenberg BA, van Dijk A, Stokkel MP, Han SH, Blijham GH, van Rijk PP. Evaluation of thrombocytopenia in patients treated with rhenium-186-HEDP: Guidelines for individual dose recommendations. J Nucl Med 1994; 35: 1423-1428.
5. Palmedo H, Rockstroh JK, Bangard M, Schliegfer K, Risse J, Menzel C, Biersack HJ. Painful multifocal arthritis: Therapy with Rhenium 186 Hydroxyethylidenediphosphonate (186 Re HEDP) after failed treatment with medication – initial results of a prospective study. Radiology 2001; 221:256-260.
6. Rodriguez-Merchan EC, Jimenez-Yzste V, Villar A, Quintana M, Lopez-Cabarcos C, Hernandez-Navarro F. Yttrium-90 synoviorthesis for chronic haemophilic synovitis: Madrid experience. Haemophilia 2001; 7, (Suppl.2), 34-35.
7. Wallny T, Brackmann HH, Semper H, Schumpe G, Effenberger W, Heß, L, Seuser A. Intra-articular hyaluronic acid in the treatment of haemophilic arthropathy of the knee. A clinical, radiological and sonographical assessment. Haemophilia 2000; 6; 566-570.
8. Wallny, T, Hess, L, Seuser, A, Zander, D, Brackmann, HH, Kraft, CN. Pain status of patients with severe haemophilic arthropathy. Haemophilia 2001; 7; 453-458.

IIIb. Monitoring of Substitution Therapy

Monitoring of Anticoagulant Therapy with the endogenous Thrombin Potential

A. Siegemund, T. Siegemund, U. Scholz, S. Petros, and L. Engelmann

Background

The endogenous thrombin potential (ETP) describes the thrombin-mediated coagulability state of the plasma. It reflects the process of thrombin formation and elimination. ETP depicts the »fire risk«, while the prothrombin fragment F_{1+2} is »a smoke detector that reports an ongoing fire« [1], i.e. the process of conversion of prothrombin to thrombin.

ETP is decreased under anticoagulant therapy independent of the class used. For an effective anticoagulation 60 to 80% of thrombin has to be inhibited.

Methods

ETP was measured as described by Wielders et al. [5] with some modifications in substrate and activator concentrations. D-Dimer and prothrombinfragment F_{1+2} were measured with Enzygnost D-Dimer and Enzygnost F_{1+2} resp. (Dade Behring Marburg GmbH).

Case report

Two weeks after immobilization because of Scheuermann's disease, a 16 year old overweight (90 kg) girl was admitted to the university hospital with a deep vein thrombosis (DVT) of the left leg extending into the inferior vena cava up to just below the confluence of the renal veins. She had been taking an oral contraceptive since 3 months. She reported history of thrombosis in the family. The patient was also suffering from allergic bronchial asthma. Laboratory investigation revealed a heterozygote prothrombin mutation 20210 GA and high concentration of factors VIII, IX and XI.

The diagnosis of DVT was made by means of Duplex ultrasonography and CT scan. The thrombus was estimated to be about 4–5 days old.

Fibrinolytic treatment with urokinase (Ukidan) in combination with aPTT-adjusted anticoagulation with unfractionated heparin was started immediately after informed consent of the parents. Antithrombin was given on days 1 and 3. Despite this management the patient developed an additional DVT in the right arm.

I. Scharrer/W. Schramm (Ed.)
32nd Hemophilia Symposion Hamburg 2001
© Springer-Verlag Berlin Heidelberg 2003

Due to further elevation of the markers of coagulation activity (prothrombin fragment F_{1+2}, D-dimer and ETP) anticoagulation was switched to the low molecular weight heparin nadroparin (Fraxiparin) adjusted to body weight. However, no improvement was observed at day 5 and 9 by means of ultrasound investigation. For this reason, anticoagulant treatment with hirudin (Refludan) was started. This was given as a bolus followed by a continuous infusion, and therapy was titrated by regular estimation of the ecarin clotting time (ECT). The ECT during the treatment period was in this case 1000 to 1700 ng/ml. This anticoagulant switch resulted in at least a recanalization of all the affected veins. The patient was then put on oral anti-coagulation.

Discussion

In the present case, fibrinolytic therapy in combination with heparin did not result in a regression of the thrombosis. Using ETP (Fig. 1) a hypercoagulability state was identified although treatment was tailored using reptilase time and aPTT (Fig. 2). Thrombolytic therapy may induce a procoagulant state with increased thrombin activity [4] as a result of the thrombin bound to fibrin (and fibrin degradation products). This thrombin is protected from inhibition by heparin. In contrast, hirudin is able to penetrate the thrombus and thus can inactivate both free and bound thrombin (Fig. 3). This effect may explain the advantage of hirudin over heparin as

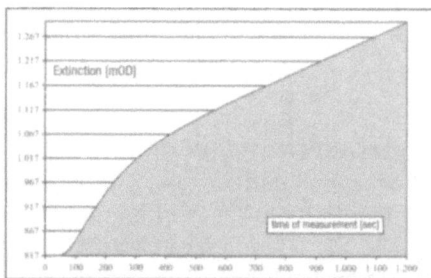

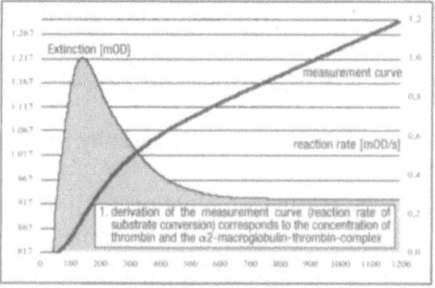
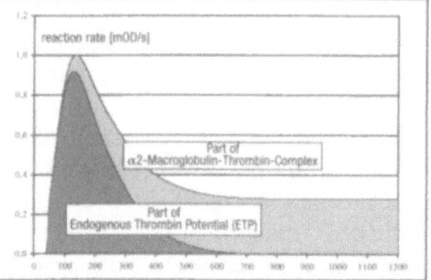

Fig. 1. Principle of ETP measurement. 1) Measurement of the thrombin generation curve; 2) Calculation of the contribution of thrombin-complex at substrate conversion according to Hemker

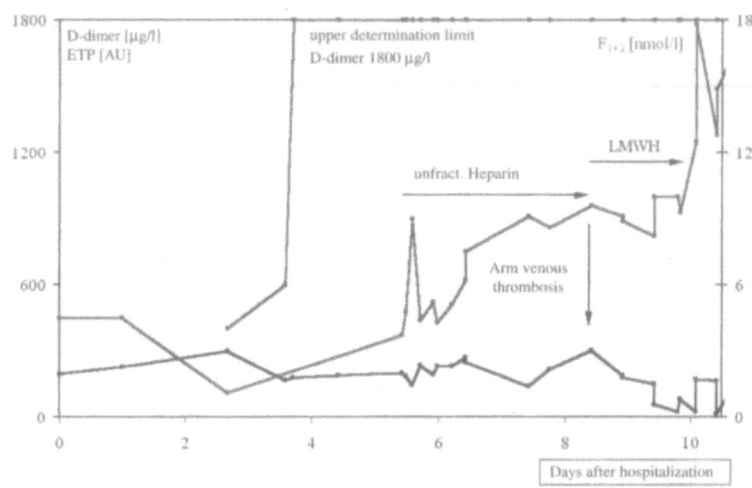

Fig. 2. ETP, D-dimer and F_{1+2} in a patient with DVT and fibrinolytic therapy

Fig. 3a, b. Comparison of the inhibitory effect of different anticoagulants.

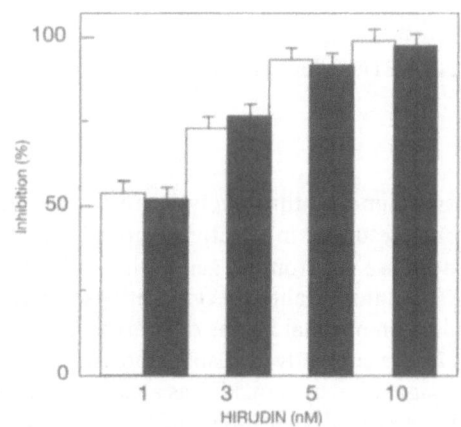

a. Comparison of the inhibitory effect of hirudin aganinst fluid-phase thrombin (open bars) and thrombin bound to soluble fibrin degradation products (closed bars). Each bar represents the mean of three separate experiments (each done in duplicate), while the lines above the bars represent the 95% CI.

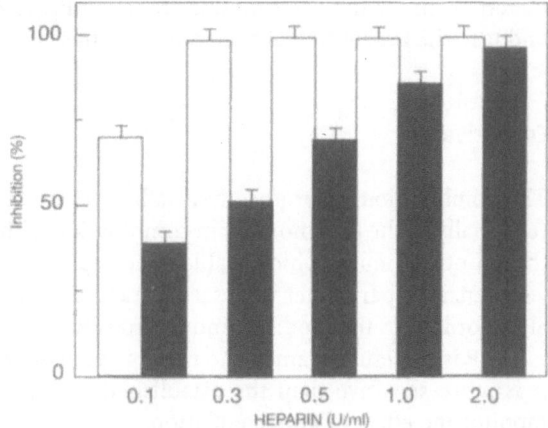

b. Comparison of the inhibitory effect of heparin against fluid-phase thrombin (open bars) and thrombin bound to soluble fibrin degradation products (closed bars). Each bar represents the mean of three separate experiments (each done in duplicate), while the lines above the bars represent the 95% CI.

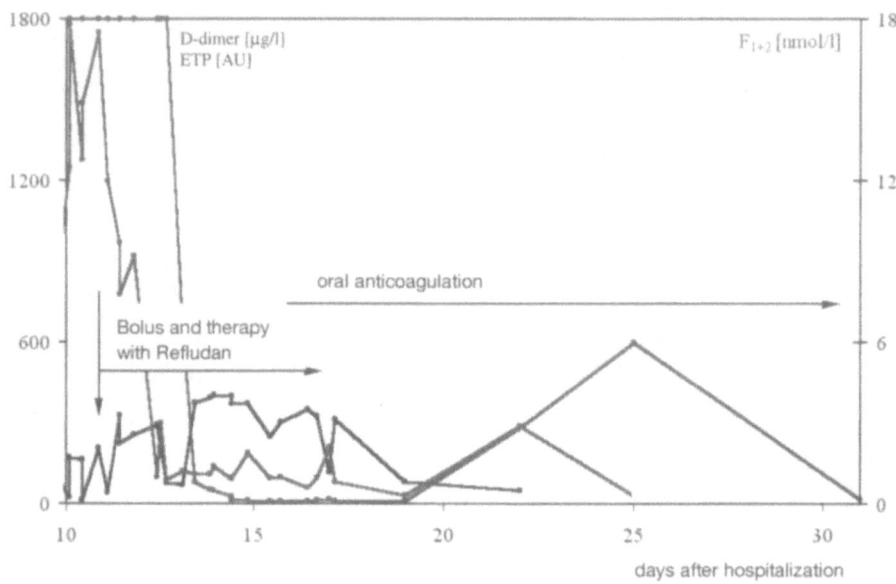

Fig. 4. ETP, D-dimer, F_{1+2} in a patient with DVT and fibrinolytic therapy

an adjunct to thrombolytic treatment. This could be demonstrated in the present case, resulting in effective venous recanalization within a short period of time and decrease in thrombin generating capacity (Fig. 4).

An important aspect in anticoagulant treatment using different regimens is finding an optimal means of control. Considering the cell-based model of hemostasis [2], the currently available laboratory methods may not give the true picture of the coagulation system. ETP as a global parameter best describes the state of hypo- and hypercoagulation independent of the anticoagulant used (Fig. 5), and we believe that it is very useful in high-risk patients in combination with the activation parameters D-dimer and prothrombin fragment F_{1+2}. However, it is still time consuming and test kits for routine use are not available.

Conclusion

The combination of prothrombin allel 20210 GA and taking oral contraceptives (especially in the first months) in combination with acquired risk factors is a strong thrombotic stimulus which is able to across the thrombosis threshold. The ETP is a very sensitive parameter to describe such patients with a high thrombosis potential (according to the modified model from Rosendaal [3] Fig 6).

ETP is a useful parameter to manage patients with a high thrombosis potential. It is more sensitive than the established methods, such as aPTT and anti-Xa, to monitor the effect of anticoagulation.

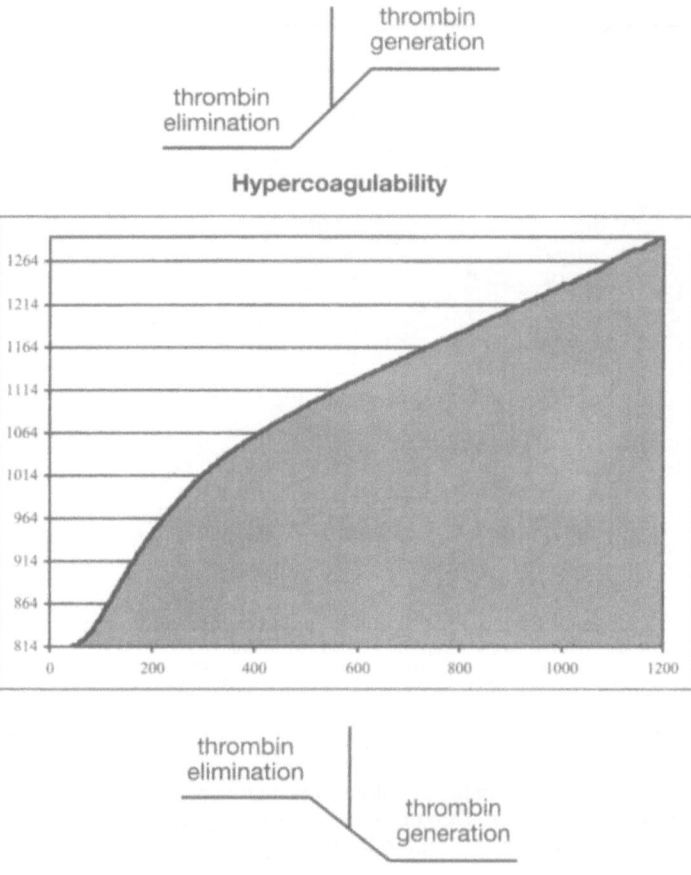

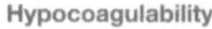

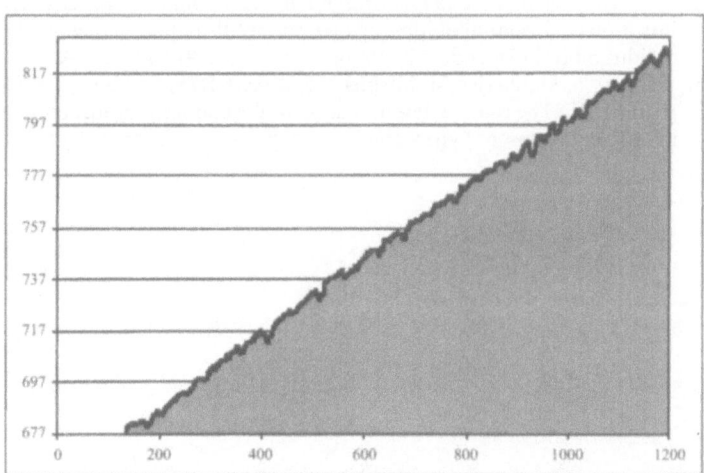

Fig. 5. ETP in patients with hyper- and hypo- coagulability

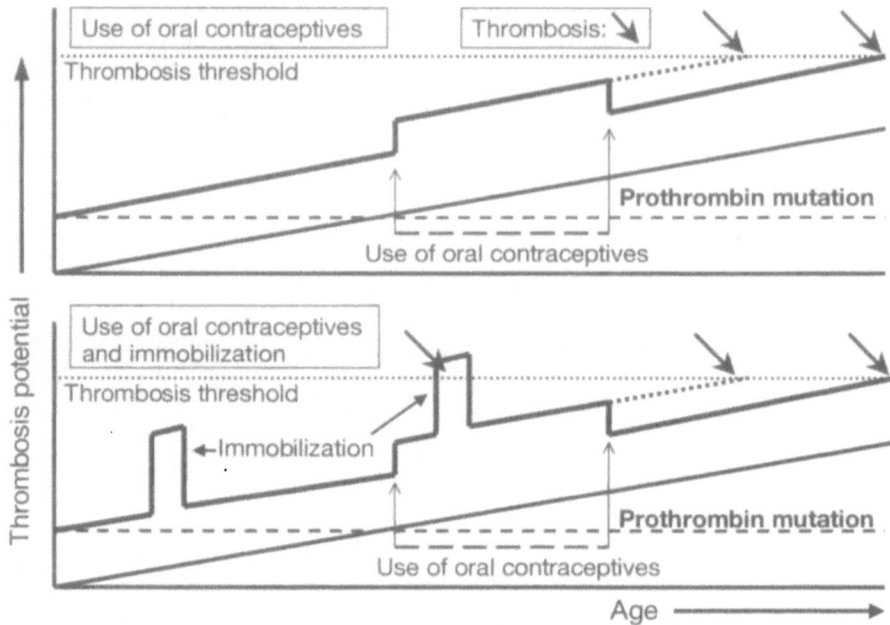

Fig. 6. Model of thrombotic risk (modified according to Rosendaal)

References

1. Hemker HC, Béguin S: Thrombin generation in plasma: its assessment via the endogenous thrombin potential. Thromb Haemost 74:134–38,1995
2. Hoffman M, Monroe DM: A cell based model of hemostasis. Thromb Haemost 85: 958–65, 2001
3. Rosendaal FR: Venous thrombosis: a multicausal disease. Lancet 353:1167–73,1999
4. Weitz JI, Leslie B, Hudoba M: Thrombin binds to soluble fibrin degradation products where it is protected from inhibition by heparin-antithrombin but susceptible to inactivation by antithrombin-independent inhibitors. Circulation 97:544–52,1998
5. Wielders S, Mukherjee M, Michiels M, Rijkers DTS, Cambus JP, Knebel RWC, Kakkar V, Hemker HC: The routine determination of the endogenous thrombin potential, first results in different forms of hyper- and hypocoagulability. Thromb Haemost 77: 629–36,1997

IV. Pediatric Hemostaseology

Chairmen:

G. AUERSWALD (Bremen)
A. H. SUTOR (Freiburg)

First thromboembolic Onset in Children carrying either the heterozygeous Factor V G1691A Mutation or the Prothrombin G20210A Variant

A. Kosch, S. Becker, K. Kurnik, K. Sudbrak, R. Schobess, R. Junker, M. Käse, and U. Nowak-Göttl

Introduction

Disorders of the hemostatic system are major causes of thrombophilia in adults. Various genetic defects in the regulation of blood coagulation and fibrinolysis predispose to thromboembolic events [1–5]. The factor V (FV) G1691A mutation and the prothrombin (FII) G20210A variant appear to be relevant not only in adult thromboembolism. However, due to the low incidence of thromboembolic events in childhood, the role of hereditary prothrombotic risk factors is still a matter of discussion [6–12]. There is still a lack of data concerning the exogenous triggering factors associated with a first thromboembolic event. Furthermore, a significantly higher incidence of thrombosis – especially renal venous thrombosis – in male neonates and infants compared to females has been described [13–15]. Therefore, a possible impact of age and gender on thromboembolic manifestations in pediatric patients is of interest.

We here present the results of a multicenter follow-up study on pediatric patients suffering from a first symptomatic thromboembolic event (TE) with respect to gender, age, site of thromboembolism and underlying triggering factors. All patients were carrying either the heterozygous FV G1691A mutation or the FII G20210A variant without further additional hereditary prothrombotic risk factor.

Patients, Materials and Methods

Ethics

The present study was performed in accordance with the ethical standards laid down in the updated Declaration of Helsinki and approved by the medical ethics committees at the Westfälische Wilhelms-University, Münster, Frankfurt, Halle and Munich, Germany.

Inclusion criteria

Children aged neonate to 18 years with a first symptomatic thromboembolic event carrying either the heterozygous FV G1691A mutation or the heterozygous FII G20210A variant not combined with further genetic prothrombotic risk factors were enrolled in the study.

I. Scharrer/W. Schramm (Ed.)
32nd Hemophilia Symposium Hamburg 2001
© Springer-Verlag Berlin Heidelberg 2003

Exclusion criteria

Children with an additional prothrombotic risk factor such as elevated lipoprotein (a) > 30 mg/dl or elevated fasting homocysteine (above the age-dependent 95th percentile), deficiency states of protein S, protein C or antithrombin were excluded. Children with a homozygous FV G1691A mutation or homozygous FII G20210A variant were also not enrolled in this study.

Study population

848 pediatric patients aged neonate to 18 years with a first symptomatic thromboembolic event were consecutively recruited and screened for hereditary prothrombotic risk factors between January 1995 and June 2001 by the participating centers. 150 patients fulfilled the inclusion criteria and were analyzed in this subgroup analysis.

Imaging methods

Ultrasonography, compression Duplex-sonography and phlebography were used to confirm deep venous thrombosis. In abdominal/pelvic thrombosis ultrasonography, computed tomography (CT) and spiral CT were performed, and in cerebral thromboembolism MRT-imaging methods including MR-angiography were the methods applied.

Assays for genotyping

The FV G1691A and FII G20210A genotypes were determined by polymerase chain reaction and analysis of restriction fragments as previously reported [2, 5]

Assays for plasma proteins

Amidolytic protein C and antithrombin activities were measured on an ACL 300 analyzer (Instrumentation Laboratory) with the use of chromogenic substrates (Chromogenix). Free protein S antigen, total protein S, and protein C antigen were measured by using commercially available ELISA assay kits (Stago). Lp(a) and ACAs (IgM and IgG) were also determined with ELISA techniques (Sigma) [9–11].

Exogenous triggering factors

The following exogenous triggering factors were documented: immobilization, surgery, trauma, central lines, steroid administration, oral contraceptives (in females) and smoking.

Statistical analysis

Statistical analysis was performed by using StatView 5 software package (SAS Institute Inc.). As non-parametric tests for evaluation and comparison of different groups the Mann-Whitney U-test was performed. To compare frequencies of thrombotic locations, triggering factors in the two study groups the chi-square test, or, if necessary Fisher`s exact test was used. The thromboembolism-free survival as a function of time was additionally analyzed according to the Kaplan and Meier method including the log-rank test. P-values < 0.05 were considered significant.

Results

With respect to the inclusion and exclusion criteria 150 of the 848 children carrying either the FV G1691A or the FII G20210A mutation were enrolled in the study. 118 of 150 patients carried the heterozygous FV mutation (78.7 %; male n = 64) and 32 children the heterozygous FII mutation (21.3%; male n = 20).

Thromboembolic onset

Table 1 shows median/range age and gender distribution of pediatric patients at the time of first thromboembolic onset carrying either the FV mutation or the FII mutation respectively. In addition, absolute numbers of acquired triggering factors as well as venous or arterial thrombosis are given. At the bottom of the Table number of patients during infancy were shown: Whereas significantly more infants were male in this age group, no difference was observed for acquired non genetic risk fac-

Table 1. Median and range age, gender distribution at the first thromboembolic onset in children carrying either the factor V mutation or the FII mutation.

	Factor V G1691A N=118	Factor II G20210A N=32	P-value
Age (median and range): all patients	4,0 (0,1-<18)	8,5 (0,1-17,7)	0,1**
Gender: male	64/118 (54,2%)	20/32 (62,5%)	0,52
Exogenous trigger	42/118 (35,6%)	12/32 (37,5%)	0,99
Number of venous thrombosis	72/118 (61,0%)	18/32 (56,3%)	0,78
Number of arterial thrombosis	46/118 (39,0%)	14/32 (43,8%)	0,78
Patients infancy*	**53/118 (44,9%)**	**8/32 (25,0%)**	**0,045***
Trigger infancy	14/53 (26,4%)	2/8 (25,0%)	1,0*

Chi-square test, *Fisher`s exact test, and ** Mann-Whitney U-test; *** venous thromboembolism only, no arterial thrombosis present in these patients

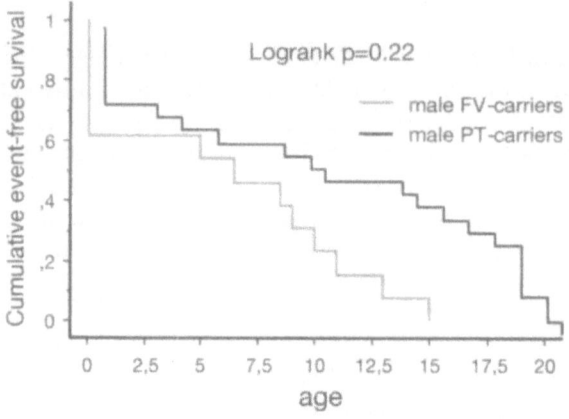

Fig. 1. Thromboembolism-free survival in the male pediatric FV-carriers compared with male PT-carriers (Kaplan-Meier-plot)

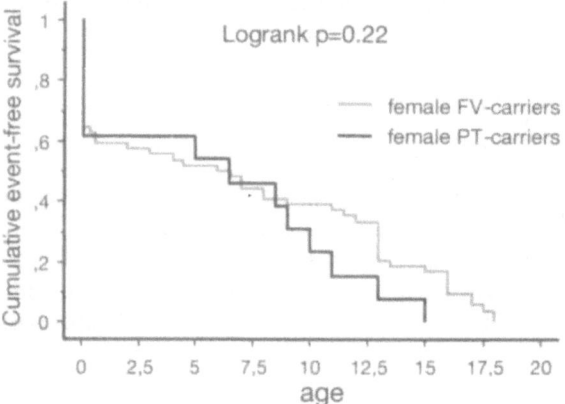

Fig. 2. Thromboembolism-free survival in the female pediatric FV-carriers compared with female PT-carriers (Kaplan-Meier-plot)

tors. The Kaplan-Meier-plot (Fig. 1) shows the thromboembolism-free survival in the male pediatric FV carriers compared with male FII patients: Boys carrying the FV mutation had a significantly shorter thromboembolism-free survival than male patients with the FII mutation (logrank: p = 0.015). The thromboembolism-free survival in the female pediatric FV carriers compared with female FII carriers is shown in Figure 2. There was no significant difference between the two groups (logrank: p = 0.22).

Localization of thrombosis

To analyze, whether the different mutations are associated with specific localization of thromboembolic events we studied the distribution of manifestation sites. Figure 3 shows the localization of thromboembolic events in the groups with factor V and prothrombin mutations. There was no statistical difference between these

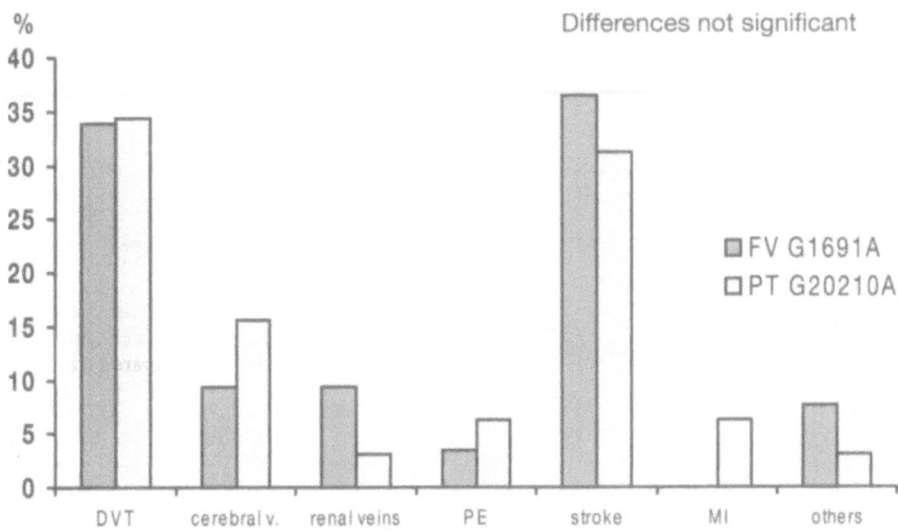

Fig. 3. Localization of thromboembolic manifestation

two groups (p=0,78: Chi-square test). The most common events were venous thromboembolism during infancy, and venous thrombosis and strokes in the remaining children > 12 months of age (Fig. 3).

Exogenous triggering factors

No statistical difference was found in patients carrying the FV mutation compared with carriers of the FII variant with respect to additionally acquired triggering factors. The most common exogenous triggering factors in both groups were central venous lines, steroid therapy and infections (Fig. 4) respectively.

Discussion

Data presented in the present subgroup analysis show that the heterozygous FV mutation as well as the heterozygous FII variant without further combination with additional prothrombotic risk factors are associated with symptomatic thromboembolic events in children with a significantly earlier first onset in male carriers of the FV gene mutation. Exogenous triggers were additionally found in more than one third of cases to contribute to thromboembolic events.

The factor V G1691A and particularly the prothrombin G20210A mutations have been shown to be highly prevalent hereditary risk factors for thromboembolic events in the white population [3–5, 16, 17]. However, few studies have focused so far on thromboembolic events in children and adolescents carrying not only the FV

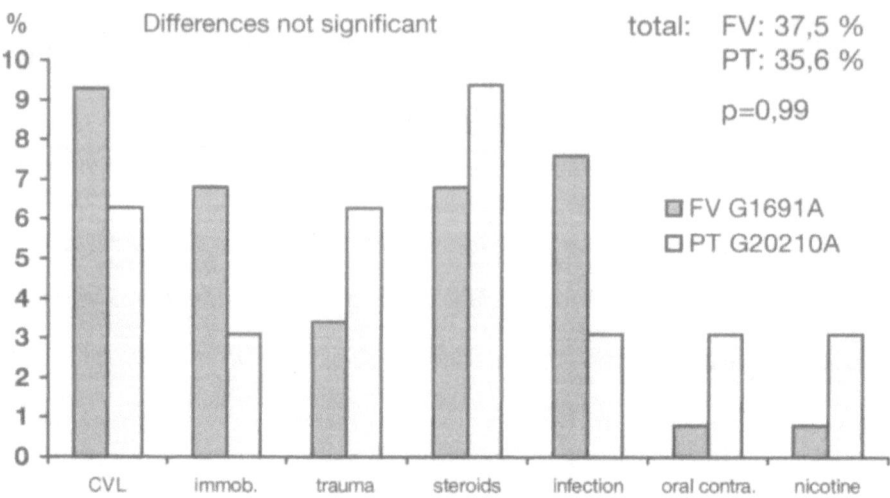

Fig. 4. Exogenous triggers in FV-carriers and PT-carriers

G1691A and FII G20210A mutations but also further inherited or acquired pro-thrombotic risk factors [6, 18, 19, 7, 9-11].

On the one hand, thrombosis during infancy and childhood has been frequent-ly discussed to be associated with non-genetic endogenous or exogenous triggering mechanisms. On the other hand, increasing data are available demonstrating that thromboembolic vascular accidents with and without exogenous triggering stimuli are also found in children with underlying genetic prothrombotic risk factors [9, 12, 20]. Since the relevance of different hereditary risk factors, mainly the heterozygous FV G1691A mutation and the FII G20210A variant without further inherited prothrombotic risk factors, for spontaneous and triggered thrombo-embolic events in pediatric patients is not clear so far, we performed the present study. To assess the possible influence of different underlying exogenous triggering factors in patients with the common heterozygous factor V mutation or the hetero-zygous FII variant this subgroup analysis was performed.

Middeldorp et al. described a yearly incidence of venous thrombosis of 0.58% in patients older than 15 years with an isolated factor V mutation in a large prospec-tive study. In 5 of 9 patients an underlying triggering factor such as hormone repla-cement therapy, oral contraceptives and surgery was present [21]. In accordance with these data we found an underlying exogenous stimuli in 37% of the patients with factor V and 36% in children carrying the FII mutation in our cohort. Although the type of exogenous triggering factors was different from those described in adults patients, both, the acquired stimuli as well as the sites of thromboembolic manifestation were not different between the two pediatric groups studied here. It is therefore assumed, that the rate of exogenous causes – and the thrombotic risk in provoked prothrombotic clinical situations – in patients carrying the two studied hereditary risk factors is equal and comparable to that observed in adult patients.

More than one third of thromboembolic events in both carrier groups occurred in the presence of such exogenous triggering factors, underlining the importance of additional acquired prothrombotic states in heterozygous FV or FII carriers not only in adults but also during infancy and childhood. In the remaining majority of symptomatic children thrombotic vascular accidents have occurred without the known transient major risks already known in adults and defined in the method part.

In addition, the presented study aimed to evaluate the possible impact of age and gender of patients on prothrombotic risk since a number of studies suggested a higher risk in male neonates and infants [13–15]. We also have found a significantly higher proportion of males in neonates with renal venous thrombosis during recently reported data of the German neonatal thrombosis registry [22]. In the total population analyzed in the present subgroup analysis of all symptomatic vascular accidents in our country we found a mild overrepresentation of males in both study groups (FV: 54,2% male, FII: 62,5% male), reaching significance in patients < 12 months of age. Interestingly, the male carriers of the FV mutation appeared to have an earlier onset of thromboembolic events than the female FV carriers: boys carrying the factor V G1691A mutation showed significantly shorter thrombosis-free survivals compared to male patients with the FII variant. However, given the relatively high prevalence of the FV mutation in the general white population the early manifestation in males may contribute to the higher proportion of male patients observed in studies focussing on thrombosis in neonates and very young children. These hypothesis is in accordance with data from Arneil et al., Schmidt et al., and Mocan et al. who observed a higher proportion of male thrombotic patients during the first year of life compared with a rather balanced gender ratio in later childhood and adolescence. However, up to now, no gender specific differences in hemostaseological parameters have been reported during the first year of life that could explain this findings. Thus, further and larger controlled multicenter international studies are necessary to clarify the open questions.

References

1. Dahlbäck B, Carlsson M, Svensson PJ. Familial thrombophilia due to a previously unrecognized mechanism characterized by poor anticoagulant response to activated protein C: prediction of a cofactor to activated protein C. Proc Natl Acad Sci U S A. 1993;90:1004–1008.
2. Bertina RM, Koeleman BPC, Koster T, Rosendaal FR, Dirven RJ, de Ronde H, van der Velde PA, Reitsma PH. Mutation in blood coagulation factor V associated with resistance to activated protein C. Nature 1994;396:64–67.
3. Lane DA, Mannucci PM, Bauer KA, Bertina RM, Bochkov NP, Boulyjenkov V, Chandy M, Dahlbäck B, Ginter EK, Miletich JP, Rosendaal FR, Seligsohn U. Inherited thrombophilia, part 1. Thromb Haemost 1996;76:651–662.
4. Lane DA, Mannucci PM, Bauer KA, Bertina RM, Bochkov NP, Boulyjenkov V, Chandy M, Dahlbäck B, Ginter EK, Miletich JP, Rosendaal FR, Seligsohn U. Inherited thrombophilia, part 2. Thromb Haemost 1996;76:823–834.
5. Poort SR, Rosendaal FR, Reitsma PH, Bertina RM. A common genetic variation in the 3'-untranslated region of the prothrombin gene is associated with elevated plasma prothrombin levels and an increase in venous thrombosis. Blood 1996;88:3698–3703.

6. Ashka I, Aumann V, Bergmann F, Budde U, Eberl W, Eckhof-Donovan S, Krey S, Nowak-Göttl U, Schobess R, Sutor AH, Wendisch J, Schneppenheim R. Prevalence of FV Leiden in children with thromboembolism.- Eur J Pediatr 1996; 155: 1009–1014.
7. Sifontes MT, Nuss R, Jacobson LJ, Griffin JH, Manco-Johnson MJ. Thrombosis in otherwise well children with the factor V Leiden mutation. J Pediatr 1996 Mar; 128(3):324–328.
8. Ehrenforth S, von Depka Prondzinski M, Aygören-Pürsün E, Nowak-Göttl U, Scharrer I, Ganser A. Study of the prothrombin gene 20210 GA variant in FV:Q506 carriers in relationship to the presence or absence of juvenile venous thromboembolism. Arterioscler Thromb Vasc Biol 1999; 19:276–280.
9. Junker R, Koch HG, Auberger K, Münchow N, Ehrenforth S, Nowak-Göttl U. Prothrombin G20210A gene mutation and further prothrombotic risk factors in childhood thrombophilia. Arterioscler Thromb Vasc Biol 1996;19:2568–2572.
10. Nowak-Göttl U, Junker R, Hartmeier M, Koch HG, Münchow N, Assmann G, von Eckardstein A. Increased lipoprotein (a) is an important risk factor for venous thrombosis in childhood. Circulation 1999;100:743–748. a
11. Nowak-Göttl U, Wermes C, Junker R, Koch HG, Schobess R, Fleischhack G, Schwabe D, Ehrenforth S. Prospective evaluation of the thrombotic risk in children with acute lymphoblastic leukemia carrying the MTHFR TT677 genotype, the prothrombin G20210A variant, and further prothrombotic risk factors. Blood 1999;93:1595–1599. b
12. Schobess R, Junker R, Auberger K, Münchow N, Burdach S, Nowak-Göttl U. Factor V G1691A and prothrombin G20210A in childhood spontaneous venous thrombosis – Evidence of an age-dependent thrombotic onset in carriers of factor V G1691A and prothrombin G20210A mutation. Eur J Pediatr 1999; 158: 105–108.
13. Arneil GC. Renal venous thrombosis. Contrib Nephrol 1979; 15:21-29.
14. Mocan H, Beattie TJ, Murphy AV. Renal venous thrombosis in infancy: long-term follow-up. Pediatr Nephrol 1991; 5(1): 45–49.
15. Schmidt B, Andrew M. Neonatal thrombosis: report of a prospective Canadian and international registry. Pediatrics 1995; 96 (5 Pt 1): 939–943.
16. Ehrenforth S, Zwinge B, Scharrer I. High prevalence of factor V R506Q mutation in German thrombophilic and normal population. Thromb Haemost 1998; 79:384--385.
17. Martinelli I, Bucciarelli P, Margaglione M, De Stefano V, Castaman G, Mannucci PM. The risk of venous thromboembolism in family members with mutations in the genes of factor V or prothrombin or both. Br J Haem 2000; 111: 1223–1229
18. Lawson SE, Butler D, Enayat MS, Williams MD. Congenital thrombophilia and thrombosis: a study in a single centre. Arch Dis Child 1999; 81: 176–178
19. Bonduel M, Hepner M, Sciuccati G, Torres AF, Pieroni G, Frontroth JP. Prothrombotic abnormalities in children with venous thromboembolism. J Pediatr Hematol Oncol 2000; 22: 66–72
20. Nowak-Göttl U, Junker R, Kreuz W, von Eckardstein A, Kosch A, Nohe N, Schobess R, Ehrenforth S; Childhood Thrombophilia Study Group. Risk of recurrent thrombosis in children with combined prothrombotic risk factors. Blood 2001; 97: 858–862
21. Middeldorp S, Meinardi J, Koopman M, van Pampus E, Hamulyak K, van der Meer J, Prins M, Büller H. A prospective study of asymptomatic carriers of the factor V Leiden mutation to determine the incidence of venous thromboembolism. Ann Intern Med 2001; 135: 322–327.
22. Nowak-Göttl U, von Kries R, Göbel U. Neonatal symptomatic thromboembolism in Germany: two year survey. Arch Dis Child Fetal Neonatal Ed 1997; 76(3):F163–167.

UFH Bolus Administration in Comparison to subcutaneous Low Molecular Weight Heparin in pediatric cardiac Catheterization

B. Roschitz, A. Beitzke, A. Gamillscheg, K. Sudi, B. Leschnik, M. Köstenberger, and W. Muntean

Introduction

Venous or arterial thrombosis after cardiac catheterization is one of the most frequent adverse events. Anticoagulation with heparin reduces this risk of thromboembolic complications during cardiac catheterization in both children and adults. Different dosages and modalities of heparin administration, from heparin bolus therapy to low-dose flush heparin, have been recommended for the pediatric cardiac catheterization laboratories.

Unfractionated heparin (UFH) is still the anticoagulant of choice for the initial treatment of thromboembolic complications as well as for thrombosis prophylaxis in the pediatric patient.

Low molecular weight heparin (LMWH) seems to offer a number of advantages over UFH in various clinical settings. In prophylactic trials LMWH were either as effective as UFH or either more effective in preventing thrombotic complications, with no detectable increase of bleeding. The few data available in pediatric patients also suggested that LMWH might be advantageous in this age group. In adults potential advantages of LMWH over UFH in heart catheterization were shown in several clinical trials. By removing the need for coagulation monitoring, LMWH might simplify the procedure while potentially also offering greater efficacy.

To study the potential of LMWH in thrombosis prophylaxis in pediatric cardiac catheterization we compared UFH bolus to LMWH subcutaneous application on their effects on markers of coagulation activation during cardiac catheterization.

Materials and methods

Patients

65 patients with congenital heart disease who underwent cardiac catheterization were included in the study. A diagnostic hemodynamic catheterization or electrophysiologic study was performed in all 65 patients, 11 had an additional interventional procedure. Vascular access was obtained percutaneously. Distal leg pulses were evaluated before and immediately after the procedure. A clinical examination took place one day after the catheterization to evaluate hemorrhage and leg pulses again.

I. Scharrer/W. Schramm (Ed.)
32nd Hemophilia Symposion Hamburg 2001
© Springer-Verlag Berlin Heidelberg 2003

Anticoagulation

Patients were treated as follows: a UFH bolus of 100 IU/kg bodyweight was administered to 40 patients (30 days to 16 years of age). No additional UFH was administered. Dosages were controlled by activated clotting time (ACT). Interventional procedures were included in this group. In 25 patients (28 days to 26 years) enoxaparin was administered subcutaneously 3 hours before catheterization subcutaneously in a dosage of 1.6 mg/ kg bodyweight in infants younger than 2 months of age and for the remaining patients in a dosage of 1mg/kg bodyweight.

Coagulation studies

Blood samples for coagulation studies were obtained before, 5 minutes and 30 minutes after puncture and at the end of heart catheterization. In children below an age of 3 years only 2 ml blood were obtained. The samples were immediately centrifuged at 3000 g for 10 minutes. Platelet poor plasma was stored in plastic tubes at -80 °C and analyzed within 1 month of storage. UFH and enoxaparin activity in plasma was determined by Coacute Heparin (Chromogenix). Thrombin generation F1+2 and D-dimer formation were analyzed by ELISA (Coachrom). *Activated Clotting time*: was performed on the Hemochron Jr ACT-LR.

Results

F1+2 generation was observed in 13 patients after UFH bolus application (mean 1,4 nmol/l; range 1,1-2,3 nmol/l). D-dimer was elevated in 3 patients. Thrombin gene-

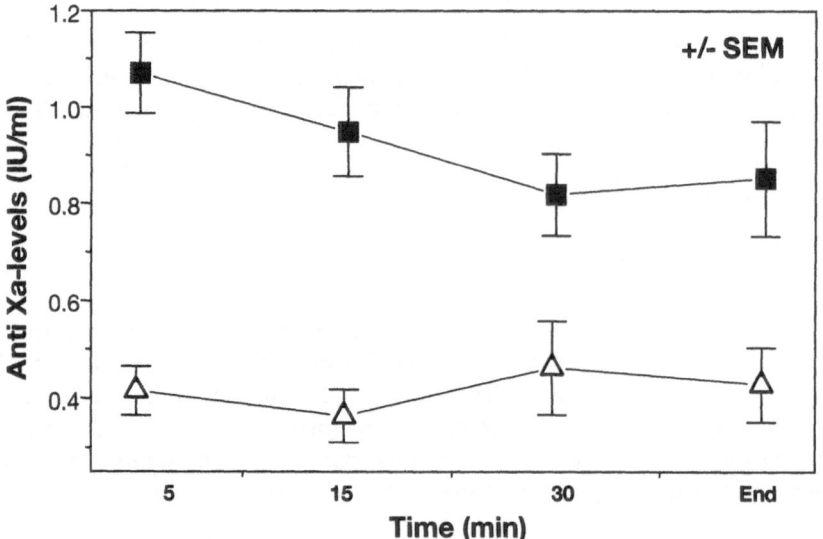

Fig. 1. Figure compares anti Xa UFH activity ■, to anti Xa enoxaparin activity △

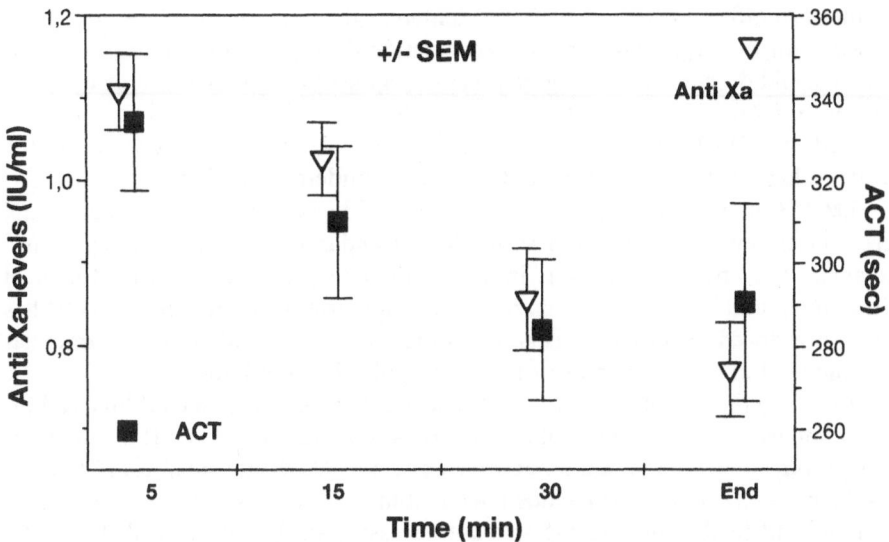

Fig. 2. Figure 2 compares ACT to anti Xa UFH activity. γACT; ⊕ anti Xa

ration was inversely correlated to age. Children at mean age of 3.19 years were at greater risk for activating while no activation was found at an age of 7.23 years. In cell-Chi Square analysis no influence of the catheterization procedure was found (q-Square 0,34; d.f.: 1). Duration of catheterization showed no influence on coagulation activation. In the enoxaparin group F1+2 generation was found in 11 patients (median 2.7 nmol/l; range 1.5-5.77). No significant difference of F1+2 generation could be found between the two groups. In the enoxaparin group no correlation of F1+2 generation to age was found. No D-dimer generation was observed in children with subcutaneous enoxaparin.

In the enoxaparin group no major complications to LMWH application occurred. No postcatheterization bleeding was observed.

In the UFH group unsightly echymoses were developed in 5 cases. One female patient, 3 months of age, developed during diagnostic cardiac catheterization lasting for 115 minutes, an arterial thrombosis. The baby girl was showing up with the lowest 30 minutes and end ACT values (180 and 168 seconds) of all 40 patients. No further UFH was administered.

Discussion

In our study a 100 IU/kg bodyweight bolus of UFH administered after arterial or venous access led to none or moderate F1+2 generation in 40 pediatric patients. But anti Xa activity of UFH varied from patient to patient. This variability is well explained by the pharmacokinetics and clinical effects of UFH and can especially be pronounced in children, depending on their physical maturity. Therefore, use of a fixed dosed UFH in pediatric cardiac catheterization, without monitoring of efficacy can result in significant overcoagulation or undercoagulation. The ACT is a quantitative assay for monitoring heparin anticoagulation during various medical procedures. To avoid over- or undercoagulation, the degree of coagulation can be determined by ACT. An ACT>210 seconds reflected adequate anti Xa UFH activity and none or moderate F1+2 generation in our study. ACT was a reliable bedside test in the heart catheterization laboratory to decide about undercoagulation

LMWH offers many advantages over standard heparin including less bleeding, greater efficacy, longer-half life, less monitoring and more predictable dosage requirements. The efficacy of LMWH in adults for both prevention and treatment of thromboembolic disease has been proved by numerous trials. Recently LMWH has been introduced for prophylaxis and treatment of venous and arterial thrombosis in children, but only a few reports have been published until now.

To clarify the role of LMWH in pediatric heart catheterization UFH bolus administration was compared with subcutaneous administration of LMWH in our study. The prophylactic level of anti Xa activity was set by Masicotte at 0.2-0.4 IU/ml and was achieved by all patients included in our study. Pharmacokinetics were very predictable and further monitoring was not necessary in the cardiac catheterization laboratory. Coagulation activation in the UFH group and LMWH group were equal, no bleeding or concomitant thrombosis was observed.

We conclude in our preliminary study that application of LMWH may be at least equally efficacious and safe during pediatric cardiac catheterization than UFH bolus therapy as determined by plasma levels and markers of clotting activation. Because of a consistent dose to plasma activity no further monitoring is necessary during cardiac catheterization. Larger clinical trials with thrombosis and bleeding as endpoint seem to be justified to show the efficacy and safety of LMWH in pediatric catheterization.

Incidence of Inhibitor Development in consecutively recruited severe Hemophilia A and B Patients – a retrospective Single Centre Study

S. Halimeh, A. Kosch, N. Bogdanova, K. Abshagen, and H. Jürgens

Introduction

Hemophilia A (HA) and B (HB) are X-linked genetic disorders resulting in deficiencies of blood coagulation factors VIII and IX. In order to prevent joint bleedings and hemophilic arthropathy in hemophilia patients, a long-term prophylactic therapy with factor VIII or IX concentrates has been suggested. This coagulation factor substitution can be complicated by the development of antibodies against factor VIII or IX (sc. inhibitors).

Based on a number of studies the incidence of antibody development in patients with severe hemophilia A (residual activity of factor VIII less than 1% of normal) has been estimated to be between 3.6% - 33% [Scharrer et al. 1993, Gilles et al. 1997]. These data suggest that up to one third of patients with severe hemophilia may develop an inhibitor sometime in their lives. However, among patients with hemophilia B, inhibitors are less frequent, affecting only 1% to 4% of the moderately and severely affected patients (Biggs et al. 1974, Ehrenforth et al. 1992). Is has been controversially discussed, whether the type of factor preparation used for substitution, namely plasma derived or recombinant concentrates, may influence the incidence of antibody development. No final prospective data are available [Kreuz, Auerswald personal correspondence]. Moreover, specific mutations in the factor VIII and IX genes like gross deletions or inversions, have been suspected to increase the risk for inhibitor development (Briet et al. 1994, Hoyer et al. 1995, Kavakli et al. 1998, Kreuz et al. 1996, Rasi et al. 1990, Scharrer et al., 1998, 1999).

Our present study aimed to evaluate the incidence of inhibitor development in relation to the type of factor substitution and type of disease causing mutations in a group of consecutively recruited patients with severe hemophilia.

Patients and methods

Patients group

We investigated the records of 87 moderately and severely affected pediatric patients with hemophilia A (n = 64) and hemophilia B (n=23) with regard to bleed-

---

* The patients enrolled in this retrospective study were treated in part by G. Kurlemann, H. Pollmann, R. Ernst, and S. Halimeh at the Department of Pediatric Hematology/Oncology of the University Hospital of Muenster

I. Scharrer/W. Schramm (Ed.)
32nd Hemophilia Symposion Hamburg 2001
© Springer-Verlag Berlin Heidelberg 2003

ing frequency and the presence of factor VIII and IX inhibitors. However in the current study we concentrate on the development of inhibitors.

The median age of the hemophilia A (HA) patients was 9.3 years (0.5–22) and of the hemophilia B (HB) 20.2 years (0.5–48).

All patients were initially treated on demand (clinically suspected joint bleeding) either with recombinant factor concentrates (rFVIII or rFIX) or plasma derived factor concentrates (pdFVIII or pdFIX). After 6 bleedings into one target joint the treatment was changed into a prophylactic regimen with weight-adapted substitution of factor concentrates 3 times a week [Pollmann et al. 1999]. Patients were treated with approximately 25 IU/kg body weight of factor VIII or factor IX concentrates respectively.

Monitoring for inhibitor development was carried out according to the Bethesda inhibitor assay [Carol et al. 1975]. Inhibitor testing was performed at least every three months in all patients during a routine visit or when patients presented with bleeding complications. Inhibitors were included in the study only if they were considered clinically relevant.

DNA Analysis

Genomic DNA from the inhibitor positive patients was extracted from peripheral blood lymphocytes as described by Miller et al. (1988). The screening for gross rearrangements in the factor VIII and factor IX gene respectively, was performed by Southern blot hybridization as described previously (Lakich et al. 1993; Anson et al. 1984; Gianelli et al. 1984).

PCR was performed on 50–100 ng of extracted DNA essentially using the amplification primers and cycling conditions described by Schwaab et al. (1997) for the factor VIII gene and by Koeberl et al. (1990) for the factor IX gene. The amplified fragments were sequenced with the Applied Biosystems (ABI) BigDye Terminator Cycle Sequencing Ready Reaction Kit according to manufacturer's instructions and sequencing reactions were analyzed on an ABI 310 automated sequencer.

Results

Treatment and inhibitors development

23 of the 87 HA patients received rFVIIIC while 17 of them received pdFVIIIC. The remaining 47 patients were initially treated with pdFVIIIC and were subsequently switched to rFVIIIC.

From the 33 HB patients two received rFIX, 22 received pdFIX and 9 were switched from pdFIX to rFIX. The individual regimen of therapy was determined by the treating physician.

Clinically relevant inhibitors have been diagnosed in four HA patients (4/87 = 4.6%) and two patients with HB (2/33 = 6.0%). Information about the age at inhibitor

Table 1. Age at inhibitors development, type of treatment and disease causing mutations identified in two HB and four HA patients inhibitor positive detected in the present study.

	Patient initials	Time between first factor substitution and inhibitor development	Type of treatment	Mutation
HA	S. T.	1 month	pdFVIII	Intron 22 Inversion
HA	F. D.	8 months	rFVIII	??c.278delT
HA	P. M.	24 months	rFVIII	c.5961delA
HA	G. V.	60 months	pdFVIII	Intron 22 Inversion
HB	N. G.	4 months	rFIX	R29X
HB	D. H.	24 months	pdFIX	R29X

development, type of the treatment and the disease causing mutation identified is listed for each patient in Table 1. Peak inhibitor levels ranged from 8 BU/ml^{-1} to a maximum of 600 BU/ml^{-1} and 17.9 BU/ml^{-1} respectively. The inhibitors occurred in all cases earlier than 60-70 exposure days.

All patients developed factor VIII or IX antigens during the first five years of factor substitution. There was no obvious relation between the type of factor concentrates used for substitution and the risk of developing an inhibitor. All inhibitors were diagnosed during the patients were treated on demand.

Mutations in the Factor VIII and Factor IX gene

All mutations identified in the group of inhibitor positive HA or HB patients are leading to disruptions of the open reading frame and truncation of the protein synthesis (Table 1).

The common intron 22 inversion in the factor VIII gene was detected in two of the analyzed patients. Furthermore, we identified two single nucleotide deletions causing shift in the reading frame and a premature stop-codon, in exon 14 (c.2781delT) and in exon 18 (c.5961delA) of the factor VIII gene (Bogdanova et al., in press).

One of the HB patients with inhibitors was shown to be hemizygous for a deletion of the complete factor IX gene. A nonsense mutation ((R29X) in exon 2 of the Factor IX gene was identified in the second HB patient. Both mutations are expected to cause lack of circulating factor IX antigen.

Discussion

The formation of inhibitors to factor VIII in patients is the most serious complication of the hemophilia therapy. Inhibitor frequency in patients with hemophilia A and B is a highly controversial issue that provoked much discussion in recent years. Data from different studies show that 3.6 to 33% of the hemophilia A (Scharrer et al. 1993, Gilles et al. 1997) and 1-4% of hemophilia B patients are prone to inhibitor development (Ehrenforth et al. 1992). In our patient group 4.6% of the HA and 6.0%

of the HB patients showed clinically relevant inhibitors, thus suggesting a relatively low incidence if this complication is compared to the reviewed data of Scharrer et al. (1993). In our study only the clinically relevant inhibitors were documented, in the literature the incidence up to 35% is reported. This discrepancy may be explained in part by the fact that in our study only clinically relevant inhibitors are included whereas some authors include patients with purely laboratory evidence of inhibitor development.

Recent studies including factor VIII mutation data in patients with severe hemophilia A gave the evidence that mutations with an increased risk for inhibitor development appear to be large multidomain deletions, nonsense mutations or iso-chromosomal intron 22 inversions (Goodeve et al. 2000, Knobe et al. 2000, Oldenburg et al. 2002, Salviato et al. 2002).

Mutations like large deletions, inversions or nonsense mutations, leading to a major loss of coding information and lack of circulating factor VIII antigen are associated with a higher risk (about 35%) to develop inhibitors than missense mutations or small deletions (4.3 and 7.4% respectively) (Schwaab et al. 1997, Goodeve et al. 2000).

In accordance with these observations, four of our six inhibitor positive patients are carrying protein truncating mutations. In two patients however, single nucleotide deletions were detected, thus giving the evidence that this type of mutations is related to a higher inhibitor prevalence than previously suggested. Most probably not only the type of mutations but also their localization in the factor VIII gene influences the predisposition to inhibitor formation.

The frequencies of inhibitor development in patients treated with virus inactivated plasma derived clotting factor concentrates compared to patients treated exclusively with recombinant FVIII results are controversially discussed [Brita et al. 1994, Kavakli et al. 1998] and no final data concerning this issue are available so far. Still, large-scale multicenter studies are warranted to clarify this clinically relevant issue. Therefore, all newly diagnosed patients should be enrolled into the ongoing German multicenter PUP-study (Kreuz et al. 2001).

References

1. Anson DS, Choo KH, Rees DJG, Gianelli F, Gould K, Huddleston JA, Brownlee GG (1984) The gene structure of human anti-hemophilic factor IX. The ENBO Journal 3, 1053-1060
2. Biggs R: Jaundice and antibodies directed against factors VIII and IX in patients treated for hemophilia or Christmas disease in the United Kindom. Br J Haematol 1974, 26(3): 313–29
3. Bogdanova N, Markoff M, Pollmann H, Nowak-Göttl U, Eisert R, Dworniczak B, Eigel A, Horst J (2002) Prevalence of Small Rearrangements in the Factor VIII Gene Among Patients with Severe Hemophilia A. Hum Mutat, in press
4. Briet E, Rosendaal FR, Kreuz W, et al: High titer inhibitors in severe hemophilia A. A meta-analysis based on eight long-term follow-up studies concerning inhibitors associated with crude or intermediate purity factor VIII products. Thromb and Haemost 1994, 72(1): 162–164
5. Briet E, Rosendaal FR: Inhibitors in hemophilia A: are some products safer? Semin Hematol 1994, 31: 11–15

6. Carol KK: A more uniform measurement of factor VIII inhibitors. Thrombos Diathes Haemorrh 1975, 34: 869

7. Ehrenforth S, Kreuz W, Scharrer I, et al: Incidence of development of factor VIII and IX inhibitors in hemophiliacs. Lancet 1992, 339(8793): 594–598.

8. Gianelli F, Anson DS, Choo KH, Rees DJG, Winship PR, Ferrari N, Rizza CR, Brownlee GG (1984) Characterization and use of an intragenic polymorphic marker for detection of carriers of hemophilia B (factor IX deficiency). Lancet, i, 239–241

9. Gilles JG, Jacquemin MG, Saint-Remy JM, et al: Factor VIII inhibitors. Thromb Haemost 1997, 78(1): 641–646

10. Goodeve AC, Williams I, Bray GL, et al: Relationship between factor VIII mutation type and inhibitor development in a cohort of previously untreated patients treated with recombinant factor VIII (Recombinate). Recombinate PUP Study Group. Thromb Haemost 20000, 83(6): 844–848

11. Hoyer LW: Why do so many hemophilia A patients develop an inhibitor? Br J Haematol 1995, 90(3): 498–501

12. Kavakli K, Gringeri A, Bader R, et al: Inhibitor development and substitution therapy in a developing country: Turkey. Haemophilia 1998, 4: 104–108

13. Knobe KE, Villoutreix BO, Tengborn LI, et al: Factor VIII inhibitors in two families with mild hemophilia A: structural analysis of the mutations. Haemostasis 2000, 30(5): 268–279

14. Koeberl DD, Bottema CDK, Ketterling RP, Bridge PJ, Lillicrap DP, Sommer SS (1990) Mutations causing hemophilia B: direct estimate of the underlying rates of spontaneous germ-line transitions, transversions and deletions in the human gene. Am J Hum Genet 47:202–217

15. Kreuz W, Escuriola-Ettingshausen C, Martinez-Saguer I, et al: Epidemiology of inhibitors in hemophilia A. Vox Sang 1996, 70(1): 2–8

16. Kreuz W, Auerswald G, Budde U, et al: Inhibitor incidence in previously untreated patients (PUPs) with hemophilia A and B - A prospective, multicenter study of the pediatric study group of the German, Swiss and Austrian Society of Thrombosis and Hemostasis (GTH). Blood 2001, ASH 2238 (abstract)

17. Lakich D, Kazaziean HH, Antonarakis SE, Gischier : Inversions disrupting the factor VIII gene as a common cause of severe hemophilia A. Nature Genet. 1993, 5:236–241

18. Manco-Johnson MJ, Nuss R, Funk S, et al: Joint evaluation instruments for children and adults with hemophilia. Haemophilia 2000, 6: 649–657

19. Miller SA., Dykes DD, Polesky HF: A simple salting procedure for extracting DNA from human nucleated cells. Nucleic Acids Res 1988, 16:1215

20. Rasi V, Ikkala E, et al: Hemophiliacs with factor VIII inhibitors in Finland: prevalence, incidence and outcome. Br J Haematol 1990, 76(3): 369–71

21. Oldenburg J, El-Maarri O, Schwaab R: Inhibitor development inhibitor correlation to factor VIII genotypes. Haemophilia 2002, 8: 23–29

22. Pollmann H, Richter H, Ringkamp H, Jürgens H: When are children diagnosed as having severe hemophilia and when do they start to bleed? A 10-year single center PUP study. Eur J Paediatr 1999; 158 (Suppl 3): 166–170

23. Salviato R, Belvini D, Are A, et al: Large FVIII gene deletion confers very high risk of inhibitor development in three related severe hemophiliacs. Haemophilia 2002, 8(1): 17–21

24. Scharrer I, Bray GL, Neutzling O: Incidence of inhibitors in hemophilia A patients - a review of recent studies of recombinant and plasma-derived factor VIII concentrates. Haemophilia 1999, 5(3): 145–154

25. Scharrer I, Neutzling O: Incidence of inhibitors in hemophiliacs. A review of the literature. Blood Coagul and Fibrinolysis 1993, 4(5): 753–758

26. Scharrer I, Neutzling O, Schwaab R, et al: Experiences with recombinant factor VIII products: development of inhibitor and immune tolerance therapy. Ann of Hematol 1998, 76. A1–A6

27. Schwaab R., Oldenburg J., Lalloz M.R., Schwaab U., Pemberton S., Hanfland P., Brackmann H.H., Tuddenham E.G., Michaelides K. Factor VIII gene mutations found by a comparative study of SSCP, DGGE and CMC and their analysis on a molecular model of factor VIII protein. Hum Genet 1997, 101(3):323–32.

V. *Free Lectures*

Chairmen:

H. LENK (Leipzig)
R. ZIMMERMANN (Heidelberg)

Factor V Inhibitor and Anti-Phospholipid Antibodies after Treatment with Ciprofloxacin

W. Miesbach, J. Vogt, D. Peez, Th. Vigh, B. Bühler, G. Ashmelash, and I. Scharrer

The development of factor V inhibitor is very rare, especially in combination with raised antiphospholipid (aPL) antibodies.

This paper presents one patient with factor V inhibitor and aPL antibodies after treatment with ciprofloxacin.

Factor V inhibitor was assayed by the Bethesda method, lupus anticoagulants were assayed according to the criteria of SSC of the ISTH [1], anti-cardiolipin antibodies were assayed by an ELISA.

Other coagulation defects like FVIII-, FII- or FVII-deficiency could be excluded.

A 85 year old patient was admitted to hospital with leftside hemiparesis and sensomotoric aphasia due to a cerebral infarction.

He was also suffering from cardiac arrhythmia, diabetes mellitus and hypertension.

He was also suffering from a stroke, 5 years ago, but had recovered quickly.

Medication with heparin and infusion (Sterofundin) was given additional to the unchanged long treatment with Benazepril 5, Pravastatin 20 and Metamizol.

After improvement of the neurological defects the patient was treated with ciprofloxacin for 8 days due to an urinary tract infection. 4 days after start of the treatment PT began to decrease and PTT was prolonged. Hemoglobin stayed for the first time at 13 g/%. 6 weeks after start of treatment with Ciprofloxacin PT decreased to 12 % and PTT was prolonged at 172 sec. Hemoglobin was 6 g/% (Fig. 1).

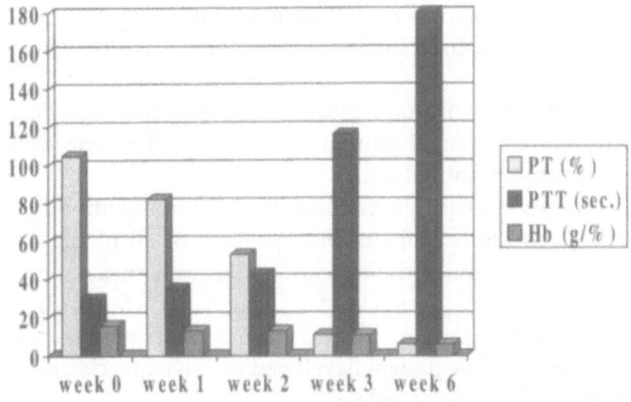

Fig. 1

I. Scharrer/W. Schramm (Ed.)
32nd Hemophilia Symposion Hamburg 2001
© Springer-Verlag Berlin Heidelberg 2003

Table 1. Coagulation system and Factor V inhibitor

	dilution	patient	normal
F V inhibitor		1156 BE	0 BE
Factor V	1 : 640	0	70–100 %
Factor V-Ag		136 %	70–150 %
Factor VII	1 : 320	0	59–114 %
Factor VII	1 : 640	128 %	59–114 %
Factor VIII-inhibitor		88.32 BE	0 BE
Factor VIII	1 : 320	0	60–150 %
Factor VIII	1 : 640	256 %	60–150 %
Factor IX	1 : 40	0	60–150 %
Factor IX	1 : 320	64 %	60–150 %
Factor IX	1 : 640	128 %	60–150 %

Table 2. Lupus anticoagulants and anti-Cardiolipin antibodies

	patient	normal
KCT	Type II	
DRVVT	pos.	
Staclot LA	pos.	0.00–7.90
PTTT	pos.	
Textarin (sec.)	114.50	21.80–29.60
IgG aCL	35.90	1.90–9.90
IgM aCL	0.30	0.90–5.90

Factor VIII could be normalized in dilutions up to 1:640. Also factor VII and factor IX were normalized in dilutions (factor II was already measured normal in dilution up to 160).

In addition, factor V inhibitor could be detected. Factor V activity could not be normalized even in dilutions up to 640. The concentration of Factor V-antigen, however was not reduced.

Lupus anticoagulants and anti-cardiolipin antibodies could also be detected.

Lupus anticoagulants were positive in all of the 4 performed tests and high levels of IgG anticardiolipin antibodies were measured (Table 2).

Changing of plasma levels of coagulation's factors began 4 days after start of treatment with ciprofloxacin and was not reversible even weeks later after terminating this therapy. The patient developed massive muscle and visceral bleedings and died from cardiovascular failure.

The extent of this coagulation imbalance could be demonstrated by ROTEG (Fig. 2).

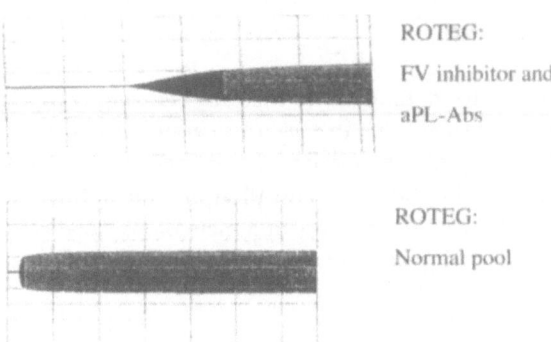

Fig. 2

Discussion

The development of factor V inhibitor is very rare, especially in combination with anti-phospholipid antibodies. The demonstrated case report shows that treatment with Ciprofloxacin may trigger the development of Factor V inhibitor and anti-phospholipid antibodies.

First changes of the coagulation system of the patient was detected 4 days after start of treatment. At this time Ciprofloxacin was the only new taken medicine. Factor V antigen was not reduced. Other coagulative defects as inhibitors of FVIII, FII or FVII were excluded.

The patient developed massive muscle and visceral bleedings and died from cardiovascular failure.

Treatment with ciprofloxacin may induce polyvalent antibodies against factor V, Anticardiolipin and with less extent against factor VIII. FVIII activity, however could be normalized in dilutions up to 640.

Until now only a few reports exist about the association of treatment with Ciprofloxacin and the development of inhibitor and anti-phospholipid antibodies.

In 1994, however the association of factor V inhibitor and lupus anticoagulants after treatment with Ciprofloxacin was detected in a 74 years old patient. But this occurrence was transient and the levels normalized after terminating treatment with Ciprofloxacin [2].

van Beek et al. reported in 1993 the occurrence of a transient FVIII inhibitor after treatment with Ciprofloxacin in a 41 years old patient with severe hemophilia A [7].

Ciprofloxacin can be involved in the pathogenesis of the acquired von Willebrand disease [3].

Some papers report a Ciprofloxacin induced Vaskulitis, without measuring anti-phospholipid antibodies [4–6].

It was striking that in these cases the clinical manifestation occurred quite early after the 3rd, 4th and 10th day after start of treatment with Ciprofloxacin and disappeared after 3 till 6 weeks after termination of treatment with Ciprofloxacin.

Conclusion

This case demonstrates massive bleeding complications after the treatment with Ciprofloxacin due to a factor V inhibitor and raised anti-phospholipid antibodies. Probably the association of treatment with Ciprofloxacin and the development of factor V inhibitor and anti-phospholipid antibodies is diagnosed to rarely. This case emphasize the necessity of a meticolous clarification of a prolonged PTT and drop of PT during and after treatment with Ciprofloxacin.

References

1. Brandt JT, Triplett DA, Alving B, Scharrer I. Criteria for the diagnosis of lupus anticoagulants: an update. On behalf of the Subcommittee on Lupus Anticoagulant/Antiphospholipid Antibody of the Scientific and Standardization Committee of the ISTH. Thromb Haemost 1995; 74:1185-90.
2. Scharrer I, Fürstenau C, Stotz D, Müller-Beißenhirtz W, Ehrenforth S, von Depka Prondzinski M, Siegert S: Auftreten eines Faktor V-Hemmkörpers und Auftreten von Lupus-Antikoagulanzien nach Ciprofloxacin. In: I.Scharrer/W.Schramm: 25 Hämophilie-Symposium Hamburg 1994, 388-92, Springer-Verlag Berlin Heidelberg 1996.
3. Castaman Rodeghiero F. (1994): Acquired transitory von Willebrand Syndrome with ciprofloxacin. Lancet 343:492
4. Choe U., Rothschild B. M., Laitman L. (1989): Ciprofloxacin-induced vasculitis. N Engl J Med 320: 257-258
5. Kanuga J., Holland C.L., Reyes R., Bielory L. (1991): Ciprofloxacin induced leukocytoplastic vasculitis with cryoglobulinemia. Ann Allergy 66-67
6. Stubbings J., Sheehan-Dare R., Walton S. (1992): Cutaneous vasculititis due to ciprofloxacin. Br Med J 305-29
7. van Beek E.J.R., Peters M., ten Cate J.W. (1993): Factor VIII inhibitor associated with ciprofloxacin. Thromb Haemostas 69(4):403

Isolated molecular Defects of von Willebrand Factor Binding to Collagen do not correlate with Bleeding Symptoms

R. Schneppenheim, T. Obser, E. Drewke, U. Gross-Wieltsch, E.G. Huizinga, F. Oyen, R.A. Romijn, A.H. Sutor, C. Wermes, and U. Budde

Background

Collagen in the subendothelium is suggested as a major binding partner of von Willebrand factor (vWF), thereby providing its function in primary hemostasis. The lack of the functionally most active vWF high molecular weight multimers in von Willebrand disease (vWd) type 2A correlates with significantly decreased vWF binding to collagen type I and III, respectively, and offers a possible explanation for the bleeding symptoms in such patients. Consequently, one would expect a similar clinical phenotype in persons with an isolated defect of vWF collagen binding (vWF:CB) but with normal vWF multimers. A mutation in the vWF A3 domain that is regarded as the major vWF:CB site [1], was recently identified in a family with mother and daughter suffering from a significant bleeding tendency [2]. However, vWF:CB seemed normal in the vWF:CB assay. Only after identification of a mutation in the vWF A3 domain and recombinant expression of the mutant protein, a reduced VWF:CB was demonstrated by the collagen binding curve [2]. Here we report on three different novel mutations in the A3 domain which do not correlate with bleeding symptoms, although they significantly decrease vWF collagen binding.

Investigated persons

Proband 1 is the mother of a Kurdish patient with severe vWd type 3. She is a heterozygous carrier of the nonsense mutation Y2292X. She never suffered from unusual bleeding or menorrhagia and three pregnancies and deliveries were uneventful. Her bleeding time was normal. Proband 2 was a healthy Turkish girl without bleeding symptoms until the age of three when she was initially diagnosed with ITP, later with aplastic anemia, currently with MDS. Thrombocytopenia <20/nl was accompanied by bleeding symptoms. Proband 3, a 14 year old Turkish girl was investigated as member of a family with thrombophilia. She had occasional epistaxis but no menorrhagia and her bleeding time was normal.

Supported by Deutsche Forschungsgemeinschaft DFG grant Schn 325/4-2

I. Scharrer/W. Schramm (Ed.)
32nd Hemophilia Symposion Hamburg 2001
© Springer-Verlag Berlin Heidelberg 2003

Methods

Phenotypic analysis included measurements of vWF:Ag, vWF:RCo, vWF:CB and vWF multimer analysis using luminescent visualization with photo-imaging. Our mutation screening concentrated on the vWF A3 domain encoded by part of exon 28 through exon 32 but was then extended to the complete coding region of the vWF gene by direct sequencing of single exons to exclude additional mutations. The effect of the identified mutations in comparison to wildtype vWF was reproduced by stable recombinant expression in 293 EBNA cells and subsequent analysis of vWF multimers and vWF:CB as previously described [3]. Recombinant mutant and wildtype vWF were compared by multimer analysis and determination of vWF:CB.

Results

In all three probands vWF:Ag, vWF:RCo and vWF multimers were normal, vWF:CB, however, was significantly impaired with 0.15, 0.10 and 0.14 U/ml relative to vWF:Ag, respectively. By screening the complete vWF coding sequence we detected three different novel heterozygous mutations – Q971H, I978T and Q999R – in the A3 collagen binding domain of vWF (Fig. 1) that significantly reduced vWF collagen binding in the three probands without clear correlation with bleeding tendency. The causal nature of these mutations was confirmed by the vWF:CB assay of recombinant mutant and wildtype vWF, respectively. Whereas multimers of mutant r-vWF were indistinguishable from wildtype r-vWF (Fig. 2), vWF:CB of mutants was significantly reduced as in the probands' plasma (Fig. 3).

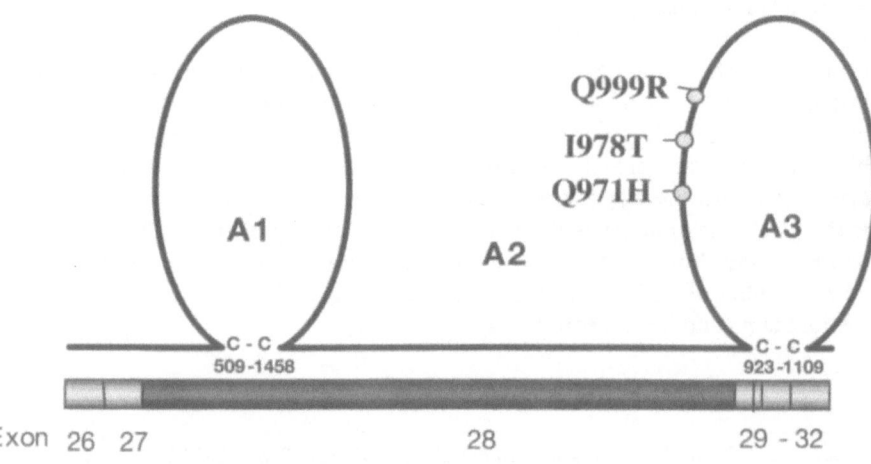

Fig. 1. Position of the three mutations in the vWF A3 domain. (Only a small part of exon 28 contributes to the A3 domain.)

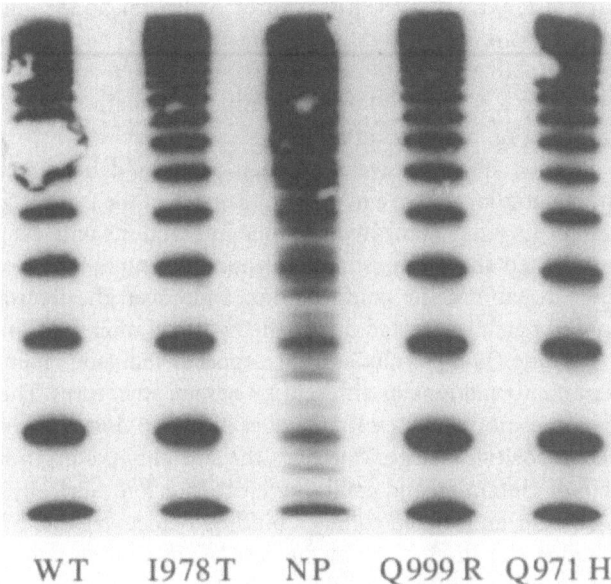

Fig. 2. Multimer analysis of recombinant wild-type (wt) and mutant vWF (rI978T, rQ999R, rQ971H) in comparison to plasma vWF (NP). High molecular weight multimers as in normal plasma and wt vWF are also seen in the mutants.

WT   I978T   NP   Q999R   Q971H

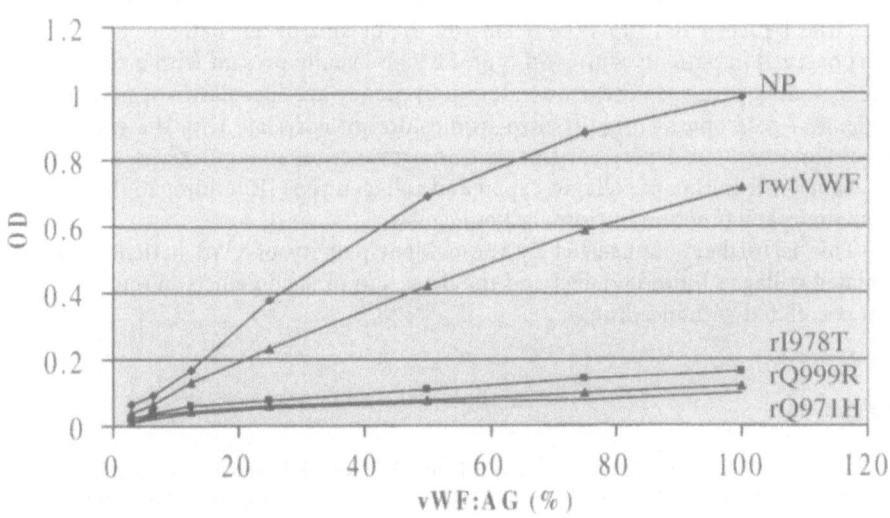

Fig. 3. Binding of type I collagen to recombinant wt (rwt-vWF) and mutant vWF (rI978T, rQ999R, rQ971H) in comparison to normal pooled plasma vWF (NP).

Discussion

The residues that are mutated in the patients are located at the front face of the A3 domain and coincide with the proposed collagen binding site [1]. Residue Q971 is buried and therefore not likely to be directly involved in collagen binding. The side chain of Q971, however, forms three hydrogen bonds with neighboring residues. Histidine can not form these hydrogen bonds. The absence of the hydrogen bonds may destabilize the conformation. Moreover, replacement of the buried side chain of Q971 by a somewhat larger histidine side chain may additionally destabilize the conformation of the A3 domain.

Residue I978 is solvent exposed and could be directly involved in collagen binding. It is located in a hydrophobic patch at the front face of the domain. The side chain of I978 has many hydrophobic interactions with neighboring residues. Upon mutation to threonine, some hydrophobic interactions can not be formed. This might destabilize the conformation. Moreover, the hydrophobic character of the exposed patch is affected due to the hydroxyl moiety of threonine.

Residue Q999 is fully solvent exposed. The side chain of Q999 is observed in many conformations in different A3 crystal structures. The amide group of its side chain does not interact with residues in the A3 domain. The mutation Q999R introduces a positive charge. Moreover, the side chain of arginine is bigger than the side chain of glutamine and could therefore interfere sterically with collagen binding.

To date, an isolated collagen binding defect was identified in only four families including our three. Only in the case of the French family an associated bleeding tendency was reported. Compared to the »French« mutation, our three mutations are certainly more severe in their impact on vWF:CB in vitro, since vWF:CB in plasma of the »French« patients seemed normal in contrast to the very low vWF:CB activities between 10 to 15 % of normal in the plasma of our patients. Such values are observed in patients with vWd type 2A who usually present with a clear bleeding tendency. Reasons for the observed discrepancy are speculative. It may be possible, that data obtained by in vitro studies do not correlate with the situation in vivo. However, our favored hypothesis is provocative and questions a clinically relevant contribution of collagen type I and collagen type III binding to the vWF A3 domain as key function in primary hemostasis.

This is further emphasized by the evident paucity of vWd patients with an isolated collagen binding defect and the detection of such defects in our probands not correlated with bleeding.

References

1. Romijn RA, Bouma B, Wuyster W, Gros P, Kroon J, Sixma JJ, Huizinga EG. Identification of the collagen-binding site of the von Willebrand factor A3-domain. J Biol Chem. 2001; 276:9985–9991
2. Ribba AS, Loisel I, Lavergne JM, Juhan-Vague I, Obert B, Cherel G, Meyer D, Girma JP. Ser968Thr mutation within the A3 domain of von Willebrand factor (vWF) in two related patients leads to a defective binding of vWF to collagen. Thromb Haemost. 2001; 86:848–854.
3. Schneppenheim R, Budde U, Obser T, Brassard J, Mainusch K, Ruggeri ZM, Schneppenheim S, Schwaab R, Oldenburg J. Expression and characterization of von Willebrand factor dimerization defects in different types of von Willebrand disease. Blood. 2001;97:2059–66.

Effects of Tissue Factor Pathway Inhibitor and Antithrombin on Thrombin Generation in Tissue Factor-activated Cord Plasma*

G. Cvirn, S. Gallistl, B. Leschnik, L. Giradi, and W. Muntean

Introduction

Despite of low concentrations of clotting factors, newborns have an excellent hemostasis. Neonates have good wound heeling and show no increased bleeding during surgery. Thus, it was the aim of our study to investigate whether low concentrations of the anticoagulatory proteins tissue factor pathway inhibitor (TFPI) and antithrombin (AT) compensate for low levels of procoagulatory proteins. In contrast to the routine determinations of clotting parameter, clotting was initiated by applying low concentrations of lipidated tissue factor (TF).

Material and Methods

Collection and preparation of plasma

Cord blood was obtained immediately following the delivery of 28 full term infants (38–42 weeks gestational age). Newborns with Apgar scores of 9 or less five minutes after delivery were excluded from the study. Blood was collected into 0.1 molar citrate using a two syringe technique, centrifuged at room temperature for 15 min at 2800 x g, pooled and stored at –70°C in propylene tubes until assayed. Pro- and anticoagulatory factors were in the normal range for neonates. In the same way plasma from 18 healthy adults was collected from the antecubital vein, prepared, and checked.

Preparation of plasma with different TFPI levels

The TFPI level of the pooled cord plasma was increased by addition of 100 µl buffer A containing 0-11 µl of human TFPI standard to 900 µl plasma. The TFPI level of the pooled adult plasma was decreased by addition of 100 µl buffer A containing 0-55 µl of rabbit anti-TFPI to 900 µl plasma.

---

* This study was supported by a grant from the »Gesellschaft zur Förderung der Gesundheit des Kindes (INVITA)«.

I. Scharrer/W. Schramm (Ed.)
32nd Hemophilia Symposion Hamburg 2001
© Springer-Verlag Berlin Heidelberg 2003

Determination of the TFPI plasma concentrations

TFPI antigen levels were determined by means of the Imubind™ Total TFPI ELISA Kit, TFPI activity was determined by means of the chromogenic assay Actichrome™ TFPI activity assay.

Activation of plasma

300 μl plasma with different TFPI and/or AT levels were incubated with 100 μl of buffer A containing lipidated recombinant human TF (0-100 pM final concentration) for 1 minute at 37°C. After subsequent incubation with 20 μl buffer A containing H-Gly-Pro-Arg-Pro-OH (Pefabloc™ FG, 1.0 mg/ml final concentration) to inhibit fibrin polymerization [1], plasma samples were activated by addition of 12 μl 0,5 M CaCl₂.

Determination of FX activation

Plasmas were prepared and activated as described above. At timed intervals 25 μl aliquots were withdrawn from the activated plasma and subsampled into 300 μl buffer C containing 0.97 mM S-2732. The reagents were prewarmed to 37°C. Amidolysis of S-2732 was stopped after 8 min by addition of 250 μl 50% acetic acid. The amount of FXa generated was quantitated by measuring the absorbency by double wave length (405–690 nm) in the Anthos microplate-reader 2001, from Anthos Labtec Instruments GmbH, Salzburg, Austria.

Determination of thrombin generation

We used a subsampling method derived from a recently described technique [2,3]. Plasmas were prepared and activated as described above. At timed intervals 10 μl aliquots were withdrawn from the activated plasma and subsampled into 490 μl buffer B containing 255 μM S-2238. The reagents were prewarmed to 37°C. Amidolysis of S-2238 was stopped after 6 min by addition of 250 μl 50% acetic acid. The amount of thrombin generated was quantitated by measuring the absorbency by double wave length (405–690 nm) in the Anthos microplate-reader 2001, from Anthos Labtec Instruments GmbH, Salzburg, Austria. The total amidolytic activity measured is caused by the simultaneous activity of free thrombin and the α 2-macroglobulin (α2-M)/thrombin complex (16). The amount of free thrombin was determined by two different methods:

a) At timed intervals, aliquots of the activated plasma were subsampled into buffer B containing heparin (20 U/ml) and AT (3.4 U/ml) to rapidly and completely inactivate free thrombin in the sample. The residual amidolytic activity was then determined as described above for the total amidolytic activity. The amidolytic activity of the a2-M/thrombin complex was substracted from the total amidolytic activity [4].

b) Free thrombin generation curves were calculated by mathematical treatment of total amidolytic activity curves using a method developed by Hemker et al. [2].

Statistical analysis

Results obtained in cord and adult plasma were compared by means of Mann Whitney U test. The effects of different concentrations of TFPI and AT on clotting time, FXa-generation, TP, and F1+2 activation were analyzed using paired t-test. The significance level of p-values was set at 5%. Calculations were performed using Winstat 3.1 (KalmiaCo.Inc., USA).

Results

Physiologic TF levels in cord and adult plasma

TF procoagulant activity levels were significantly higher in adult plasma (22.6 ± 1.8 pM) than in cord plasma (9.5 ±1.1 pM, p<0.001).

Effect of varying initiator concentrations on clotting time in cord and adult plasma

The effect of lipidated TF on clotting time was studied over a wide range of initiator concentration (Fig. 1). Cord plasma, physiologically containing approximately 9.5 pM TF, clotted within 10 minutes after addition of CaCl$_2$. When the TF content of the pooled cord plasma was decreased by applying anti-human TF, clotting did not occur within 20 min after addition of CaCl$_2$ at TF concentrations below 6 pM. When the TF concentration in cord plasma was successively elevated by addition of the purified protein, the clotting time was dose-dependently shortened. In adult

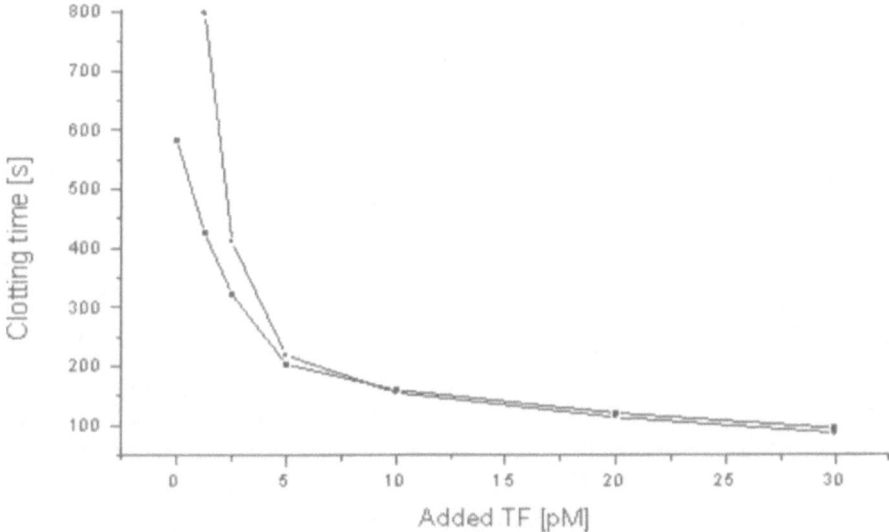

Fig. 1. Effect of addition of various amounts of lipidated TF on clotting time in cord (•) and adult plasma (■). Results shown are expressed as means (n=5).

plasma, physiologically containing approximately 22.6 pM TF, clotting did not occur within 20 min after addition of CaCl$_2$. Only when 2.5 pM TF were externally added, the plasma clotted within 10 minutes. Further successively elevation of the TF content by addition of the purified protein resulted in dose-dependently shortened clotting times. When less than 10 pM lipidated TF were added, cord plasma clotted significantly earlier than adult plasma (323 ± 6 vs. 411 ± 7 s, p<0.05, after addition of 2.5 pM lipidated TF). When more than 10 pM lipidated TF were added, adult plasma clotted slightly, but not significantly earlier than cord plasma (114 ± 4 vs. 121 ± 4 s, after addition of 20 pM lipidated TF).

Effect of varying initiator concentrations on thrombin generation in cord and adult plasma

Thrombin generation curves in both cord and adult plasma were monitored when high and low (e.g. 20 and 2.5 pM) amounts of lipidated TF were added. When activated by administration of 20 pM lipidated TF, significantly less thrombin was generated in cord plasma compared to adult plasma: the area under the thrombin generation curve, the thrombin potential (TP), was approximately 64% of adult value (298 ± 15 vs. 468 ± 19 nM.min, p<0.01, Fig. 2A). To the contrary, when activated by administration of 2.5 pM lipidated TF, thrombin generation started earlier in cord plasma and the TP was approximately 88% of adult value (291 ± 14 vs. 329 ± 16 nM.min, p<0.01, Fig. 2B).

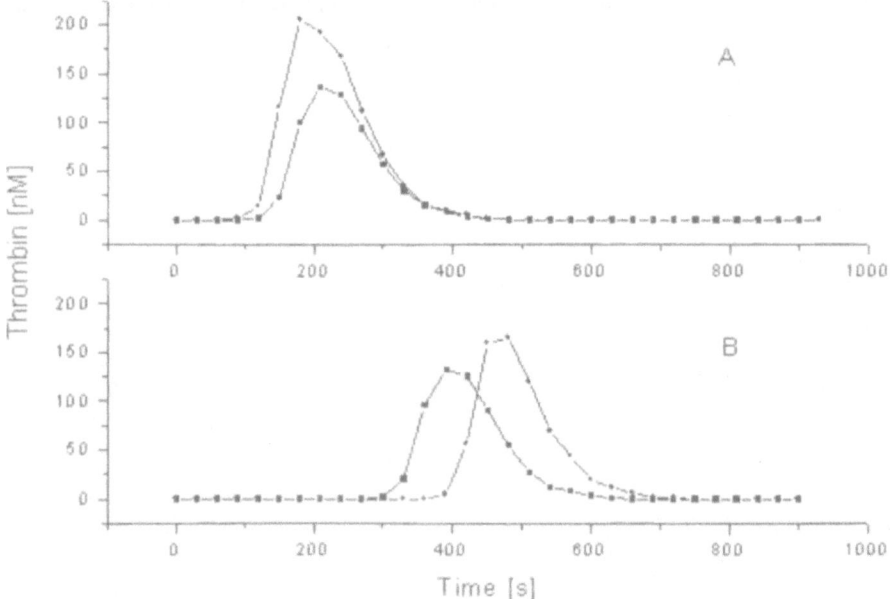

Fig. 2. Effect of administration of 20 pM (A) or 2.5 pM lipidated TF (B) on thrombin generation in cord (■) and adult plasma (•). Results shown are expressed as means (n=5).

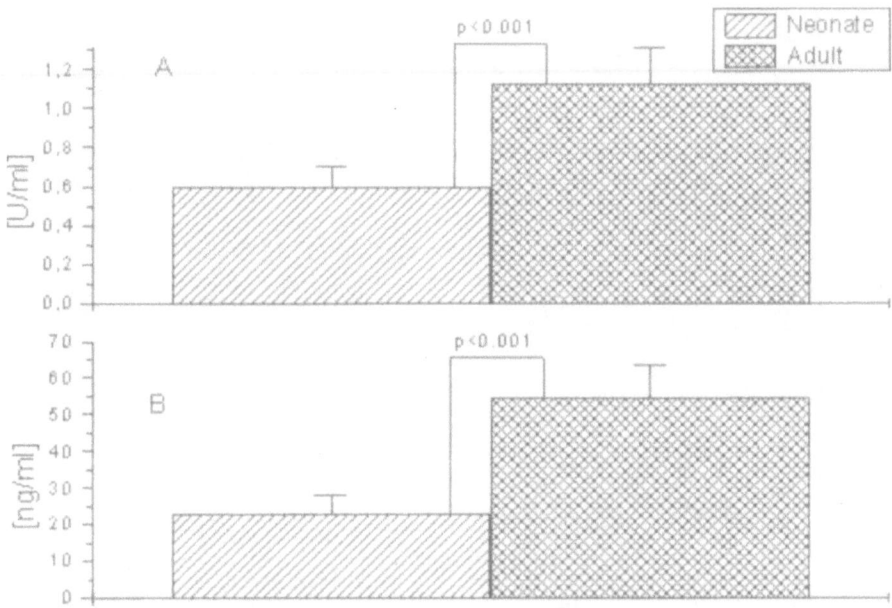

Fig. 3a, b. a) Physiologic TFPI activity levels. Each bar represents the mean ± 1 SD of 28 (cord plasma) and 18 (adult plasma) measurements. b) Physiologic TFPI antigen levels. Each bar represents the mean ± 1 SD of 28 (cord plasma) and 18 (adult plasma) measurements.

Physiologic TFPI levels in cord and adult plasma

TFPI activity levels determined by activity assay were significantly higher in adult plasma than in cord plasma (1.24 ± 0.16 vs. 0.81 ± 0.09 U/ml; p<0.01, Fig. 3A). Accordingly, TFPI antigen levels determined by ELISA were also significantly higher in adult plasma (54.53 ± 10.63 ng/ml) than in cord plasma (23.24 ± 3.96 ng/ml; p<0.01, Fig. 3B).

Effect of the simultaneous raise of TFPI and AT in cord plasma to the respective adult values on thrombin generation by varying initiator concentrations in cord plasma

When activated by addition of 100 pM lipidated TF, the TP was decreased by approximately 29% compared to cord plasma containing TFPI and AT at neonatal levels (246 ± 17 vs. 347 ± 22 nM.min, p<0.01, Fig. 4A). This effect was more pronounced when lower amounts of lipidated TF were applied: when activated by administration of 30 pM lipidated TF, the TP was decreased by approximately 32% (207 ± 11 vs. 300 ± 18 nM.min, p<0.01, Fig. 4B), and when activated by addition of 2.5 pM lipidated TF, the TP was decreased by approximately 38% (180 ± 11 vs. 291 ± 14 nM.min, p<0.01, Fig. 4C) compared to cord plasma containing TFPI and AT at neonatal levels. Correspondingly, lag phases until the onset of thrombin generation were dose-dependently prolonged when TF concentrations were successively decreased.

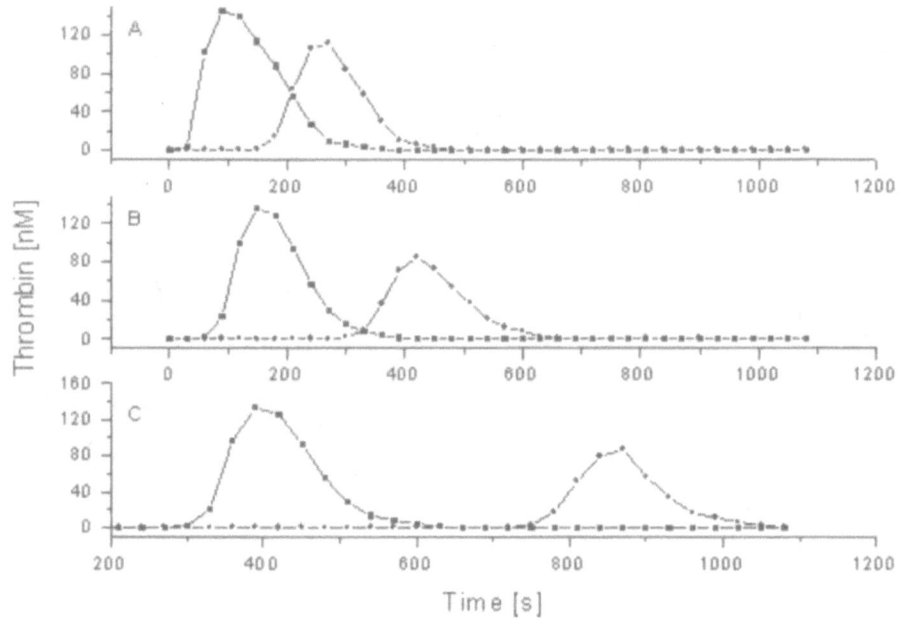

Fig. 4. Thrombin generation in cord plasma containing physiological amounts of TFPI and AT (■), and in cord plasma containing TFPI and AT at adult level (●), respectively, in the presence of 100 (A), 30 (B), and 2.5 (C) pM lipidated TF as initiator of coagulation. Results shown are expressed as means (n=5).

Effect of raising TFPI and/or AT to adult value on FXa- and thrombin generation in cord plasma activated by 2.5 pM lipidated TF

Raising TFPI, AT or both TFPI and AT to adult levels resulted in significantly suppressed FXa-peak values compared to cord plasma containing physiological amounts of inhibitors (6.94 ± 0.33, 5.99 ± 0.44, and 5.06 ± 0.24 vs. 9.02 ± 0.58 nM, $p<0.01$, Fig. 5A). Correspondingly, the raise of TFPI, AT and of both inhibitors resulted in significant suppression of the TP (227 ± 9, 197 ± 10, and 180 ± 11 vs. 291 ± 14 nM.min, $p<0.01$, Fig. 5B).

Discussion

Under a mild stimulus, cord plasma clots earlier than adult plasma, and, correspondingly, FXa- and FIIa-generation start earlier. Since we have shown in the present study that the levels of TFPI and AT have a marked influence on FXa- and FIIa-generation, we conclude that the physiologic low levels of this two inhibitors allow sufficient thrombin generation in cord plasma and thus prevent newborns from bleeding tendency.

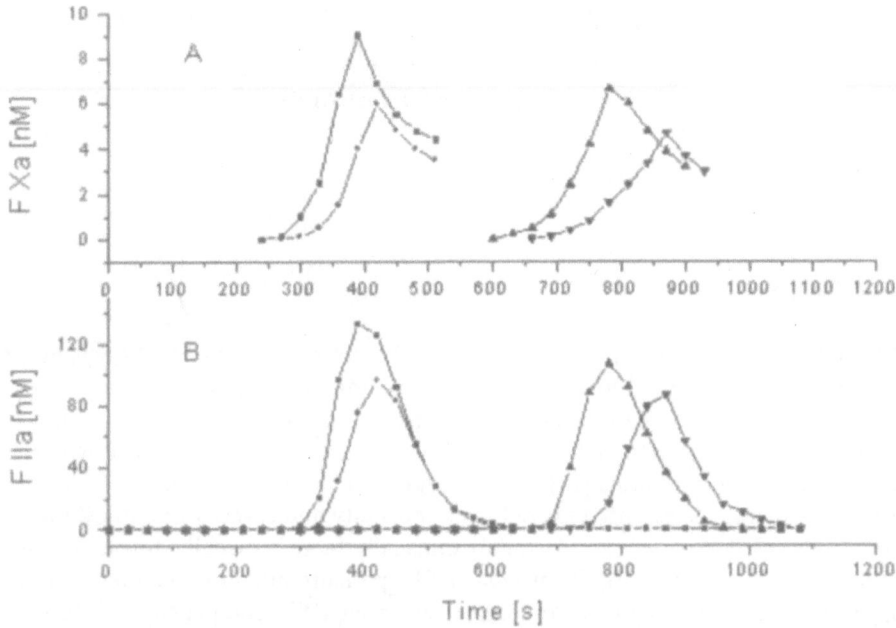

Fig. 5. FXa (A) and FIIa-(B)-generation in cord plasma with physiological amounts of TFPI and AT (■), TFPI at adult level (▲), AT at adult level (●), and both inhibitors at adult level (▼), respectively. 2.5 pM lipidated TF were applied to initiate coagulation. Results shown are expressed as means (n=5).

References

1. Rijkers D-T-S, Wielders S-J-H, Beguin S, Hemker H-C. Prevention of the influence of fibrin and alpha 2-macroglobulin in the continuous measurement of the thrombin potential: implications for an endpoint determination of the optical density. Thromb Res. 1998;89:161–169.
2. Hemker H-C, Wielders S, Kessels H, Beguin S. Continuous registration of thrombin generation in plasma, its use for the determination of the thrombin potential. Thromb Haemost. 1993;70:617–624.
3. Wielders S, Mukherjee M, Michiels J, et al. The routine determination of the endogenous thrombin potential, first results in different forms of hyper- and hypocoagulability. Thromb Haemost. 1997;77:629–636.
4. Andrew M, Schmidt B, Mitchell L, Paes B, Ofoso F. Thrombin generation in newborn plasma is critically dependent on the concentration of prothrombin. Thromb Haemost. 1990;63:27–30.
5. Hemker H-C, Willems G-M, Beguin S. A computer assisted method to obtain the prothrombin activation velocity in whole plasma independent of thrombin decay processes. Thromb Haemost. 1986;56:9–17.

Early and rapid Diagnosis of acute TTP by Measuring Activity of von-Willebrand Factor cleaving Metalloprotease (ADAMTS13): A Case Report

M. Böhm, C. Betz, I. Stier-Brück, and I. Scharrer

Introduction

Thrombotic thrombocytopenic purpura (TTP) was first described by Moschcowitz [15] and is characterized by thrombocytopenia, microangiopathic hemolytic anemia, neurological signs and occasionally renal impairment and fever. In practice, diagnosis of TTP is often delayed, since less than 40% of patients present with the classic pentad of symptoms [13]. Early recognition and rapid initiation of plasma-exchange therapy is essential for reducing mortality and severity of clinical manifestations [4]. Moake et al. [14] found unusually large molecular forms of von-Willebrand Factor (vWF) in the plasma of TTP-patients and proposed them to have a pathogenic role in the formation of microvascular vWF- and platelet-rich thrombi, which are found in the microcirculation of patients with acute TTP [14, 15]. vWF is released from endothelial cells as large multimers, which are cleaved by a combination of reductase and metalloprotease in normal plasma [6, 16]. More recently, several investigators reported deficiency of a specific metalloprotease, which cleaves vWF at the Tyr842-Met843 peptide bond in patients with congenital or acquired TTP [1, 2, 7–10, 17–19]. Based on partial amino acid sequence and genome-wide linkage analysis of pedigrees with congenital TTP, this vWF cleaving protease (vWFcp) was recently identified as a new member of the ADAMTS (a disintegrin and metalloproteinase with thrombospondin type I motif) family and designated ADAMTS13 [5, 9, 11]. We present a case, where rapid estimation of vWF cleaving protease activity of ADAMTS13 facilitated early diagnosis of a TTP-relapse in a male patient.

Methods

For determination of vWFcp activity we diluted plasma samples with low ionic TRIS buffer including 12,5 mM $BaCl_2$ and 1 mM PefaBloc SC (Roche, Germany) followed by 5 minutes incubation at 37°C for activation of the protease. A protease-free [1] vWF concentrate (gift from LFB, France) was added and digested in the presence of urea over night. The residual ristocetin cofactor activity (RCo) was assessed with a commercial test from Dade Behring, Germany. By plotting samples of serial dilutions of a normal human plasma pool (80 healthy adult subjects, 40F/40M) against RCo the Calibration Curve was obtained and used to assess the vWFcp

I. Scharrer/W. Schramm (Ed.)
32nd Hemophilia Symposion Hamburg 2001
© Springer-Verlag Berlin Heidelberg 2003

activity of the samples (expressed in % of normal). Determination of vWF-Ag was done by an home made Elisa with DAKO rabbit anti-human vWF for coating a microtiter plate and DAKO peroxidase-conjugated rabbit anti-human vWF for detection. Platelet count, hemoglobin (Hb), lactate dehydrogenase (LDH) and CRP were assayed according to conventional laboratory techniques.

Case report

The previously healthy male patient suffered onset of TTP in January 2000 at the age of 35 years. He was admitted to the hospital with thrombocytopenia (platelet count: 36/nl) and anemia (Hb: 8g/dl). With evidence of schistocytes TTP was diagnosed and plasmaexchange with FFP was initiated 10 days after initial symptoms. The patient suffered two severe seizures and clinical remission was only achieved after two months stationary care with 48 sessions of plasmaexchange. Retrospective estimation of vWcp activity showed severe vWFcp deficiency of <6.25% prior to plasmaexchange therapy (Fig. 1). The patient stayed for 16 months in clinical remission with mild reduction of vWcp activity of 46 and 60% (Fig. 1).

He visited our ambulance in August 2001 after an gastrointestinal infection and with massive swelling in the right knee (suspected Reiter-Syndrome). The patient was without fever or clinical symptoms indicating an acute episode of TTP. Laboratory data showed hemoglobin, lactate dehydrogenase and vWF-Ag within the normal range, no schistocytes in the peripheral blood smear, moderate increase of CRP and mild thrombocytopenia (Table 1). Notably, vWFcp activity was not detectable (<6.25%). Consequently, we examined the patient two days later and found significant increase of lactate dehydrogenase to 400 U/ml, distinct decrease of platelet count to 35/nl and persistent vWFcp deficiency of <6.25%. vWF-Ag was within the normal range and schistocytes could not be detected (Table 1). We thus diagnosed a relapse of TTP without schistocytes and clinical symptoms. The patient was admitted to stationary care and plasmaexchange with FFP was instituted on

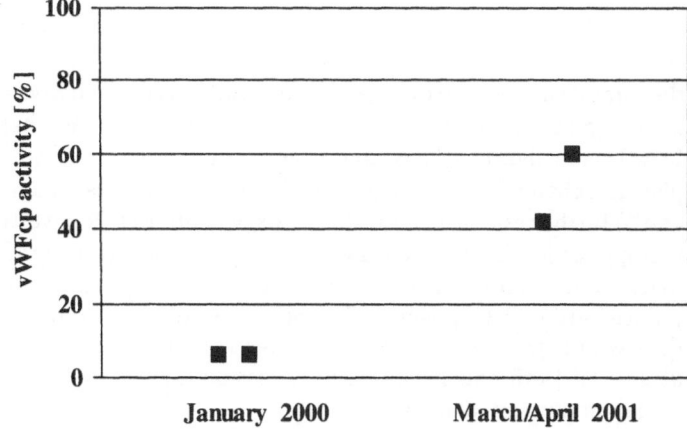

Fig. 1. vWF cleaving protease activity for the patient during index episode (January 2000) and during remission (March/April 2001)

Table 1. Laboratory data in August 2001 on presentation (day 1) and two days later.

	Day 1	Day 3	Normal range
Hb [g/dl]	14.4	14.1	14–18
LDH [U/ml]	232	400	<240
Platelet count [/nl]	80	35	150–400
Schistocytes	negative	negative	
CRP [mg/dl]	2.0	1.5	<0.8
vWF-Ag [%]	114	128	82–138
vWFcp activity	<6.25	<6.25	58–134

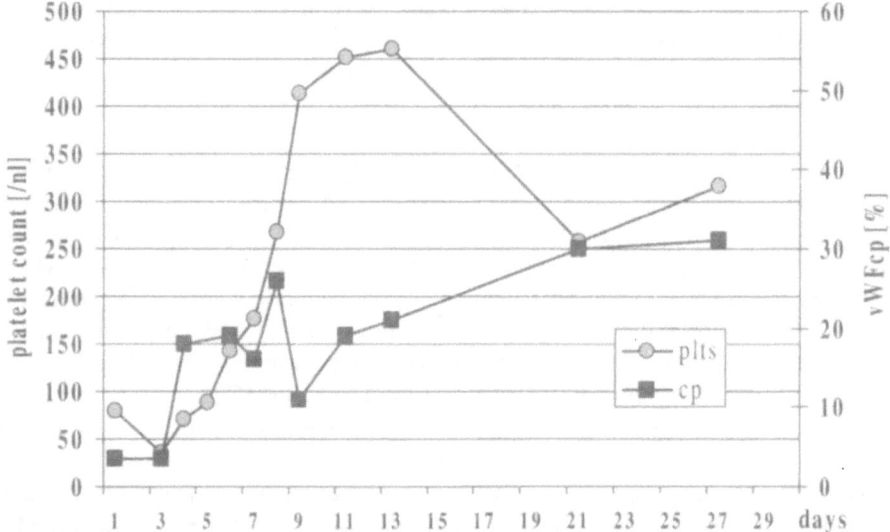

Fig. 2. Course of vWF cleaving protease activity and platelet count during relapse of TTP in August 2001. The patient received 8 sessions of plasmaexchange on day 3, 4, 5, 6, 7, 8, 9 and 11.

the same day. The course of platelet count and vWFcp activity are depicted in Figure 2. vWFcp activity increased after first session of plasmaexchange from <6.25% to 23%. Lactate dehydrogenase and platelet count normalized after 1 and 4 sessions of plasmaexchange, respectively. Detection of schistocytes on day 6 (no data for day 4 and 5) further established the diagnosis of acute TTP. To investigate the response to therapy, the levels of vWFcp and vWF: Ag before and directly after a session of plasmaexchange were determined (Fig. 3). Each treatment raised vWFcp by 15–44% and reduced vWF: Ag by 22–60%. The patient was discharged from the hospital after 10 days with 8 sessions of plasmaexchange without suffering any clinical features of acute TTP. Until now he stayed in remission for 4 months with mild deficiency of vWFcp activity of 30 to 64%.

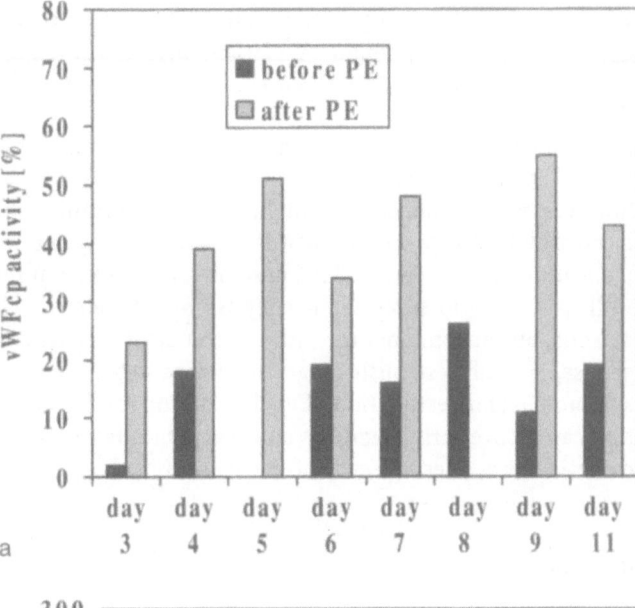

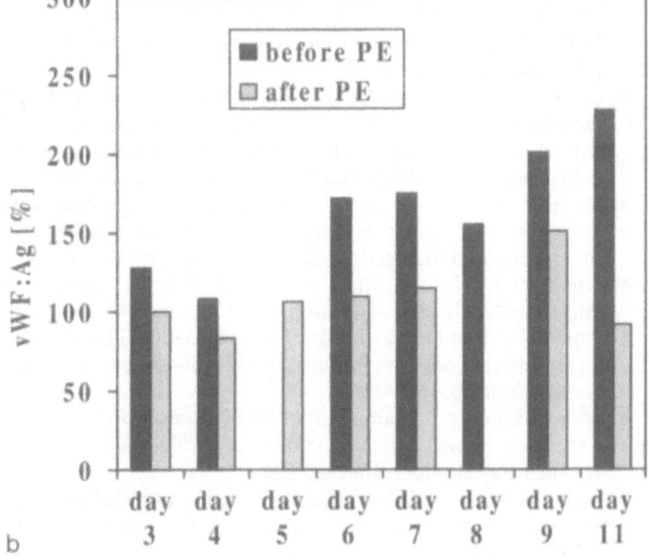

Fig. 3a, b. Effect of plasmaexchange therapy on vWFcp activity (a) and vWF-Ag (b). Blood samples were collected directly before and after each plasma-exchange session, except for two sessions, where samples were not drawn before (day 5), respectively after plasma-exchange (day 8).

Discussion

We demonstrate for the first time, that decrease of vWFcp can indicate a relapse before the occurrence of severe thrombocytopenia, elevated lactate dehydrogenase level, fragmentation of erythrocytes and clinical symptoms. The decrease of protease activity might be due to the preceded infection of the patient, as vWFcp activity has been shown to be reduced during acute inflammation [12]. Since inflammation is a well-known trigger for TTP, it can be speculated, that the associated decrease of vWFcp activity might be causally involved in triggering the acute episode. Retrospective analysis of vWFcp activity demonstrated for another TTP-patient a decrease of vWFcp activity from 20% to <6.25%, which was followed by thrombocytopenia, elevated lactate dehydrogenase level and schistocytes two weeks later. Severe vWFcp deficiency does not necessarily lead to an acute episode of TTP [1], however vWFcp deficiency might be a significant risk factor for relapse [3]. Decrease of vWFcp activity, as it is illustrated here, does not indispensably lead to clinical manifestation of TTP. Therefore, decrease from normal or mildly reduced vWFcp activity to severe deficiency is not sufficient for the diagnosis of an acute episode, but in combination with the course of platelet count and lactate dehydrogenase, it might establish diagnosis before detection of schistocytes and clinical symptoms. Thus, estimation of vWFcp during routine check-ups or in case of infection can secure early diagnosis hence rapid initiation of plasma exchange, which is essential for accelerated cure of the acute episode.

References

1. Allford SL, Harrison P, Lawrie AS, Liesner R, Mackie IJ, Machin SJ (2000) Von-Willebrand factor-cleaving protease activity in congenital thrombotic thrombocytopenic purpura. Br J Haematol 111: 1215–1222
2. Barefoot J, Costa E, Guar M, Barreirinho MS, Isvarlal P, Robles R, Gerritsen HE, Lämmle B, Furlan M (2001) Ten years of prophylactic treatment with fresh-frozen plasma in a child with chronic relapsing thrombotic thrombocytopenic purpura as a result of a congenital deficiency of von-Willebrand factor-cleaving protease. Br J Haematol 113: 649–651
3. Böhm M, Krause M, Vigh T, Scharrer I (2001) Von-Willebrand Factor-cleaving protease activity in TTP using a new method based on the positive correlation between vWF multimeric size and Ristocetin Cofactor activity. Blood: 98 (11): Abstract 130
4. Chemnitz J, Schulz A, Diehl V, Söhngen D (2001) Thrombotisch-thrombozytopenische Purpura (Moschcowitz-Syndrom). Med Klin 96: 343–350
5. Fujikawa K, Suzuki H, McMullen B, Chung D (2001) Purification of human von-Willebrand factor-cleaving protease and its identification as a new member of the metalloproteinase family. Blood 98: 1662–1666
6. Furlan M, Robles R, Lämmle B (1996) Partial purification and characterization of a protease from human plasma cleaving von-Willebrand factor to fragments produced by in vivo proteolysis. Blood 10, 4223–4234
7. Furlan M, Robles R, Solenthaler M, Lämmle B (1998) Aquired deficiency of von-Willebrand factor-cleaving protease in a patient with thrombotic thrombocytopenic purpura. Blood 91: 2836–2846
8. Furlan M, Robles R, Galbusera M, Remuzzi G, Kyrle PA, Brenner B, Krause M, Scharrer I, Aumann V, Mittler U, Solenthaler M, Lämmle B (1998) Von-Willebrand factor-cleaving protease in thrombotic thrombocytopenic purpura and the hemolytic-uremic syndrome. N Engl J Med 339: 1578–1584
9. Gerritsen HE, Robles R, Lämmle B, Furlan M (2001) Partial amino acid sequence of purified von-Willebrand factor-cleaving protease. Blood 98: 1654–1661
10. Häberle J, Kehrel B, Ritter J, Jürgens H, Lämmle B, Furlan M (1999) New strategies in diagnosis and treatment of thrombotic thrombocytopenic purpura: case report and review. Eur J Pediatr 158: 883–887

Early and rapid Diagnosis of acute TTP

11. Levy GG, Nichols WC, Lian EC, Foroud T, McClintick JN, McGee BM, Yang AY, Siemieniak DR, Stark KR, Gruppo R, Sarode R, Shurin SB, Chandrasekaran V, Stabler SP, Sabio H, Bouhassira EE, Upshaw JD, Ginsburg D, Tsai HM (2001) Mutations in a member of the ADAMTS gene family cause thrombotic thrombocytopenic purpura. Nature 413: 488–494
12. Mannucci PM, Canciani MT, Forza I, Lussana F, Lattuada A, Rossi E (2001) Changes in health and disease of the metalloprotease that cleaves von-Willebrand factor. Blood, 98: 2730–2735
13. McCrae KR, Bussel JB, Mannucci PM, Remuzzi G, Cines DB (2001) Hematology (Education Program Book): 282–305
14. Moake JL, Rudy CK, Troll JH, Weinstein MJ, Colannino NM, Azocar J, Seder RH, Hong SL, Deykin D (1982) Unusually large plasma factor VIII: von-Willebrand factor multimers in chronic relapsing thrombotic thrombocytopenic purpura. N Engl J Med 307: 1432–1435
15. Moschcowitz E (1924) Hyaline thrombosis of the terminal arterioles and capillaries: a hitherto undescribed disease. Proc NY Pathol Soc 24: 21–24
16. Tsai HM (1996) Physiologic Cleavage of von-Willebrand Factor by a Plasma Protease is dependent on its conformation and requires Calcium ion. Blood 10: 4235–4244
17. Tsai HM (2000) High titers of inhibitors of von-Willebrand factor-cleaving metalloproteinase in a fatal case of acute thrombotic thrombocytopenic purpura. Am J Hematol 65:251–255
18. Tsai HM, Lian EC (1998) Antibodies to von-Willebrand factor-cleaving protease in acute thrombotic thrombocytopenic purpura. New Engl J Med 339: 1585–1594
19. Tsai HM, Rice L, Sarode R, Chow TW, Moake JL (2000) Antibody inhibitors to von-Willebrand factor metalloproteinase and increased binding of von-Willebrand Factor to platelets in Ticlopidine-associated thrombotic thrombocytopenic purpura. Ann Intern Med 132: 794–799

Prions and the Safety of Plasma Proteins: Preventive Measures and Research Activities

T.R. KREIL

Introduction

With the BSE epidemic in the United Kingdom, and more recently – although orders of magnitude less pronounced – elsewhere [for recent information see http://www.oie.int], and then the corresponding new infectious disease entity of man, variant Creutzfeldt-Jakob disease (vCJD), questions about the safety of therapeutically important plasma proteins with respect to a potential prion transmission were raised. Specifically, for plasma-derived proteins a potential exposure to variant CJD was considered a concern, and for recombinant proteins a potential BSE exposure through the use of bovine excipients during their manufacture.

Ample clinical evidence suggests, however, that neither CJD nor vCJD can be transmitted through blood, blood products or plasma derivatives [1]. Also, for none of the natural transmissible spongiform encephalopathy (TSE) diseases, i.e. BSE, CJD, vCJD etc., has the presence of infectivity in plasma been unambiguously demonstrated [2]. More recently, using two of the most sensitive methods currently available, vCJD infectivity and the corresponding abnormal prion protein, PrP^{vCJD}, could be demonstrated in human brain, tonsil and spleen samples, but not in buffy coat or plasma [3, 4]. Only in a few experimental studies in laboratory rodents has prion infectivity been demonstrated in plasma, however at only 20 infectious units (iu) per ml during clinical stages of diseases, and ten times less than that during the pre-clinical stage [5], i.e. the one of potential relevance for a plasma/ blood donor.

A number of preventive measures have nevertheless been implemented to further enhance the safety margins of plasma proteins.

Recombinant proteins

The European Commission by means of their Directive 1999/82/EC of September 8, 1999, has required the certification of compliance of all bovine excipients with the relevant EMEA guidance [6] through the European Directorate for the Quality of Medicines (EDQM). The criteria evaluated during the process are the
- animal's country of origin: Countries are classified according to geographic BSE risk (GBR) in the order of increasing risk from level 1 to level 4.
- bovine tissue used: Different bovine tissues are categorized according to their infectivity content, with levels of risk increasing from level IV to level I.

I. Scharrer/W. Schramm (Ed.)
32nd Hemophilia Symposion Hamburg 2001
© Springer-Verlag Berlin Heidelberg 2003

– validated prion removal capacity of the manufacturing process: Here, the starting materials for down-scaled versions of the respective manufacturing process steps are spiked with model prion infectivity and it's reduction after completion of the process determined.

Plasma-derivatives

Despite the merely theoretical risk of a prion transmission through plasma derivatives, a number of donor exclusion criteria have been put in place to further enhance the safety margins of plasma as the starting material for these products. Most drastically, plasma from the UK is not any more used for manufacture of derivatives, by which measure alone the exposure to >96% of all vCJD cases which have occurred globally and to >99.9% of all BSE cases has been excluded. In addition,
– persons with Creutzfeldt-Jakob disease and persons with this disease in their families,
– persons with an indication of variant Creutzfeldt-Jakob disease and persons with this disease in their families,
– recipients of dura mater grafts or cornea transplants,
– persons who have been treated with human pituitary growth hormone
– persons who have resided in the UK 6 months or more cumulatively from 1980 through 1996, and
– persons who have undergone brain surgery do not qualify as plasma donors.

In addition, and probably more significantly, an increasing number of experimental studies using model prions spiked into plasma or plasma product intermediates have demonstrated that the manufacturing processes of plasma derivatives have an intrinsic capacity to remove prion infectivity from final products into waste fractions [7–10].

Despite all these re-assuring aspects, any product which would be realized to contain a vCJD contribution would – in agreement with regulatory requirements in both Europe [11] and the US [12] – be destroyed. In a situation where the wealth of clinical experience that we enjoy in relation to CJD is not yet available for the newer disease entity vCJD, this precautionary principle is followed to – if anything – err on the right side.

Research activities

To enhance our understanding of vCJD and the theoretical risk of a prion transmission through plasma-derivatives, Baxter has several years ago initiated a CJD/vCJD transmission study in a non-human primate model, the squirrel monkey. In contrast to other studies, the closer physiological relationship between humans and primates will provide a more relevant insight into the pathogenesis of these diseases as compared to the currently available studies in rodent models. Also, the lower species barrier – as compared to the one between humans and rodents – is anticipated to provide a more sensitive detection of infectivity in vCJD/CJD samples. Within the study, 80 animals are put to use to primarily answer two fundamental questions:

1. Is blood during the extended incubation periods of vCJD / CJD in these primates infectious, and if so – are the levels any different between experimental vCJD/CJD?
2. What are the relative concentrations of infectivity in the brain and – if at all present – buffy coat and plasma of vCJD/CJD patients ?

These two main goals are embedded into a setting including numerous controls and calibrators for the experimental models. While the positive control animals for the vCJD and the CJD infected arms of the study have started to develop the respective diseases, results for the two main targets may, however, due to the direct correlation between infectivity titers and incubation times, not be available for some time.

Summary

There is currently no clinical or firm laboratory evidence to suggest any risk for a prion transmission through blood or blood products, and thus the risk is considered theoretical. Still, a number of precautionary measures have been established to increase the safety margins of these products. In parallel, industry-driven studies are under way to solidify on understanding of prion diseases, and especially the least well known vCJD, particularly in relation to blood product safety.

References

1. WHO Weekly Epidemiological Record [December 14, 2001] 50: 398
2. Brown P. et al., J. Lab. Clin. Med. [2001] 137: 5
3. Bruce M. et al., Lancet [2001] 358: 208
4. Wadsworth J. et al., Lancet [2001] 358: 171
5. Brown P. et al., Transfusion [1999] 39: 1169
6. EMEA/410/01: Note for Guidance on Minimizing the Risk of Transmitting Animal Spongiform Encephalopathy Agents via Medicinal Products
7. Foster et al., Vox. Sang. [2000] 78: 86
8. Lee et al., J Virol Meth [2000] 84: 77
9. Lee et al., Transfusion [2001] 41: 449
10. Rohwer / Baxter & ARC, internal reports
11. CPMP/201/98: CPMP Position Statement on New Variant CJD and Plasma-derived Medicinal Products
12. FDA – 8. 9. 1998: Guidance for Industry: Revised Precautionary Measures to Reduce the Possible Risk of Transmission of Creutzfeldt-Jakob Disease (CJD) and New Variant Creutzfeldt-Jakob Disease (nvCJD) by Blood and Blood Products

VI. Poster

VIa. Clinic and Casuistic

Transmission of Parvovirus B19 by Heat-treated Coagulation Factor Concentrates

J. Blümel, I. Schmidt, W. Effenberger, H. Seitz, H. Willkommen, H.-H. Brackmann, J. Löwer, and A.M. Eis-Hübinger

Introduction

Transmission of enveloped viruses by blood products prepared from pooled plasma has fortunately become an extremely rare event due to the efficacy of the applied virus inactivation procedures. The inactivation procedures are, however, much less effective against non-enveloped viruses such as human parvovirus B19 (B19) [for review, 1; 2]. Consequently, B19 infections in association with administration of plasma-derived products are still reported until now [3, 4].

In September 1999, acute B19 infection was diagnosed by routine blood evaluation in two hemophilic children being treated at the university hospital of Bonn. Because B19 DNA was detected in all blood products recently administered to the children, viral transmission by the products could not be excluded. To clarify the causal relationship between product administration and B19 infection, DNA sequencing of the B19 genomes isolated from the patients and the coagulation products was performed. The results show that the administered products have to be considered as source of the B19 infection in both children.

Patients, Materials and Methods

Patient A was a 16-month-old African boy, patient B a 5-year-old Caucasian boy. Both children suffered from severe hemophilia A and were undergoing treatment for elimination of anti-factor VIII antibodies. The blood products used for therapy and their administered amounts are given in Table 1 and Table 2.

B19 IgG and IgM antibodies were tested by an enzyme immunoassay using viral protein 2 as antigen (Biotrin, Dublin).

The sera of the hemophiliacs and the administered blood products were tested for B19 DNA by polymerase chain reaction (PCR) as described previously [5]. For quantitative analysis of B19 DNA in the coagulation products, and in the patients' sera primers were TP1 (B19 nucleotide (nt) 2030 to 2048; sequence according [6]) and TP2 (nt 2171 to 2151). The probe (nt 2050 to 2071) was 5' fluorescent-labelled with FAM (6-carboxyfluorescein) and 3' labelled with TAMRA (6-carboxytetramethylrhodamine). PCR was performed (2 min at 50°C, 10 min at 95°C, (15 sec at 95°C, 30 sec at 60°C) 45 cycles) using 0.5 U uracil-N-glycosylase and 1 U of Ampli TaqGold™ polymerase (PE Applied Biosystems, Weiterstadt) on an ABI PRISM 7700

I. Scharrer/W. Schramm (Ed.)
32nd Hemophilia Symposion Hamburg 2001
© Springer-Verlag Berlin Heidelberg 2003

Table 1, 2. Coagulation factor therapy, B19 serological and PCR results from patient A (Table 1) and patient B (Table 2). The amount of B19 DNA administered until the day of detection of seroconversion is given. n. d. = not determined

Table 1. Patient A (16 months, male)

			Therapy			Laboratory values		
			Product A	Product B, lot-3		IgG	IgM	PCR
September	10, 1999	9 a.m.	20 ml	9.2 ml	September 10, 1999	–	–	–
	10, 1999	8 p.m.	40 ml	4.6 ml	(10 a.m.)			
	11, 1999	9 a.m.	20 ml	13.8 ml				
	11, 1999	8 p.m.	20 ml	9.2 ml				
	12, 1999	9 a.m.	20 ml	9.2 ml				
	12, 1999	8 p.m.	20 ml	9.2 ml				
	13, 1999	9 a.m.	20 ml	9.2 ml				
	13, 1999	8 p.m.	20 ml	9.2 ml				
	14, 1999	to	------					
September	22, 1999			156.4 ml	September 22, 1999	+	+	+ (ca. 10^3 geq/ml)
				--------	September 29, 1999	+	+	+
	Sum		180 ml	230 ml	January 25, 2000	+	–	–

Product A: 8.6 x 10^6 geq/ml   180 ml contain 1.6 x 10^9 geq
Product B, lot-3: 4.3 x 10^4 geq/ml   230 ml contain 9.9 x 10^6 geq

Table 2. Patient B (5 years, male)

		Therapy			Laboratory values		
					IgG	IgM	PCR
1998–1999:		Product B	May	14, 1996	–	–	n.d.
		(4 lots, B19 PCR: negative)	August	28, 1996	–	–	n.d.
			February	9, 1999	–	–	–
June 22, 1999 – July 17, 1999:		Product B, lot-0					
		(B19 PCR: negative)					
July 17, 1999 – September 14, 1999:		Product B, lot-1	September 7, 1999		+	+	+ (6 x 10^8 geq/ml)
		(B19 PCR: positive; 4.0 x 10^3 geq/ml)					
Since September 14, 1999:		Product B, lot-3	December 15, 1999		+	–	–
		(B19 PCR: positive; 4.3 x 10^4 geq/ml)					

Product B, lot-1: 966 ml applicated = 3.9 x 10^6 geq

(Applied Biosystems, Weiterstadt). For external standard, serial dilutions of a linearized plasmid was used [7].

For DNA sequence analysis, 2701 nucleotides of the B19 genome were amplified by nested PCR. Primers for the amplification regions NS1-C, DeltaV, VP1/VP2, and VPC [8], and a DNA fragment from nt 2537 to 4019 [9], and PCR conditions were as described. For DNA sequencing, PCR products were purified using the QIAquick

Gel Extraction Kit (Qiagen, Hilden). Approx. 50 ng PCR product were added to the cycle sequencing reaction using the AmpliTaq FS BigDye Terminator Kit (Applied Biosystems). Sequencing primers (10 pmol each) and annealing temperature were the same as those used for generation of the PCR products. Twenty-five cycles each consisting of 10 sec denaturation at 96 °C, 5 sec annealing, and 2 min elongation were performed. Electrophoresis was done using an ABI sequencing apparatus (Applied Biosystems).

For comparison, the genomes of two B19 strains isolated in Bonn from one child with erythema infectiosum (Bn9) and one child with flu-like illness (Bn10) one month before and one month after seroconversion of the hemophiliacs, and the genomes of two epidemiologically unrelated B19 isolates (amniotic fluid from Regensburg, Germany (No. 11); B19 DNA-containing blood donation (No. 12)) were also sequenced.

Results

In September 1999, seroconversion to B19 IgG and IgM antibodies and viremia were detected by routinely performed screening procedures in two children undergoing immune tolerance therapy because of development of anti-factor VIII antibodies. Typical symptoms of B19 infection were not recognized and retrospective revision of the erythrocytes and thrombocytes counts was not indicative. Prior to seroconversion, both patients had been treated with the same factor VIII product (product B). However, different lots were used (patient A lot –3; patient B lot –1). Additionally, patient A received one lot of an activated prothrombin complex concentrate for four days (product A). B19 DNA was found in all three coagulation factor preparations by PCR. The amounts of the coagulation factor products administered to patient A is shown in Table 1, those administered to patient B in Table 2.

To elucidate whether B19 infection was transmitted through blood product treatment, sequence analysis of the B19 genomes isolated from the patients' sera and the coagulation products was performed. For comparison with B19 strains circulating at that time in the general population, two B19 genomes (Bn9, Bn10) isolated in Bonn from two non-hemophilic children one month before and one month after seroconversion of the hemophiliacs, resp. were also sequenced. In addition, two epidemiologically unrelated B19 strains were included in the sequence analysis (No. 11, No. 12). Sequence data were compared with the nucleotide sequence of the B19-Au isolate [6] and the B19-Wi isolate [10].

DNA analysis of about half of the B19 genome (2701 nucleotides) revealed that the sequence found in patient A and that found in the product A were identical. Furthermore, there was no difference between the isolate from patient B and that from product B, lot –1 (Fig. 1). In contrast, the sequence detected in product B, lot –3, which was also given to patient A within the respective time period, clearly differed from that detected in the blood of patient A. The sequence data from product B, lot –3, revealed ambiguities in 11 nucleotide positions. Most probable, these ambiguities were caused by the presence of multiple B19 strains within the plasma pool. As expected, analysis of the plasma subpools used for production of product

Nt	Strain Au	Strain Wi	Patient A	Product A	Patient B	Product B, lot -1	Product B, lot -3	Bn9	Bn10	No. 11	No. 12	Aa exchange
1978	G	G	G	G	G	G	G	A	A	A	G	V - F
2086	G	G	G	G	A	A	G	A	G	G	G	G - F
2096	T	T	C	C	C	C	C	C	T	T	C	F —S
2107	C	T	C	C	C	C	C	C	C	C	C	P —S
2145	A	A	A	A	G	G	A	A	G	G	G	--
2244	A	A	A	A	A	A	G	A	G	G	G	--
2268	G	C	C	C	C	C	C	C	C	C	C	--
2352	A	G	A	A	A	A	A	A	G	G	G	--
2453	A	G	A	A	A	A	A	A	A	A	A	K - E
2527	A	G	A	A	A	A	A	A	A	A	A	--
2594	A	T	A	A	A	A	A	A	A	A	A	N —Y
2624	G	A	G	G	G	G	G	G	G	G	G	D —N
2736	G	G	G	G	G	G	G/A	G	A	A	A	S —N
2762	A	A	G	G	A	A	A	G	A	A	A	--
3172	G	T	G	G	G	G	G	G	G	G	G	--
3182	T	C	T	T	T	T	T	T	T	T	T	S —P
3187	C	C	C	C	C	C	T	C	T	T	T	--
3212	A	A	A	A	A	A	A	A	G	A	A	Y —A
3223	T	C	T	T	T	T	T	T	T	T	T	--
3307	G	A	G	G	G	G	G	G	G	G	G	--
3355	C	T	C	C	C	C	C	C	C	C	C	--
3415	A	A	A	A	A	A	G	A	A	A	A	--
3454	T	T	T	T	T	T	C	T	C	C	C	--
3538	G	G	G	G	G	G	G/A	G	A	A	A	--
3541	A	A	G	G	G	G	A	G	A	A	A	--
3544	G	G	G	G	G	G	G/A	G	A	A	A	--
3562	A	A	A	A	A	A	A/C	A	C	C	C	--
3625	G	G	A	A	A	A	A/G	A	G	G	G	--
3685	A	A	A	A	A	A	G	A	A	G	G	--
3691	A	B	A	A	A	A	A	A	A	A	A	--
3715	T	C	T	T	T	T	T	T	T	T	T	--
3778	T	C	T	T	T	T	T	T	T	T	T	--
3787	T	T	T	T	T	T	T	T	C	T	T	--
3809	T	A	A	A	A	A	A	A	A	A	A	S —T
3817	T	T	T	T	T	T	C	T	C	C	C	--
3865	A	A	A	A	A	A	A	A	A	A	A	--
3901	C	C	C	C	C	C	T	C	T	T	T	--
3913	T	T	T	T	T	T	T/C	T	C	T	C	--
3988	C	T	C	C	C	C	T	C	T	T	T	--
4039	T	T	T	T	T	T	T	T	C	T	T	--
4041	A	A	A	A	A	A	G	A	G	G	G	D —S
4081	T	T	T	T	T	T	A	T	T	A	A	Y —N
4090	A	A	A	A	A	A	A	A	A	A	A	Q —R
4105	C	C	C	C	C	C	C	C	T	C	C	--
4132	A	A	G	G	G	G	A	T	A	A	A	--
4135	C	C	C	C	C	C	T/C	C	T	T	T	--
4162	C	T	C	C	C	C	C	C	C	C	C	--
4165	A	A	A	A	A	A	A	A	C	A	A	--
4192	G	A	A	A	A	A	G	A	G	G	G	--
4198	T	T	T	T	T	T	A/T	T	A	A	A	--
4207	C	C	C	C	C	C	T/C	C	T	T	T	--
4216	C	C	C	C	C	C	T/C	C	T	T	T	--
4258	A	A	A	A	G	G	A	A	A	A	A	--
4282	T	T	T	T	T	T	T	T	G	T	T	--
4300	C	T	C	C	C	C	T/C	C	T	T	T	--
4303	T	C	T	T	T	T	T	T	T	T	T	--
4486	T	T	T	T	G	G	T	T	T	T	T	--
4522	A	A	A	A	A	A	C	A	C	C	C	--
4567	T	G	T	T	T	T	T	T	T	T	T	--
4591	T	T	T	T	C	C	T	C	T	T	T	--
4609	G	G	T	T	T	T	G	T	T	T	T	--
4642	A	A	A	A	G	G	A	A	A	A	A	--

Fig. 1. Sequencing results. Listed are all nucleotide (nt) positions with variations in at least one of the investigated B19 genomes. Dark-shaded box: variation in only one of the genomes, light-shaded box: variation in more than one genome. Last column shows the resulting amino acid (aa) variation in respect to B19 reference strain Au [6]. Amino acids are given by the one-letter code.

B, lot –3, showed B19 DNA in 7 out of 8 subpools. The B19 DNA contamination in the subpools was in the range of 10^3 to 10^8 genome equivalents (geq)/ml.

The DNA sequence of the B19 isolate from patient A/product A, and the sequence of the isolate from patient B/product B, lot –1, were clearly different from each other, and also differed by 4 to 43 nucleotides from the genomes from the five sequenced isolates as well as from the sequences of the reference strains Au [6] and Wi [10].

Quantitative PCR analysis of product A showed 8.6 x 10^6 genome equivalents B19 DNA per ml. Patient A received a total of 180 ml of product A, thus a total amount of 1.6 x 10^9 geq of B19 DNA was administered. Product B, lot –1, contained 4.0 x 10^3 geq per ml. Patient B was treated over a period of 52 days with 966 ml of this product resulting in a total amount of 3.9 x 10^6 geq B19 DNA administered before detection of seroconversion.

Discussion

The sequence identity between the isolates obtained from the hemophilic children and the blood products indicates that the two cases of B19 infection were acquired through treatment with the activated prothrombin complex concentrate (product A/patient A) and the coagulation factor VIII product (product B, lot –1/patient B), respectively.

Product A was highly contaminated with B19 DNA (8.6 x 10^6 geq/ml) and infection was transmitted by this product within a four-day treatment period. Although detection of B19 DNA does not necessarily indicate viral infectivity, experimental data and theoretical considerations concerning the efficiency of commonly used procedures to inactivate non-enveloped viruses suggest a high probability of infectious B19 being present in preparations with such high concentrations of B19 DNA. The virus inactivation method applied to product A was vapor heating for 10 h at 60°C, followed by one 1 h at 80°C. In contrast, B19 DNA contamination of product B, lot –1,.was low (4.0 x 10^3 geq/ml). Nevertheless, the viral inactivation procedure applied to this product, i.e. dry heat for 72 h at 80°C, was also not sufficient to eliminate viral infectivity.

Recently, it has been observed during a clinical trial with solvent detergent (S/D)-treated plasma that lots contaminated with $10^{7.5}$ to $10^{8.5}$ geq/ml were infectious while lots with low B19 DNA contamination ($\leq 10^{3.5}$ geq/ml) were not [11]. Probably, the loss of infectivity of the low contaminated lots was due to the presence of neutralizing antibodies in the plasma and not to S/D treatment which should be without effect on B19 infectivity. However, conclusions drawn from S/D treatment studies can not be applied to these of heat treatment although heat treatment may have a certain effect against non-enveloped viruses.

The cases of B19 infection reported here occurred without clinical symptoms. Nevertheless, B19 can cause long-lasting, severe or life-threatening diseases such as chronic arthropathy, aplastic crisis, myocarditis, hepatitis, hydrops fetalis, or intrauterine death [for review 12, 13]. Although some of these clinical scenarios may be rare events, physicians must be aware of the potential risk concerning B19 transmission by blood derivatives. However, to avoid transfusion-associated B19 infections further progress is needed to improve the technology for viral inactivation and removal as well as the methods for measurement of their efficiency. In addition, research on the benefit of both donor selection and B19 screening procedures are required to ensure the safety of blood.

References

1. Azzi A, Morfini M, Mannucci PM (1999): The transfusion-associated transmission of parvovirus B19. Transfus Med Rev 13: 194-204
2. Schmidt I, Blümel J, Seitz H, Willkommen H, Löwer J (2001) Parvovirus B19 DNA in plasma pools and plasma derivatives. Vox Sang 81: 228-235
3. Hino M, Ishiko O, Honda K-I, Yamane T, Ohta K, Takubo T, Tatsumi N (2000) Transmission of symptomatic parvovirus B19 infection by fibrin sealant used during surgery. Br J Haematol 108: 194-195
4. Koenigbauer UF, Eastlund T, Day JW (2000) Clinical illness due to parvovirus B19 infection after infusion of solvent/detergent-treated pooled plasma. Transfusion 40: 1203-1206
5. Eis-Hübinger AM, Sasowski U, Brackmann HH, Kaiser R, Matz B, Schneweis KE (1996) Parvovirus B19 DNA is frequently present in recombinant coagulation factor VIII products. Thromb Haemost 76: 1120
6. Shade RO, Blundell MC, Cotmore SF, Tattersall P, Astell CR (1986) Nucleotide sequence and genome organization of human parvovirus B19 isolated from the serum of a child during aplastic crisis. J Virol 58: 921-936
7. Mori J, Beattie P, Melton DW, Cohen BJ, Clewley JP (1987) Structure and mapping of the DNA of human parvovirus B19. J Gen Virol 68: 2797-2806
8. Hemauer A, von Poblotzki A, Gigler A, Cassinotti P, Siegl G, Wolf H, Modrow S (1996) Sequence variability among different parvovirus B19 isolates. J Gen Virol 77: 1781-1785
9. Johansen JN, Christensen LS, Zakrzewska K, Carlsen K, Hornsleth A, Azzi A (1998) Typing of European strains of parvovirus B19 by restriction endonuclease analyses and sequencing: identification of evolutionary lineages and evidence of recombination of markers from different lineages. Virus Res 53: 215-223
10. Blundell MC, Beard C, Astell CR (1987) In vitro identification of a B19 parvovirus promoter. Virology 157: 534-538
11. Brown KE, Young NS, Alving BM, Barbosa LH (2001) Parvovirus B19: implications for transfusion medicine. Summary of a workshop. Transfusion 41: 130-135
12. Cohen B (1995) Parvovirus B19: an expanding spectrum of disease. BMJ 311: 1549-1552
13. Cherry JD (1999) Parvovirus infections in children and adults. Adv Pediatr 46: 245-269

Course of a severe Hemophilia A.
Successful Immune Tolerance Therapy (ITT) ten Years after Inhibitor Development

A. Grunske, E. Holfeld, and D. Möbius

Introduction

Inhibitor development is a serious complication of replacement therapy in hemophilia A. Depending on the type of factor VIII gene lesion 5–30 % of patients with severe hemophilia A are affected [1]. Increased morbidity and costs of care associated with this complication require inhibitor eradication and reinstitution of specific replacement prophylaxis. Several concepts of ITT, mainly based on daily application of high doses of factor VIII-concentrates, are approved and often successful [2]. Because of enormous costs of ITT it seems helpful to determine circumstances in patient's history which point to a successful outcome or therapy failure. For prediction of a successful outcome the time between inhibitor development and the beginning of ITT and the number of factor VIII-exposure-days seem less important (not significant) than maximum inhibitor level before and during ITT. These levels correlate negatively with the success of ITT [3].

In some cases the use of central venous access devices (CVAD) for treatment of hemophilia is required. The common problems of using CVADs in hemophilia include bleeding episodes, extravasation, allergic reaction to factor concentrates and, predominantly, catheter-associated infections. The infection rate in patients with factor VIII inhibitors is much higher than in patients without this immune response. [4,5].

Case report

We report a case of severe hemophilia A. The boy was born in 1981 and had no affected family members. The younger sister was identified as a conductor of factor VIII gene lesion. After acute bleeding on the lingual frenulum 1982 the diagnosis of hemophilia A was made. In the following years numerous bleedings occurred in different joints, skin, kidneys and muscles. In former East Germany factor VIII concentrates were not available. Episodes of acute bleedings were treated with cryoprecipitates, fresh frozen plasma and, by way of exception, FEIBA. In 1983 a prophylaxis with cryoprecipitates was begun for some months without any benefit. In 1984 factor VIII inhibitors occurred for the first time (140 BU/ml), a sufficient ITT was not available at this time. After application of factor VIII concentrate because of an acute bleeding in 1990 a maximum inhibitor level of 556 BU/ml was detected.

I. Scharrer/W. Schramm (Ed.)
32nd Hemophilia Symposion Hamburg 2001
© Springer-Verlag Berlin Heidelberg 2003

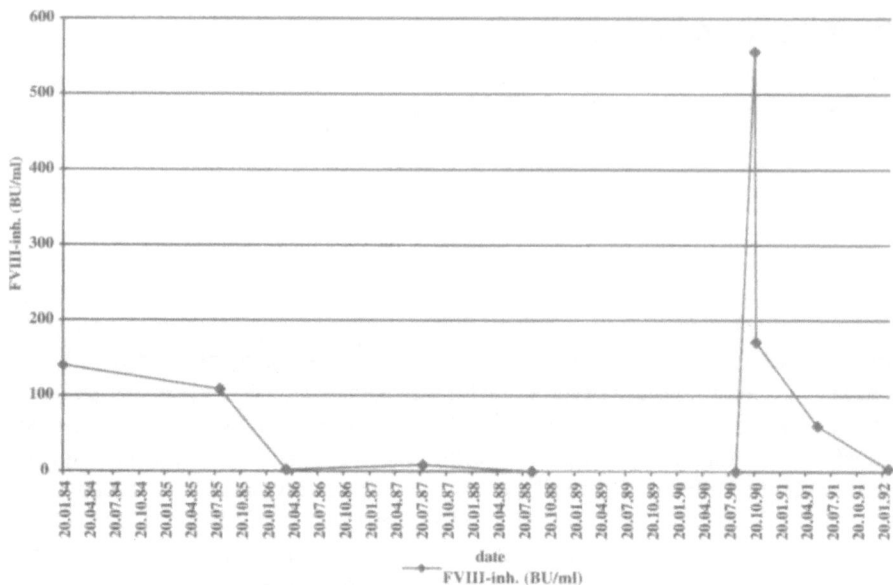

Fig. 1. Factor VIII inhibitor levels before ITT

In 1992 ITT with 200 IU factor VIII concentrate/kg/d was initiated. 9 months later the dose was increased to 350 IU/kg/d. This increased dose and a single application of IVIG had no effect on the occurrence of bleedings and the persistently low inhibitor level (1–10 BU/ml). 6 months later we changed to lower doses (35 IU/kg/d). However, after a severe kidney bleeding occurred some weeks later we decided to continue the ITT with 330 IU/kg/d for one week, 200 IU/kg/d for the following 3 weeks and 75 IU/kg/d in the following time in combination with

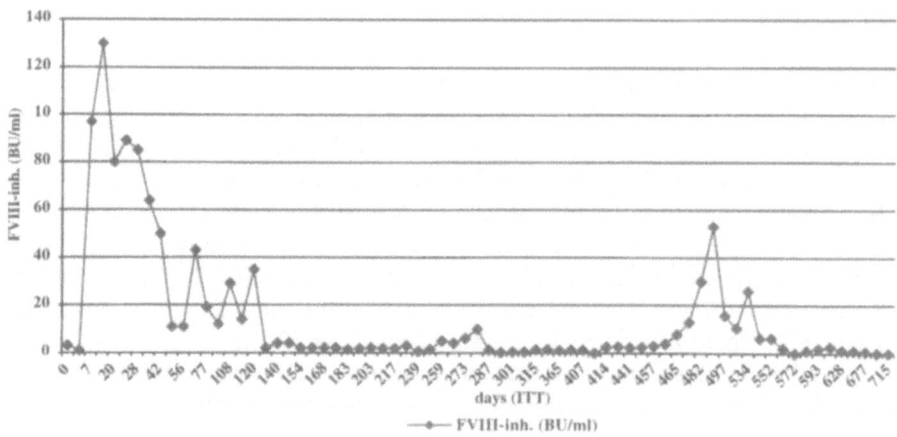

Fig. 2. Inhibitor level during ITT

cyclophosphamide (400 mg on day 1 and 2, then 80 mg/d for 3 months) and IVIG (0.4 g/kg/d on 3 days every 4 weeks for 6 months).

In January 1994 no factor VIII inhibitors were detected, but the factor VIII recovery still remained pathologically (the recovery nearly normalized in the following years). The replacement therapy was continued with 60 IU/kg/d and gradually reduced to 25 IU/kg/every second day in 1999. In the genetic analysis 1997 a large deletion in the factor VIII gene was found. It is responsible for the complete deletion of the A1- and probably of parts of the A2-domain of factor VIII protein.

In 2000 our patient left the pediatric care without serological signs of hepatitis B, hepatitis C or HIV infection.

Accompanying problems/secondary diagnoses:
1. Multiple CVAD-infections, several revisions of PortaCath, associated bleedings, i. v.-antibiotic treatment.
2. Hyposomia, diagnosis of growth hormone deficiency in 1994; a treatment with growth hormone was refused by the parents.
3. Muscular atrophia on legs because of muscle bleedings and immobilization.

Conclusions

The type of mutation of factor VIII gene of our patient predisposes for development of factor VIII inhibitors, his individual risk for this complication is probably greater than 30 %. The trial of ITT many years after development of inhibitors may be successful. This was confirmed by the results of the ITT-register in 1997 [3]. The high maximum inhibitor levels before (556 BU/ml) and during ITT (130 BU/ml) in our case did not diminish the final success of the ITT. The possibly helpful immune modulation with cyclophosphamide and IVIG can not be evaluated conclusively.

References

1. Schwaab, R., Brackmann, H.-H., Meyer, C., Seehafer, J., Kirchgesser, M., Haack, A., Olek, K., Tuddenham, E. G. D., Oldenburg, J.: Haemophilia A: Mutation Type Determines Risk of Inhibitor Formation, Thrombosis and Haemostasis, 1995 Dec, 74 (6), 1402−6
2. Di Michele, D. M.: Immune tolerance: a synopsis of the international experience. Haemophilia (1998), 4, 568–573
3. Lenk, H., Kertzscher, F., Bartsch, M. et al.: Immuntoleranztherapie bei Hämophilie A und B – Ergebnisse des ITT-Registers 10/1997, in: Scharrer, I., Schramm, W. (Hrsgg.), 28. Hämophilie-Symposion Hamburg 1997, Berlin, Heidelberg 1999, 219–225
4. McMahon, C., Smith, J., Khair, K., Liesner, R., Hann, I. M., Smith, O. P.: Central venous access devices in children with congenital coagulation disorders: complications and long-term outcome, British Journal of Haematology, 2000, 110, 461–468
5. van den Berg, H. M., Fischer, K., Roosendaal, G., Mauser-Bunschoten, E. P.: The use of the Port-A-Cath in children with haemophilia – a review, Haemophilia (1998), 4, 418–420

Increased Resistance to activated Protein C and Protein C Deficiency in the same Family

B. Maak, F. Bergmann, L. Kochhan, F.H. Herrmann, W. Schröder, and S. Hutschenreiter

Introduction

Today we have certain knowledge about a number of hereditary factors which change the hemostatic balance of their carriers towards a tendency to develop venous thrombo-embolism. Typically the first manifestation occurs frequently without any recognizable cause at a young age and in the majority of cases as thrombotic occlusion of the deep veins of the lower extremities. Pulmonary embolizations as life-threatening complications may be observed in young patients. Furthermore a marked tendency to recurrent thrombotic events exists.

The above-mentioned factors include deficiencies of antithrombin III, protein C and protein S.

In 1993 we got information about the so-called resistance to activated protein C (aPCR) as a cause of hereditary thrombophilia [3]. The aPCR doesn't represent a deficiency of any protein involved in the process of coagulation and/or fibrinolysis but is caused by a point mutation (G 1691 A) in the gene encoding for coagulation factor V [1]. As the consequence, an amino acid substitution Arg → Gln in position 506 of the factor V molecule results. The cleaving rate of this altered factor V by activated protein C is therefore markedly reduced and a hyper-coagulable state results.

The aPCR is the risk factor with the highest prevalence in northern and middle European countries and is practically not present in regions outside Europe [5]. Therefore it seems likely that within the European countries combinations of aPCR with other risk factors exist. From the theoretical point of view, individuals bearing two or more inherited or also acquired risk factors should be prone to an increased severity of the clinical course.

As an example for this assumption we present the results of an extended family study. The index patient was a 20 year old man who died from a pulmonary embolization after a short course of illness. We investigated a total of 36 family members, his parents an his brother included.

Case report

The index patient (III/9, Fig. 1), a 20 year old man, died after a short period of difficulties with breathing. The postmortem examination revealed multiple pul-

I. Scharrer/W. Schramm (Ed.)
32nd Hemophilia Symposion Hamburg 2001
© Springer-Verlag Berlin Heidelberg 2003

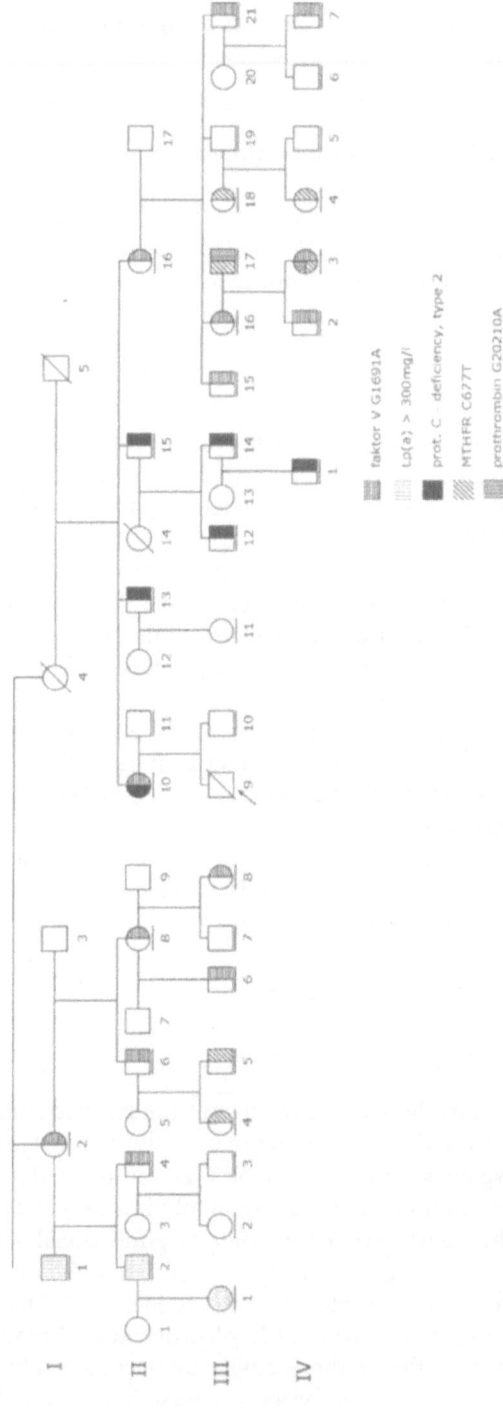

Fig. 1. Pedigree of the family. The arrow denotes the index case. Underlined symbols: Investigated family members. Half-filled symbols indicate the heterozygous state of the different mutations detected (see symbols). Deceased individuals are characterized by a diagonal line through the boxes or circles. Generations are indicated by roman numerals.

monary embolizations as the cause of death. By microscopic investigation, aneurysms of pulmonary arteries as signs of a longer lasting disease process were demonstrated.

Approximately eight weeks before the catastrophic event a swelling of the left leg was noticed and a thrombosis of the deep veins was supposed. However, this diagnosis was not confirmed by ultrasonographic examination and therefore anticoagulant treatment was not instituted.

In the family of the young man there are three members with well proven vascular complications: I/2, II/4 and II/10. In two other family members (II/8 and II/15) suspected thrombosis was not yet confirmed.

Methods

Prothrombin time, aPTT, aPCR, and the activities of proteins C and S were measured with reagents from IL according to the recommendations of the manufacturer. The protein C assays were completed by an amidolytic and immunologic method (radial immunodiffussion).

For the detection of the mutation in the protein C gene total DNA of all protein C deficient patients was extracted from whole blood using micro spin columns (Quiagen, Hilden, Germany). Exons of the protein C gene were amplified by polymerase chain reaction (PCR) using primers (without restriction endonuclease sites) and conditions previously described [4]. PCR products were sequenced directly using the Big Dye Terminator Cycle Sequencing kit (Perkin Elmer Applied Biosystems, Foster City, USA) and analyzed using an automated DNA sequencer (ABI PRISM/377 DNA Sequencer; Applied Biosystems, Weiterstadt, Germany).

Primers used for sequencing were the same as those used for PCR amplification.

The detection of the mutation G 1691 A in the factor V gene was performed as described by Bertina et al. [1]. The polymorphisms in the MTHFR-gene and in the prothrombin gene were analyzed according to Kluijtmans et al. [6] and according to Poort et al. [8].

Results

36 family members were investigated (underlined symbols in Fig. 1). In the mother (II/10) of the deceased young man (III/9) the increased aPCR was caused by the heterozygous state for the factor V Leiden (G 1691 A). Her protein C values were 50% (coagulation assay), 72% (amidolytic assay) and 2.37 mg/l (antigen concentration). This constellation represents a dysfunctional protein C (protein C deficiency type II). As the cause of protein C deficiency, the mutation Gly 350 (GGG) → Arg (AGG) in exon 9 of protein C gene was identified. The first thrombotic event in this woman occurred at an age of 32 years during oral contraceptive use. Contrary to the findings from the mother, completely normal results with respect to well known thrombotic risk factors were obtained from the father (II/11) and the brother (III/10) of the young man.

Two brothers (II/13, II/15) of the mother are protein C deficient, two children and the grandson from one of the brothers also have low protein C activities and normal concentrations of protein C antigen. In all cases (II/13, II/15, III/12, III/14, IV/1) the same mutation in exon 9 of protein C gene was detected. II/15 reported on recurrent swellings of his right leg some years ago: ultrasonographic studies excluded residual thrombosis.

The sister (II/16) of II/10 is heterozygous for the factor V mutation (G 1691 A) and four pregnancies were uneventful with regard to thrombotic events. Three out of four children are carriers of the same mutation. The husband (III/17) of her daughter (III/16) was identified as heterozygous for the mutations in the prothrombin gene (G 20210 A) and in the MTHFR-gene (C 677 T). The daughter (IV/3) of this married couple, now eight years old, is heterozygous for these three mutations.

The parents of II/10 are no longer alive. However, an aunt (I/2) was available for an investigation. This woman suffered from a cerebral infarction and a residual palsy exists until now. She was identified as a heterozygous carrier of the factor V mutation G 1691 A. From her first marriage with I/3 two children (II/6 and II/8) exist, both are heterozygous for the factor V mutation G 1691 A. The woman (II/8) reported on repeatedly occurring swellings of her right leg. By ultrasonographic examinations however, no thrombotic occlusions or signs of previously occurring thrombosis were detected. The offspring of two marriages of II/8 are in good health at present. Two (III/6 and III/8) are heterozygous for the factor V mutation G 1691 A. At the time of investigation III/8 was pregnant. The pregnancy and the puerperium were without thrombotic complications.

The second marriage of I/2 (with I/1) resulted in two children, both males. The older of these brothers (II/4) was found to be heterozygous for the factor V mutation G 1691 A. Some years ago he suffered from a posttraumatic thrombosis of his left leg. The thrombosis was confirmed by ultrasonographic examination. The other young man (II/2) exhibited an elevated Lp(a) concentration (917 and 961 mg/l); currently he is in good health. The same is true for his father (I/1) and his daughter, a three year old girl. Both have high concentrations of Lp(a) (539 and 769 mg/l respectively).

Conclusions

- The unexpected death of a 20 year old man caused by pulmonary embolizations seems to be the result of one or more inherited thrombotic risk factors. This assumption could not be proven directly because the pathologist saved no material appropriate to perform the corresponding investigations.
- In our opinion it seems important to clarify the reasons for this catastrophic event because the great majority of the relatives is at a young age, that means under 50 years. Especially the parents desired an investigation of their other boy who is two years older than his brother.
- In the mother of the deceased young man we found heterozygosity for the factor V mutation G 1691 A and protein C deficiency. The combination of these two factors bears an increased risk of developing thrombosis [9].

- In the father and also in the brother of the deceased young man we were unable to demonstrate any of the well known risk factors (aPCR, deficiencies of proteins C and S, antithrombin III deficiency, mutation G 20210 A in the prothrombin gene, hyperhomocysteinemia).
- To be based on the results obtained from the parents and the brother we may speculate that the deceased young man had an increased resistance to activated protein C or he was protein C deficient or both or he has had nothing of all. The last possibility seems rather unlikely at present. We believe that the young man was heterozygous for the factor V mutation G 1691 A and also for the protein C deficiency. This assumption is in accordance with the results published by Koeleman et al. [7]. These authors demonstrated that in individuals who were heterozygous for factor V mutation G 1691 A and protein C deficiency the thrombosis rate was higher than in patients bearing only one of the defects. In addition the first thrombosis of such individuals occurred also at a younger age.
- The identification of inherited thrombotic risk factors in a great number of currently asymptomatic individuals will be helpful for the prompt institution of an efficient prophylaxis during situations bearing an increased thrombosis risk.
- Investigations regarding currently identified candidate genes that are able to modify the thrombosis risk [2] should be used in the future to specify the risk in patients with known mutations.

Summary

The results of a study from 36 members of a family with different thrombotic risk factors are presented.

The index patient was a 20 year old man who died after a short course of difficulties with breathing. The postmortem examination revealed multiple pulmonary embolizations as the cause of death. In the mother of the young man heterozygous states for the factor V Leiden and protein C deficiency were detected. Father and brother of the index patient showed no thrombotic risk factors. In 15 family members heterozygosity for factor V Leiden was found, three out of these 15 persons are victims of vascular occlusions. Five out of the 36 individuals investigated are protein C deficient, in one of them a possible thrombotic event was noticed. In two family members the mutation in the prothrombin gene was demonstrated and in three other individuals elevated Lp(a) levels were detected. The mutation in the MTHFR gene is often associated with slightly elevated homocysteine levels and therefore possibly responsible for arterial complications. This mutation was present in four family members, an eight year old girl shows the MTHFR-mutation (C 677 T) in combination with the mutations in the factor V gene and the prothrombin gene. The prothrombin gene mutation and the MTHFR gene mutation were found also in the girl's father who is asymptomatic at present.

References

1. Bertina RM, Koeleman BPC, Koster T, Rosendaal FR, Dirven RJ, de Ronde H, van der Velden PA, Reitsma PH (1994) Mutation in blood coagulation factor V associated with resistance to activated protein C. Nature 369: 64-67
2. Bertina RM (2001) Genetic approach to thrombophilia. Thromb Haemostas 86: 92-103
3. Dahlbäck B, Carlsson M, Svensson PJ (1993) Familiar thrombophilia due to a previously unrecognized mechanism characterized by poor anticoagulant response to activated protein C: prediction of a cofactor to activated protein C. Proc Natl Acad Sci USA 90: 1004-1008
4. Doig RG, Begley CG, Mc Grath KM (1994) Hereditary protein C deficiency associated with mutations in exon IX of the protein C gene. Thromb Haemostas 72: 203-208
5. Herrmann FH, Koesling M, Schröder W, Altman R, Jimenez-Bonilla R, Lopaciuk S, Perez-Requejo JL, Sing JR (1997) Prevalence of factor V Leiden mutation in various populations Genet Epidemiol 14: 403-411
6. Kluijtmans LAJ, van den Heuvel LP, Boers GHJ, Frosst P, Stevens EMB, van Oost BA, den Heijer M, Trijbels FJM, Rosen R, Bloom HJ (1996) Molecular genetic analysis in mild hyperhomocysteinemia: a common mutation in the methylenetetrahydrofolate reductase gene is a genetic risk factor for cardiovascular disease. Am J Hum Genet 58: 35-41
7. Koeleman PBC, Reitsma PH, Allaart CF, Bertina RM (1994) Activated protein C resistance as an additional risk factor for thrombosis in protein C deficient families. Blood 84: 1031-1035
8. Poort SR, Rosendaal FR, Reitsma PH, Bertina RM (1996) A common genetic variation in the 3'-untranslated region of the prothrombin gene is associated with elevated plasma prothrombin levels and an increase in venous thrombosis. Blood 88: 3698-3703
9. Seligsohn U, Zivelin A (1997) Thrombophilia as a multigenic disorder. Thromb Haemostas 78: 297-301

A Life-threatening Cardiomyopathy following Port-a-Cath Infection under Immune Tolerance Therapy

G. Wiegand, R. Rauch, W. Effenberger, H.-H. Brackmann, and M. Hofbeck

Introduction

For elimination of inhibitors against factor VIII immune tolerance therapy (Bonn-or Malmö-protocol) is mainly used. It requires intravenous injections twice daily up to several months – while in early infancy antibodies mostly appear within the first 36 days of treatment [6]. Therefore, in patients with inhibitors or on prophylactic treatment, Port insertion is increasingly recommended (Fig. 1). We describe a particularly complicated case.

Case report

We report on an 18-year-old patient, in whom severe hemophilia A (factor VIII < 1%) was diagnosed at the age of 5 years following an accident with fractured thigh and compartment syndrome. He was substituted with plasma derived factor VIII. After 28 days of treatment a high anti-factor VIII inhibitor (>1000 Bethesda Units, BU) had established. Immune tolerance therapy was initiated and poor venous access required the implantation of a Port system at the age of 9 years. Following surgery with perioperative antibiotic prophylaxis serious septicemia with disseminated intravascular coagulation and cardiac insufficiency developed. Ultrasound excluded abscess

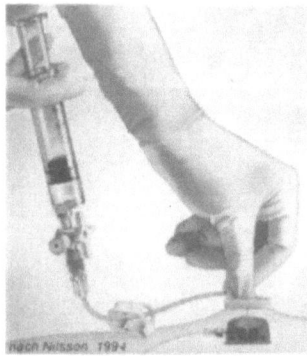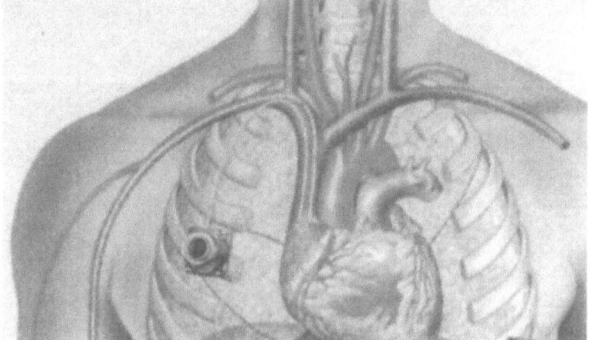

Fig. 1. Port-a-cath in situ

I. Scharrer/W. Schramm (Ed.)
32nd Hemophilia Symposion Hamburg 2001
© Springer-Verlag Berlin Heidelberg 2003

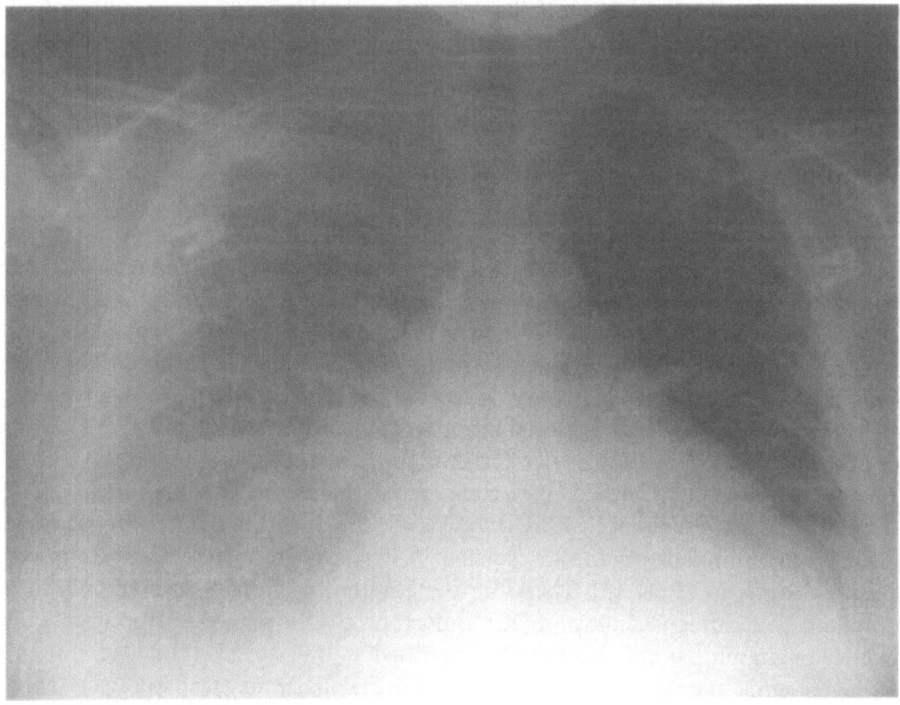

Fig. 2. Considerable cardiomegaly with pulmonary edema and large bilateral pleural effusions

formation or a thrombosis at the catheter tip. Despite enlarged antimicrobial therapy with cefotaxim, teicoplanin and imipenem the Port had to be removed after 26
days due to persistent fever, suspecting a catheter-related infection. Therapy with
digitalis and diuretics initially improved cardiac insufficiency, but a dilative cardiomyopathy with cardiac arrhythmia developed, probably due to myocarditis.
Repeatedly performed blood cultures were negative. Because of the patient's bad
general condition the immune tolerance therapy had to be stopped and on-demand
treatment with FEIBA (Baxter) was started. With progressive cardiac insufficiency
and pulmonary hypertension a combined heart-lung transplantation at the age of 18
was the only option. It was rejected as cardiac and hemostatic problems further worsened: the cardiomyopathy led to generalized (increase in body weight > 20 kg) and
pulmonary edema (Fig. 2) and an almost uncontrollable ventricular arrhythmia (Fig.
3); the anti-FVIII inhibitors are still high (195 BU) at present.

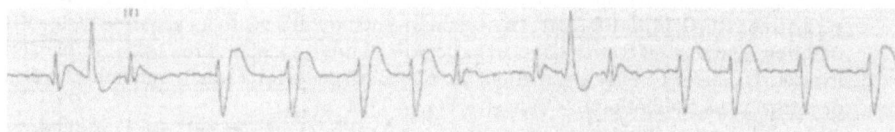

Fig. 3. Polymorphic ventricular extrasystoles on the basis of atrial flutter

Mutation analysis for hemophilia A revealed the intron 22 inversion; furthermore the patient was shown to be heterozygous for the activated protein C resistance (R506Q).

Discussion

Besides skin necrosis and thrombosis bacterial colonization represents the main risk of Port-a-caths. In large studies the incidence of infections is specified with 0.21–0.5 per 1000 device days [5, 7, 12]. With that, it is much lower than for catheters, which penetrate the skin (2.4–2.77/1000 d) [5, 11]. In general, Ports remain in place for long periods of time, depending on the underlying disease (>400d in hemophiliac children [12]). The short episode of 26 Port-days in our patient with perioperative antibiotic prophylaxis suggests bacterial infection at or early after surgery.

Patients needing a Port device for immune tolerance therapy seem to have a higher rate of infection with 50–80% compared to those without inhibitors [3, 9, 15]. This may be a consequence of the frequency with which the devices are accessed [2]. The predominant organisms isolated in Port-related bacteremia were gram-positive coccis in 65.5% [5]. Therefore some authors generally recommend flush solutions containing vancomycin [13]. Unfortunately, the pathogen responsible for septicemia in our patient could not be identified.

Bacteremia in totally implantable devices occasionally may lead to cardiac colonization. In almost all cases the endocardium is concerned [16]. A life-threatening dilative cardiomyopathy on the basis of a generalized cardiac involvement as in our inhibitor patient has not been described yet. However, there are two reports of successful cardiac transplantations in hemophiliacs with inhibitors [1, 14]. These patients had lower inhibitor titers prior to surgery.

Two findings of the mutation analysis partly explain the clinical course in our patient. First, the extent of inhibitor formation can be attributed to the intron 22 inversion, associated with a 7 to 10 times higher inhibitor prevalence than less severe molecular gene defects [10]. Second, the late detection of severe hemophilia A in our patient – 5 years of age versus 9 month in severe hemophiliacs reported by Ljung et al. [8] – was probably due to the heterozygous FV Leiden mutation, which has been shown to cause a milder clinical presentation of the disease [4]. It may have delayed the diagnosis of hemophilia for several years and now has to be taken into account, when anticoagulation for atrial flutter is performed.

References

1. Bontempo FA, Lewis JH, Spero JA, Ragni MV, Kiss JE, Petroski CJ, Thompson ME, Hardesty RL, Kormos RL, Griffith BP. Heart transplant in a hemophiliac with an acquired factor VIII inhibitor: Synthesis of factor VIII:C in pericardial fluid. Transplant Proc 1988; 20: 790–791.
2. Brincker H, Saeter G. Fifty-five patient years' experience with a totally implanted system for intravenous chemotherapy. Cancer 1986; 57: 1124–1129.
3. Collins PW, Khair KS, Liesner R, Hann IM. Complications experienced with central venous catheters in children with congenital bleeding disorders. Br J Haematol 1997; 99: 206–208.

4. Ghosh K, Shetty S, Mohanty D. Milder clinical presentation of haemophilia A with severe deficiency of factor VIII as measured by one-stage assay. Haemophilia 2001; 7: 9–12.
5. Groeger JS, Lucas AB, Thaler HT, Friedlander-Klar H, Brown AE, Kiehn TE, Armstrong D. Infectious morbidity associated with long-term use of venous access devices in patients with cancer. Ann Intern Med 1993; 119: 1168–1174.
6. Kreuz W, Escuriola-Ettingshausen C, Martinez-Saguer I, Gungor T, Kornhuber B. Epidemiology of inhibitors in haemophilia A. Vox Sang 1996; 70: 2–8.
7. Laffer U, Dürig M, Bloch HR, Zuber M, Stoll HR. Implantable catheter systems. Experience with 205 patients. Dtsch Med Wochenschr 1989; 114: 655–658.
8. Ljung R, Petrini P, Nilsson IM. Diagnostic symptoms of severe and moderate haemophilia A and B. A survey of 140 cases. Acta Paediatr Scand 1990; 79: 196–200.
9. Ljung R, Van Den Berg M, Petrini P, Tengborn L, Scheibel E, Kekomaki R, Effenberger W. Port-A-Cath usage in children with haemophilia: experience of 53 cases. Acta Paediatr 1998; 87: 1051–1054.
10. Oldenburg J, Brackmann HH, Schwaab R. Risk factors for inhibitor development in hemophilia A. Haematologica 2000; 85: 7–13.
11. Salzman MB, Rubin LG. Intravenous catheter-related infections. Adv Pediatr Infect Dis 1995; 10: 337–368.
12. Santagostino E, Gringeri A, Muça-Perja M, Mannucci PM. A prospective clinical trial of implantable central venous access in children with haemophilia. Br J Haematol 1998; 102: 1224–1228.
13. Schwartz C, Henrickson KJ, Roghmann K, Powell K. Prevention of bacteremia attributed to luminal colonization of tunneled central venous catheters with vancomycin-susceptible organisms. J Clin Oncol. 1990; 8: 1591–1597.
14. Sheth S, Dimichele D, Lee M, Lamour J, Quaegebeur J, Hsu D, Addonizio L, Piomelli S. Heart transplant in a factor VIII-deficient patient with a high-titre inhibitor: perioperative management using high-dose continuous infusion factor VIII and recombinant factor VIIa. Haemophilia 2001; 7: 227–232.
15. Van Den Berg HM, Fischer K, Roosendaal G, Mauser-Bunschoten EP. The use of the Port-A-Cath in children with haemophilia – a review. Haemophilia 1998; 4: 418–420.
16. Weidmann B, Hanseler T, Jimenez C, Niederle N. Tricuspid endocarditis by implantable venous access. J Clin Oncol 1994; 12: 1103–1105.

Therapy and Prophylaxis of Bleeding Symptoms in a Patient with Acquired Factor X-Deficiency due to Systemic Amyloidosis (AL-Amyloidosis)

R. Klamroth, and Ch. Heinrichs

Background

A number of cases of acquired factor X deficiency have been reported in patients with systemic amyloid light-chain amyloidosis [3,4]. The underlying mechanism could be an absorption of factor X to the amyloid fibrils and rapid clearance of factor X by the amyloid in vasculature and tissues [2]. The incidence of Factor X deficiency varies from 2% to 50%. According to case reports patients with factor X levels less than 10% showed severe or fatal bleeding [1,5].

Anamnesis

In September 1999 a 67-year-old patient (169cm, 65kg) from Dessau was transferred to our hemophilia care center after severe posttraumatic oral hemorrhage. There was no history of preexisting diseases. Appendectomy was performed in 1957 without complications. Clinical examination was without pathological findings except two old skin hematomas on both legs. The patient reported that they have been present since one month.

Initial laboratory findings

Serum natrium, serum kalium, creatinine, ASAT, ALAT, γ-GT, alkaline phosphatase, bilirubin, red cell count, white cell count and platelet count were in normal range.

PT	19%	(70–100)		Factor II	95%	(70–120)
aPTT	66sec	(26–36)		Factor V	122%	(70–140)
TT	15sec	(16–21)		Factor VIII	140%	(70–150)
Fibrinogen	5,8g/l	(2,0–3,5)		Factor IX	169%	(70–120)
Factor X	3%	(70–120)		Factor XIII	124%	(70–140)

Lupus anticoagulant was negative, aPTT in plasma mixing remained negative after one hour incubation. Bleeding time (Ivy) and closure time (PFA 100, Dade Behring) were not prolonged.

I. Scharrer/W. Schramm (Ed.)
32nd Hemophilia Symposion Hamburg 2001
© Springer-Verlag Berlin Heidelberg 2003

Diagnosis and primary therapy

Via rectum biopsy an amyloid light chain amyloidosis (AL) was diagnosed. A hematological disease associated with disturbed immunglobuline production was not found.

In January 2000 an autologous stemcell transplantation was performed after high-dose chemotherapy with 300 mg melphalan. This procedure was well tolerated.

Bleeding complications

We observed six intramuscular hemorrhages requiring therapy with 240 kIU (4.8 mg) recombinant factor VIIa (NovoSeven) followed by continuous therapy with tranexamic acid.

Since October 2000 we observed three episodes with gastrointestinal bleedings, which could be managed by infusion of 320 kIU (7.2 mg) factor VIIa and 2 to 4 units packed red cells. Duration of hospital stays was five to ten days.

Amyloidosis

Despite of stem cell transplantation there was a progression of amyloidosis with incorporation of amyloid fibrils in heart muscle cells, in liver cells and renal parenchym cells, clinically leading to severe heart and liver insufficiency.

Laboratory findings November 2000

Elevation of creatinine, ASAT, ALAT, γ-GT, alkaline phosphatase and bilirubin.

PT	7%	(70–100)	Factor II	99%	(70–120)
aPTT	102sec	(26–36)	Factor V	115%	(70–140)
TT	18sec	(16–21)	Factor VII	61%	(70–120)
Fibrinogen	4.8g/l	(2.0–3.5)	Factor IX	37%	(70–120)
Factor X	<1%	(70–120)			

Acute bleeding complication

In January 2001 the patient was admitted to hospital in Dessau with severe epistaxis. Despite of primary successful therapy with recombinant factor VIIa combined with local treatment epistaxis started again within 24 hours. The patient needed 8 units of packed red cells and three times infusion of 240 kIU Factor VIIa within four days. Due to recurrency of epistaxis the patient was transferred to our hemophilia care center.

Therapy

We started intravenous infusion of activated prothrombincomplex-concentrate (FEIBA) two times 3000 IU per day for three days and initiated immunological therapy with high dose immunoglobulin (0.4g/kg BW for 3 days) and prednisolone (100 mg intravenous for 5 days). With this strategy bleeding could be stopped while factor X-activity remained undetectable.

Prophylaxis

To prevent recurrent bleeding complications requiring packed red cells transfusion and hospitalization prophylactic treatment was necessary. We chose to give FEIBA three times 2000 IU per week in combination with low molecular weight heparin (1750 IU Reviparin) s.c. to avoid thromboembolic complications. In addition with three times 1g tranexamic acid per day there was no recurrent hemorrhage. No additional transfusion of packed red cells was necessary. Due to progression of amyloidosis the patient died in May 2001 of terminal liver and renal disease.

Comments

In two reports factor X deficiency was described in 8.7% and 14% of patients with AL amyloidosis. 50% of this patients had moderate to severe bleeding complications [1,5]. Factor X activity lower than 2% was not described.

This case report shows that acute bleeding complications due to factor X deficiency in patients with AL amyloidosis can be successfully treated with recombinant factor VIIa as an initial treatment. Recurrent bleeding can be avoided by prophylactic therapy with factor eight bypassing agents like FEIBA.

References

1. Choufani EB, Sanchorawala V, Ernst T, Quillen K, Skinner M, Wright DG, Seldin DC: Acquired factor X deficiency in patients with amyloid light-chain amyloidosis: incidence, bleeding manifestations and response to high dose chemotherapy. Blood 97 (2001), 1885–1887
2. Furie B, Voo L, McAdam K, Furie BC: Mechanism of factor X deficiency in systemic amyloidosis. MEJM 1981 (304), 827–831
3. Greipp PR, Kyle RA, Bowie EJW: Facor X deficiency in primary amyloidosis. NEJM 1979 (39), 1050–1053
4. Howell M: Acquired factor X deficiency associated with systemic amyloidosis – a report of a case. Blood 1963 (21), 739–745
5. Mumford AD, O'Donnell J, Gillmore JD, Manning RA, Hawkins PN, Laffan M: Bleeding symptoms and coagulation abnormalities in 337 patients with AL amyloidosis. Br J Haematol 110 (2000), 454–60

Is there a Correlation between vWF-cleaving Protease-Activity, vWF:Ag, Clinical Course and Number of Relapses in 15 Patients with TTP?

U. Mosebach, M. Böhm, M. Krause, Th. Vigh, and I. Scharrer

Introduction

The thrombotic thrombocytopenic purpura (TTP), first described by Moschcowitz in 1924 [6], is a rare disease, characterized by microangiopathic hemolytic anemia, thrombocytopenia, neurological symptoms, renal dysfunction and fever. The mortality of the disease was reduced from 90% to 10–20% by modern treatment like plasmapheresis, steroids and chemotherapy [2, 7]. The etiology of the disease is not understood, however endogenous predisposition like disorder of vWF-hemostasis [4, 5, 8] and exogenous triggers like infection, pregnancy, drugs, contraceptive agents [3] are reported to precede acute TTP. 10 to 36% of patients experience one or more relapses occurring up to 8 years after the initial episode [1]. For that reason the clarification of the causing mechanism, especially for these patients, is very important. Recent research indicates an important role of vWF:Ag and vWF-cleaving protease (vWFcp) in the pathogenesis of TTP [3, 4, 8], however the exact pathomechanism remains unclear. We describe the retrospective study of the course of the disease for 15 TTP-patients observed between 1982 and 2001 considering vWF-cleaving protease activity and vWF:Ag. The question is, whether there is a correlation between vWFcp activity, vWF:Ag, clinical course and number of relapses.

Methods

We analyzed the stationary and ambulant case reports from 1982–2001. The case material included 9 female and 6 male patients, who were treated in our hospital. The diagnosis of TTP resulted from the common characteristics (hemoglobin, schistocytes, lactate dehydrogenase (LDH), platelet count [2]). Most patients were treated with plasmapheresis against FFP usually until normalization of platelet count and LDH-Level.

vWF:Ag was measured by ELISA with antibodies from Dako, Denmark.

Until 1998 vWFcp activity was measured by Prof. Furlan, Bern, after that in our own laboratory using a modified method of Furlan et al [4].

I. Scharrer/W. Schramm (Ed.)
32nd Hemophilia Symposion Hamburg 2001
© Springer-Verlag Berlin Heidelberg 2003

Results

5 of 9 female and 3 of 6 male patients showed at least 1 relapse, all together were 22 relapses documented. One female patient died during first episode. The mean age at first episode was 30.2 years for females (range 13–52) and 44.8 years for males (range 34–54). The mean body–mass–index was 25.8 (females) and 25.5 (males).

6 of 9 female and 4 of 6 male patients were smokers (mean 25.8 and 38.8 cigarettes/day).

In 18 occurrences of TTP (10 patients, 9 index episodes, 9 relapses) vWFcp activity in **acute stage** were tested. In 16 cases we found activity < 6.25%, 1 patient showed an activity of 25% during first episode and relapse. The majority of patients (n=9), where data about vWFcp activity during **first episode** exist, demonstrate during **remission** moderately decreased or normal vWFcp activities, 1 patient showed a non measurable vWFcp activity (Fig. 1). From 6 patients we have no value of vWFcp activity during **first episode**. 2 of these patients have not measurable, 2 moderately decreased and 1 normal cp-activity during remission. Patients without relapse had distinctly lower vWFcp activity in remission than patients with relapse (33.3% vs. 78.3%). The risk of relapse increased with low cp-activity in remission (Fig. 2). One patient died, therefore we have no value.

Looking at vWFcp activity in remission regarding the duration of the acute stage (number of plasmaphereses) we found no clear correlation between low vWFcp activity and exceptionally long lasting treatment (Table 1).

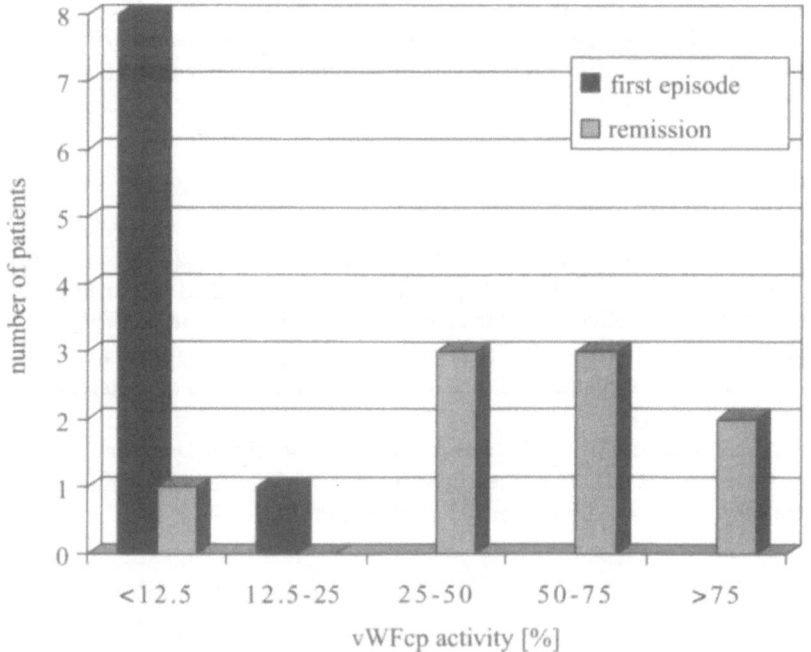

Fig. 1. vWFcp activity during first episode and remission

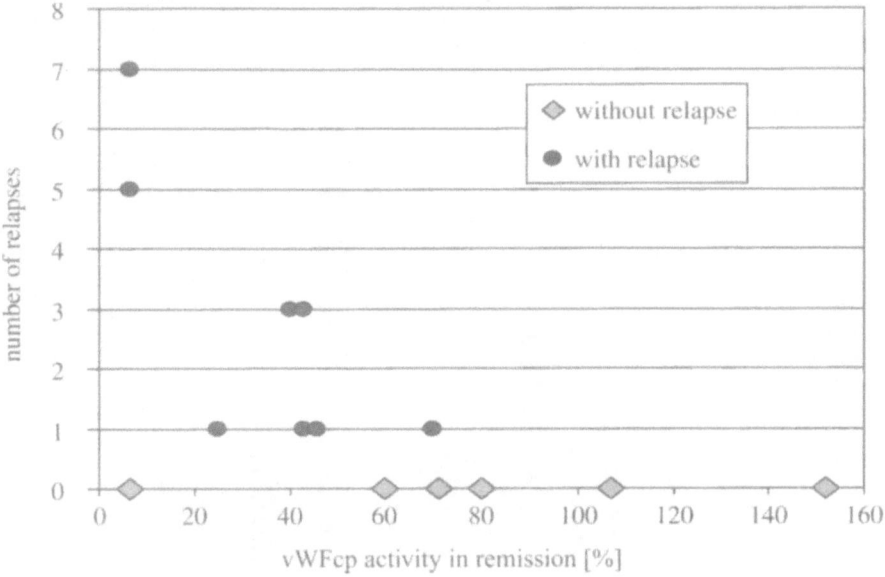

Fig. 2. Correlation of vWFcp activity in remission and number of relapses

Table 1. Association between vWFcp activity in remission and number of plasmaphereses for therapy of first episode and relapse of TTP

vWFcp activity in remission	Number of PP first episode	Number of PP relapses
< 12.5% n=3 patients	30 / 41 / 0	50 / 12 / 4 4 / 0
12.5–25% n=1 patient	20 >25–50%	8
>25–50% n=4 patients	48 / 20 / 5 0	8 / 7 / 7 / 7 6 / 6 / 5 / 0
>50–75% n=3 patients	37 / 19 / 5	15
>75% n=3 patients	86 / 28 / 21	

vWF:Ag (normal range: 82–138% of normal) during first episode was continuously higher than during relapse and there again higher than during remission. Figure 3 shows the vWF:Ag-level during first episode, relapse and remission for 5 patients with intermittent TTP. The mean concentration during first episodes was 264%

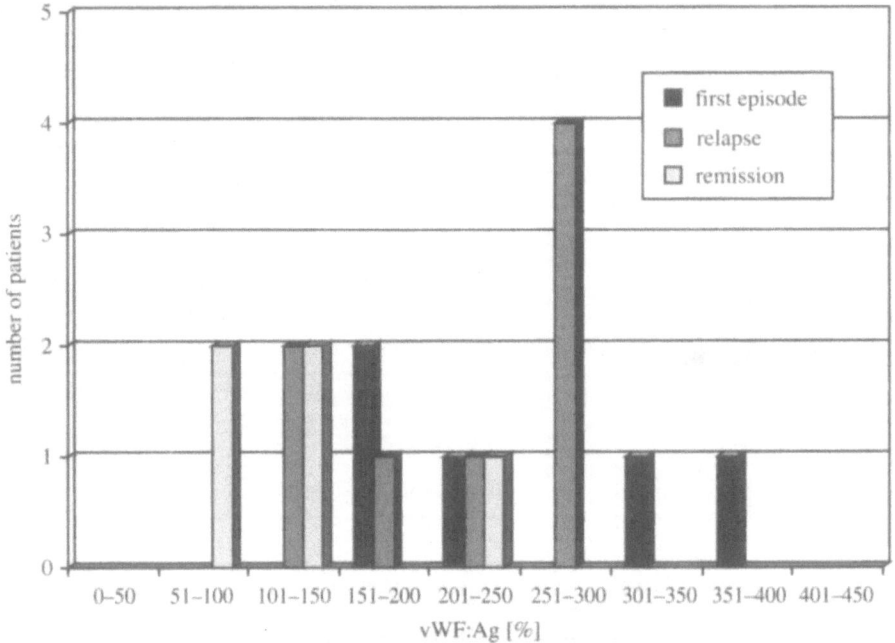

Fig. 3. vWF:Ag during first episode, relapse and remission (data from 5 patients with 8 relapses)

compared to 213% during relapses and 124.6% in remission. The values of 3 patients were incomplete, so we could not take them into account.

The first episodes (n=14) showed a more severe clinical picture than the relapses (n=15) with lower platelet count and higher LDH-level (Fig. 4).

In patients without relapses (n=6) we found a mean vWF:Ag-concentration of 243% in acute episode compared to 117.8% in remission. Looking at all 8 patients with relapses their mean vWF:Ag-concentration in remission was 133.8%.

No clear correlation was detected between high vWF:Ag-concentration in acute episode and an exceptionally long PP-treatment. We found especially in episodes with a treatment of more than 30 plasmaphereses only moderately increased or normal values of vWF:Ag (Table 2).

Summary

Retrospectively we examined the clinical course for 15 TTP-patients observed between 1982–2001, specifically in consideration of vWF:Ag-concentration and activity of vWF cleaving protease. The duration of the acute episode does not depend on vWF:Ag level during the acute episode nor on vWFcp activity in remission. At this stage no clear prediction is possible about the length of essential treatment regarding these parameters. The courses of relapses were clearly shorter and more favorable than the courses of first episodes, probably due to earlier time of

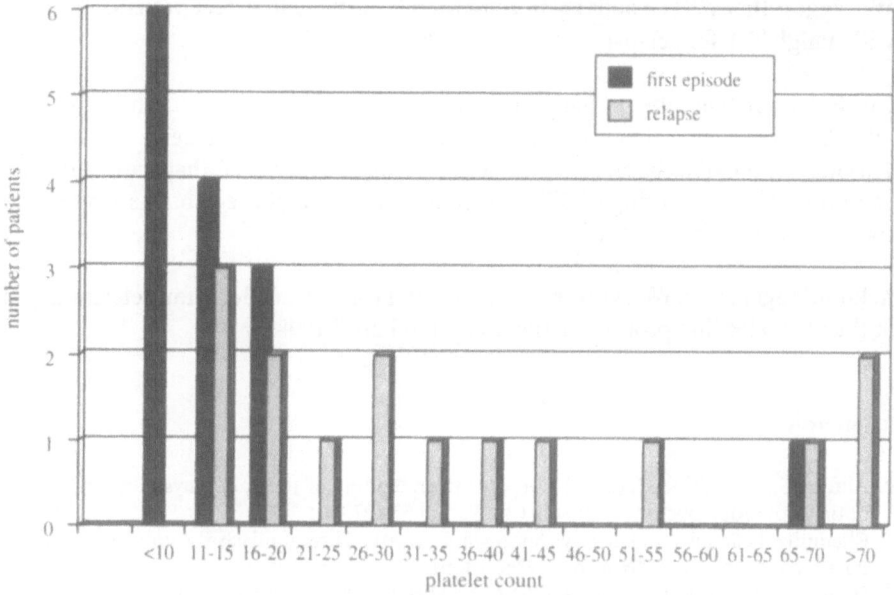

Fig. 4. Lowest platelet count during first episode and relapse

Table 2. Association between vWF:Ag during acute episode and number of plasmaphereses

0 PP	1–10 PP	11–20 PP	21–30 PP	>30 PP
3 occurrences of 2 patients	8 occurrences of 6 patients	5 occurrences of 5 patients	3 occurrences of 3 patients	4 occurrences of 4 patients
250%	128%	279%	320%	199%
234%	260%	754%	276%	109%
228%	267%	234%	411%	132%
	107%	397%		154%
	135%	270%		
	269%			
	168%			
	264%			
Ø=237.3%	Ø=206.5%	Ø=386.8%	Ø=335.6%	Ø=148.5%

diagnosis and adequate therapy. Our data indicate a correlation between decreased vWFcp activity in remission and the occurrence of relapse. Patients with relapses compared to patients without relapses had a distinct decreased vWFcp activity in remission. Also the frequency of relapses seems to increase with decreased vWFcp activity in remission.

We suggest that vWFcp activity in remission is suitable to detect patients with a high risk for relapse

Due to the small number of patients we are not able yet to comment, whether a high vWF:Ag-level during first episode and remission favors the incidence of relapses. This may be possible, because we know according to experience, that acute infection can promote the releasing of TTP, but also other acute-phase-proteins may play a role. To evaluate this we need further investigations.

Acknowledgements. We express our thanks to Prof. Furlan, Bern, for determination of the vWF-cleaving protease activity executed until 1998.

References

1. Allford, S.L., Machin, S.J. (2000) Current understanding of the pathophysiology of thrombotic thrombocytopenic purpura. J Clin Pathol 53:497–501
2. Chemnitz, J., Schulz, A., Diehl, V., Söhngen, D. (2001) Thrombotisch-thrombozytopenische Purpura (Moschcowitz-Syndrom). Med Klinik 96:343–350
3. Douglas B. Cines, Barbara A. Konkle, Miha Furlan (2000) Thrombotic Thrombocytopenic Purpura: A Paradigm Shift ? Thromb Haemost 84: 528–535
4. Furlan, M., Robles, R., Galbusera, M., Remuzzi, G., Kyrle, P.A., Brenner, B., Krause, M., Scharrer, I., Aumann, V., Mittler, U., Solenthaler, M., Lämmle, B. (1998) Von-Willebrand factor-cleaving protease in acute thrombotic thrombocytopenic purpura. N Engl J Med 339:1578–1584
5. Moake, J.L., Chow, T.W., (1998) Increased von-Willebrand factor binding to platelets associated with impaired vWF breakdown in thrombotic thrombocytopenic purpura J Clin Apheresis 13:126–132
6. Moschcowitz, E. (1924) Hyaline thrombosis of the terminal arterioles and capillaries: a hitherto undescribed disease. Proc N Y pathol Soc 4:21–24
7. Rock, G., Shumak, K., Buskard, N., Blanchette, V., Kelton, J., Nai, R., Spasoff, R. (1991) Comparison of plasma exchange with plasma infusion in the treatment of thrombotic thrombocytopenic purpura. Canadian Apheresis Study Group. N Engl J Med 325:393–397
8. Tsai, H.M., Chun-Yet, E. (1998) Antibodies to von-Willebrand factor cleaving protease in acute thrombotic thrombocytopenic purpura. N Engl J Med 339:1585–1594

Life-Threatening Hemorrhage in a Patient with Red Cell Antibodies – Effective Blood Coagulation with rFVIIa

E. Strasser, B. Neidhardt, P. Klein, R. Zimmermann, J. Ringwald, J. Zingsem, V. Weisbach, and R. Eckstein

Introduction

Life-threatening gastrointestinal hemorrhage in Crohn's disease is rare but well recognized and represents about 1% of the cases for hospital admissions in Crohn's disease. Patients with ileocolic location of disease are more likely to have severe hemorrhage and may require resection of the small bowel, which is the most frequently performed intestinal resection (53%) in this disease [1].

The following report describes a severe gastrointestinal hemorrhage of a young female patient with Crohn's disease after resection of the ileocoecum. Clinical management and blood supply was complicated by the rare blood group of the patient (BG 0, ccddee) and the occurrence of irregular red cell antibodies.

Case report

A 23-year-old female with a history of Crohn's disease since 1989 was admitted to the hospital with symptoms of anorexia and malnutrition (body weight: 38 kg). Endoscopically a stenosis affecting the ileocoecal region and fistula formations between the proximal small bowel (jejunum) and the colon ascendens were diagnosed. Laparotomy including resection of the fistula formations and the distal half of the small bowel comprising the ileocoecum followed by an ileocolic anastomosis was performed.

The postoperative course of the patient was complicated by massive lower gastrointestinal hemorrhage: the hemoglobin level dropped from 9.4g/dl (preoperative blood count) to 3.4g/dl in a short postoperative period. There was no hint for specific coagulation disorders in personal or family history. In this emergency situation the patient received 10 units of red cell concentrates and 5 units of fresh frozen plasma within 6 hours followed by a substitution of coagulation components, 1200 IE PPSP, 1250 IE Factor XIII and 1 plateletpheresis concentrate. After normalization of coagulation parameters (PT 59%, INR 1.36, aPTT 40s, platelet count 117000/µl) the patient was still bleeding heavily assuming the therapy was ineffective. Additional supply with red blood cell concentrates was difficult due to the rare blood group (0 ccddee) and existing red cell antibodies (Anti-E and Anti-Lu^a). Concerning the young age of the female patient the application of Rhesus positive red cell concentrates (e.g. 0 Cc D.ee) which are more commonly available was

I. Scharrer/W. Schramm (Ed.)
32nd Hemophilia Symposion Hamburg 2001
© Springer-Verlag Berlin Heidelberg 2003

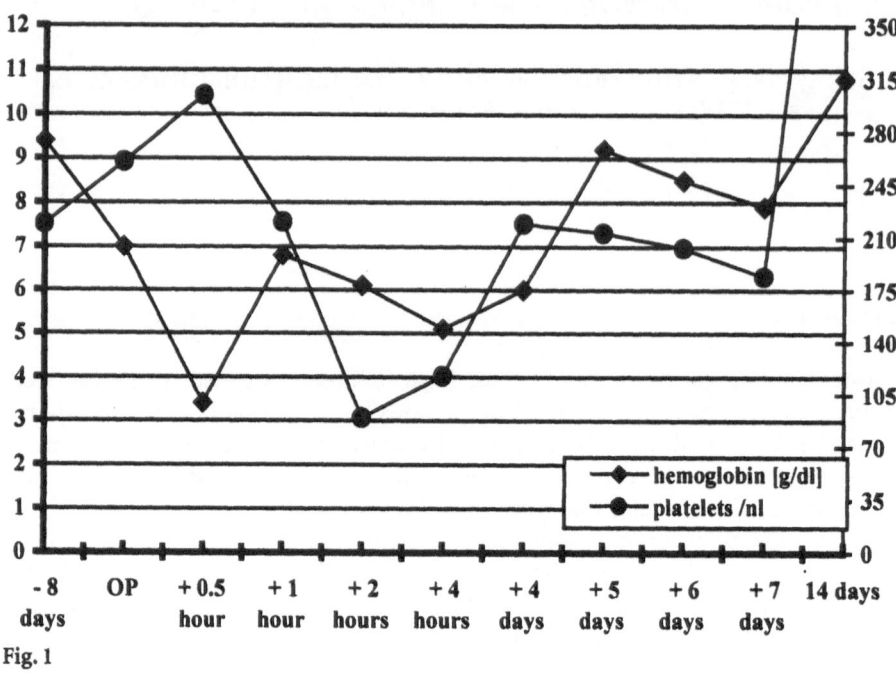

Fig. 1

strictly avoided. Alternatively the patient received a bolus of rFVIIa (NovoSeven) in a dose of 60µg/kg body weight followed by a continuous infusion of rFVIIa in a dose of 30 µg/kg body weight for another two hours. The hemorrhage was staunched immediately and the further clinical course of the patient was straightforward – no further heavy bleeding occurred. The blood count of the patient showed increasing hemoglobin and platelet levels (Fig. 1). Two days later the patient was released from the ICU. Due to a febrile reaction a second look operation was performed two weeks later where only old hematoma was removed and surgical reasons for bleeding could be excluded; the patient was released from the ICU after two days.

Summary

Life-threatening gastrointestinal hemorrhage may occur at any age or stage of Crohn´s disease [1]. In this case report a young female with Crohn´s disease suffered from intractable postoperative hemorrhage of the lower gastrointestinal tract which was successful treated with rFVIIa (NovoSeven). Although rFVIIa was developed for therapy of hemorrhage associated with inhibitor to coagulation factors, rVIIa was an effective treatment in this patient with profuse intraabdominal bleeding.

According to an increasing number of case reports, rFVIIa is an approved therapy for coagulation-inhibitor that has nowadays emerged as an effective treatment of intractable hemorrhage, surgical bleeding and multitransfusion syndrome which are characterized by a complex consumptive coagulopathy [2–4]; further studies are in progress to investigate the optimal dosing regimen to treat profusely bleeding patients.

The therapeutic mechanism of rFVIIa is probably based on the factor VIIa-TF (tissue factor)-complex overcoming the inhibitory effect of factor VII on thrombin generation [5]. Regarding the dose of rFVIIa administered or the target FVII:C levels achieved, treatment intensity alone does not appear to provide the full explanation for discrepant outcomes of different studies on this field and therefore remain a matter of ongoing debate [6].

Conclusion

1. rFVIIa (NovoSeven) is an effective therapy in the postoperative management of profuse abdominal hemorrhage in Crohn´s disease that has failed to respond to conventional coagulation therapy.
2. rFVIIa is an useful hemostatic agent in patients with intractable bleeding and irregular red cell antibodies where sufficient compatible red cell concentrates are not readily available in case of an emergency.
3. Dosing regimen: in the present case life-threatening profuse bleeding can be controlled by a rFVIIa-therapy consisting of bolus application and short-time infusion.

References

1. Cirocco W.C., Reilly J.C., Lawrence C.R. Life-Threatening Hemorrhage and Exsanguination from Crohn´s Disease. Dis Colon Rectum 1995; 38:85–95.
2. White B., McHale J., Ravi N., et al. Successful use of recombinant factor VIIa (NovoSeven) in the management of intractable post-surgical intra-abdominal haemorrhage. Br J Haematol 1999; 107: 677–678.
3. Kenet G, Walden R, Eldad A, Martinowitz U. Treatment of traumatic bleeding with recombinant factor VIIa. Lancet 1999;354(9193):1879.
4. Vlot AJ, Ton E, Mackaay AJ, Kramer MH, Gaillard CA. Treatment of a severely bleeding patient without preexisting coagulopathy with activated recombinant factor VII. Am J Med 2000;108(5):421–3.
5. Van´t Veer C., Mann K.G. The regulation of the Factor VII-Dependent Coagulation Pathway: Rationale for the Effectiveness of Recombinant Factor VIIa in Refractory Bleeding Disorders. Seminars in Thrombosis and Hemostasis 2000; 26(4): 367–372.
6. Ewenstein B.M. Continuous Infusion of Recombinant Factor VIIa: Continue or not? Thromb Haemost 2001; 86:942–44.

Liver Transplantation
in a HIV/HCV coinfected Hemophilia A Patient

W. Mondorf, C. Mondorf, M. Malagó, and C. E. Broelsch

Introduction

A 36-year-old patient with severe haemophilia A and HIV/HCV coinfection received liver transplantation (LTX) on January 26th, 2001 at the University Hospital of Essen in Germany. As two major centers rejected transplantation because of HIV infection, the pros and cons of LTX in patients with haemophilia A and HIV/HCV coinfection were analyzed according to pre- and postoperative laboratory data and clinical results (Table 1) as well as according to a specific questionnaire presented to the propositus (Table 2). In addition the patient gave a short comment of his experiences 7 months following transplantation (Table 3). LTX occurred without complications after bolus injection of recombinant Factor VIII (Recombinate, Baxter).

Table 1. Laboratory results before and 3 as well as 7 months after LTX

	(normal value)	pre-LTX	post-LTX 3rd month	post-LTX 7th month
PTT	(28–41 seconds)	59*	54	41
TP	(75–100 %)	61	84	88
Fibrinogen	(200–400 mg/dl)	163	271	217
Antithrombin	(75–100 %)	40	110	133
Protein C	(75–100 %)	46	70	115
Factor VII	(70–100 %)	32	n.d.	145
Factor VIII	(75 – 150 %)	20*	50	88
GPT	(<28 U/l)	91	172	118
GOT	(<26 U/l)	64	166	90
Gamma-GT	(<20 U/l)	250	368	139
Thrombocytes	(150–450 x 1000/μl)	26	92	74
Erythrocytes	(4.2–6.3 x Mill/μl)	3.80	4.05	4.29
Hemoglobin	(12–16 g/dl)	15,1	14.3	16.9
Leukocytes	(4–10 x 1000/μl)	1.9	4.3	5.2
CD4	(550–1550/μl)	233	345	722
CD8	(300–800/μl)	200	833	1895
CD4/CD8 ratio	(>1.0)	1,6	0,4	0,4
HIV-Load#	(<20 copies/ml)	<20	<20	<20

* = daily factor VIII prophylaxis; # = HIV therapy pre- and post-LTX with Lamivudine + Stavudine + Effavirenz; n.d. = not done

I. Scharrer/W. Schramm (Ed.)
32nd Hemophilia Symposion Hamburg 2001
© Springer-Verlag Berlin Heidelberg 2003

Table 2. Questionnaire presented to the propositus 7 months following LTX (positive answers are bold)

1. In comparison to before LTX I feel
   much better   a little better   unchanged   a little worse   much worse

2. My physical capacity in comparison to before LTX is now
   much better   **a little better**   unchanged   a little worse   much worse

3. My mental capacity in comparison to before LTX is now
   much better   a little better   **unchanged**   a little worse   much worse

4. In future I expect my general health to be
   much better   a little better   unchanged   a little worse   much worse

5. Due to HIV I now expect
   much more   a little more   **unchanged**   a little less   much less
   ...complications

6. Prior to LTX my daily job activity was
   none   **less than 3 hours**   3–6 hours   above 6 hours

7. Seven months after LTX my daily job activity is now
   none   **less than 3 hours**   3–6 hours   above 6 hours

8. The number of tablets in comparison to before LTX is now
   much less   a little less   **equal**   a little more   much more

9. The side effects of my daily medications are now
   much less   a little less   **equal**   a little more   much more

10. The end of factor VIII substitution therapy I consider to be
    a great relief   some relief   no real change

11. The danger of bleeding I consider now to be
    much less   a little less   equal   a little more   much more

12. Having a second choice for LTX I would
    definitely do not   probably do not   probably do   **definitely do**   ....decide for LTX

13. Other patients in a similar situation I would give the advice
    for LTX   against LTX   nothing and leave their own choice

Table 3. Personal comment of propositus (translated from German)

»*One additional comment to the questionnaire: I have never considered factor VIII therapy as a great burden; however without needing to inject I feel a great relief. I now have much less pain in my joints. I believe, whatever prophylaxis one can infuse it can not compete with a »continues prophylaxis« of a new liver. Seven months after LTX I personally expected more complications. However this might be different in others. Because the number of leucocytes have doubled and thrombocytes have trippled a 50% increase of CD4-helper cells resulted in spite of immuno-suppression. No signs of cold or other infections let me expect a good prognosis. Due to longer waiting periods for LTX I would recommend an early enrollment for other patients and consider this as a new opportunity and not as final emergency.*«

Summary

Seven months following LTX quality of live has increased markedly in the hereby presented patient. A prolonged life expectance can be anticipated due to improved liver function and decreased bleeding tendency as a result of elevated leukocyte and thrombocyte counts. A positive surprise is the patients comment of less joint pain in spite of unchanged hemophilic arthropathy. If this is also true for other haemophilia patients following LTX this may develop as a new objective towards gene therapy as well.

From a clinical perspective bleeding risk is markedly reduced due to nearly normal factor VIII and thrombocyte levels as well as a presumable reduction of blood pressure in esophageal varacies. CD4-Helper cells increased significantly after LTX. However, at the same time a decrease of CD4/CD8 ratio was measured. CD4 count alone may therefore not be appropriate for HIV staging or subsequent decision whether or not immunfunction is sufficient for later LTX. Due to a CD4 count of above 700 following liver transplantations the risk of opportunistic infections is low at this time. According to these preliminary results LTX should be considered in a subgroup of haemophilia patients with advanced liver cirrhosis in spite of HIV infection.

Dysfibrinogenemia following after Snake Bite

M. Krause, J. Bojunga, D. Mebs, and I. Scharrer

Introduction

A 35 year old snake breeder was bitten on the left foot by a middle American pit viper Crotalus durissus dryinas which had escaped.

Crotalus durissus dryinas is about 1.5 m long and one of the most dangerous of the 7 known subspecies found in Guyana, Surinam, French Guyana and north-east Brazil. The venom is myotoxic, proteolytic hemorrhagic, neurotoxic and produces edema [5]. Initial paralysis can occur within 30 minutes to one hour (usually after 6 hours), and appears as ptosis, with disturbances of vision and of swallowing [2, 3, 8]. There is no antiserum, neither is there any report for the effectiveness of Mexican or Brazilian polyvalent antisera for Crotalus durissus species [6, 8, 10}.

Clinical effects of the toxin

Neurotoxicity can appear as paralysis of ocular muscles i.e. ptosis, visual disturbances, double vision, mydriasis; disturbances of taste and smell, facial muscle paralysis, occasionally dysphagia, weakness of the extremities and respiratory muscles as well as possible somnolence. Resolution of ptosis can take up to 4 days [2, 6, 8].

Myotoxic effects are characterized by generalized muscle pain and rhabdomyolysis with increased creatinine kinase levels and myoglobinuria 13 to 24 hours after the bite [6].

Blood clotting disturbances can be disseminated coagulopathy (DIC), disturbances of fibrinolysis, and thrombocytopenia [8,10]. Hemorrhagic symptoms vary in intensity and duration.

Generalized symptoms such as nausea, vomiting, melaena and hematemesis have been reported [6].

Nephrotoxic effect can appear in the first 48 hours as acute renal failure, usually due to rhabdomyolysis [6].

Clinical course

Swelling and cyanotic skin changes appeared locally at the site of the bite. About 7 hours after the bite, prothrombin time (PT) in % fell to 48% (INR: 1.77); the mini-

I. Scharrer/W. Schramm (Ed.)
32nd Hemophilia Symposion Hamburg 2001
© Springer-Verlag Berlin Heidelberg 2003

mal level of 16% (INR: 5.39) was reached at 14 hours post envenomation. Thrombin time was 89 sec (normal 0–20 sec), and the reptilase time > 120 sec (normal <20 sec) with a partial thromboplastin time of 63 sec (normal 31–42 sec). Fibrinogen levels (Clauss) were <17 mg/dl (normal 150–450 mg/dl), the heat fibrinogen <120 mg/dl (normal 200 to 400 mg/dl) and the immunological fibrinogen 215 mg/dl (normal 205 to 439 mg/dl). Plasminogen activity dropped to 35% (normal 71 to 116%) with plasminogen antigen levels remaining at normal levels. The D-dimer was 0.4 mg/dl (normal 0.1 to 0.5 mg/dl) with antithrombin and thrombocytes counts within the normal range.

Substitution was instigated and a total of 12 units fresh frozen plasma, 8 g fibrinogen and aprotinin (Trasylol) 200,000 units/hour over a total of 4 hours.

Normal PT, thrombin time and fibrinogen levels (Clauss) were achieved after 81 hours (Fig. 1).

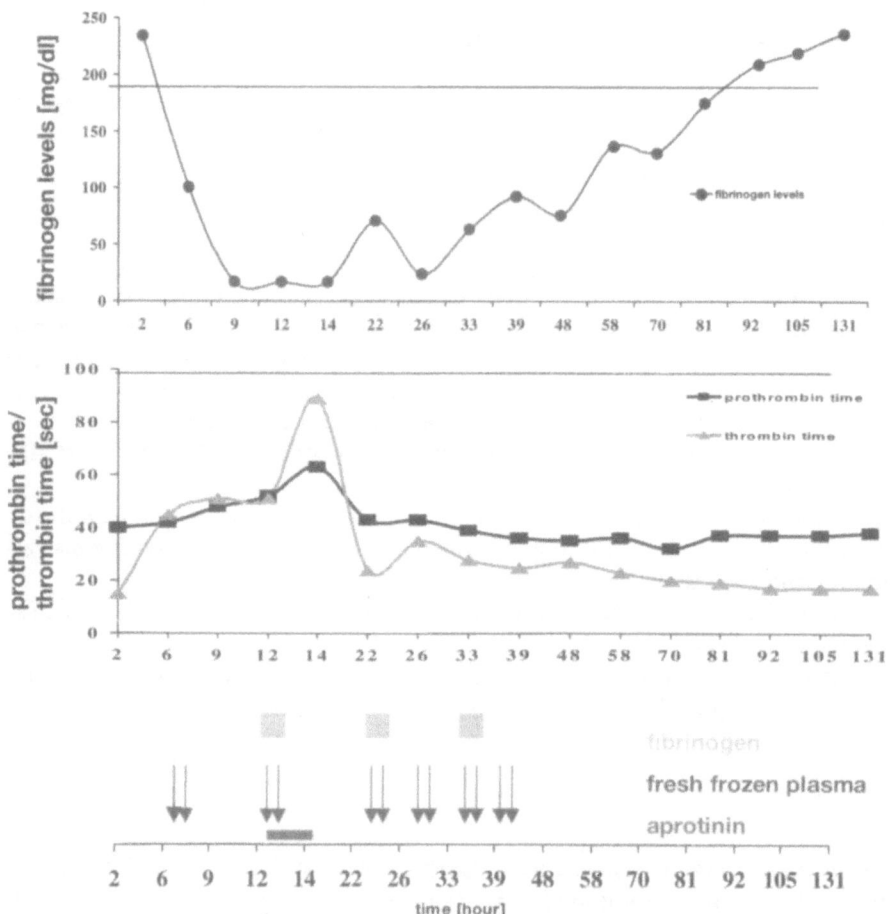

Fig. 1. Clinical course

Creatinine kinase (CK) levels started to rise after 6 hours with a maximum of 997 U/l (normal 80U/l) after 27 hours. These parameters returned to normal within 100 hours (creatinine levels normal). The myoglobulin concentration reached a peak of 491 ng/ml (normal 60 ng/ml) after 17 hours. The lactate dehydrogenase rose to 268 U/l (normal 240 U/L) and the GOT 42 U/l (normal 18 U/l) were both marginally raised.

Microhematuria was present as part of the increased hemorrhagic tendency but hemoglobin levels remained unchanged. The patient did not report nausea and did not vomit. Incomplete right bundle branch block appeared 82 hours after envenomation (Fig. 2 a+b).

Discussion

The poison from the middle American pit viper Crotalus durissus dryinas contains proteolytic enzymes which affect intravascular clotting and can lead to edema extending to myo- and neurotoxicity [3]. This is a serin protease with thrombin-like effect changing fibrinogen to fibrin by fibrinogenolytic peptides. In vitro, these thrombin-like proteases lead to clotting in the presence of calcium ions although a DIC can be induced in vivo. Comparative studies on the biological activities of venoms of three subspecies of the south American pit viper Crotalus durissus on various experimental animals demonstrated that the venoms have a thrombin-like activity with no subsequent activation of prothrombin and/or Factor X [13]. This could be confirmed in further studies on Crotalus durissus subspecies [4, 11, 14].

There are only a very few recorded cases of hemorrhagic diatheses; a few of the victims with afibrinogenemia or DIC died [1, 12]. The pathophysiological effects of viper venom on the clotting system has been well researched, and is typically that of defibrination (9). There has been less undertaken on the appearance of a dysfibrinogenemia after envenomation with Crotalus durissus subspecies.

The diagnosis of dysfibrinogenemia could be made in our patient based on the discrepancy between the fibrinogen level of <17 mg/dl (Clauss) and immunological fibrinogen of 215 mg/dl, as well as the extremely prolonged reptilase time. As D-dimers were not found and as plasminogen activity was reduced, it must be presumed that marked fibrinogenolysis had occurred.

Hemorrhage is not normally a characteristic of dysfibrinogenemias; clinical evidence of bleeding can be anticipated with a fibrinogen level of <50 mg/dl (Clauss).

Although fibrinogen fell to < 17 mg/dl, microhematuria was the only sign of bleeding in this case. Serious bleeding problems were prevented by the supportive therapy combination of fresh frozen plasma, fibrinogen and aprotinin.

Edema at the site of envenomation has been reported, irrespective of the dose, within 30 mins and is said to resolve within 5 hours [13]. However this was not seen in our patient. Also according to previous reports, myotoxic effects peaked at 3 hours prolonged to 9 hours with return to normal after 24 hours [13]. We saw a rise in CK with maximal level at 27 hours with no evidence of rhabdomyolysis. Myotoxic effects were shown by an incomplete right bundle branch block at a CK level of 883 U/l with no symptoms or sign of tropinin T. This has not been described in the literature.

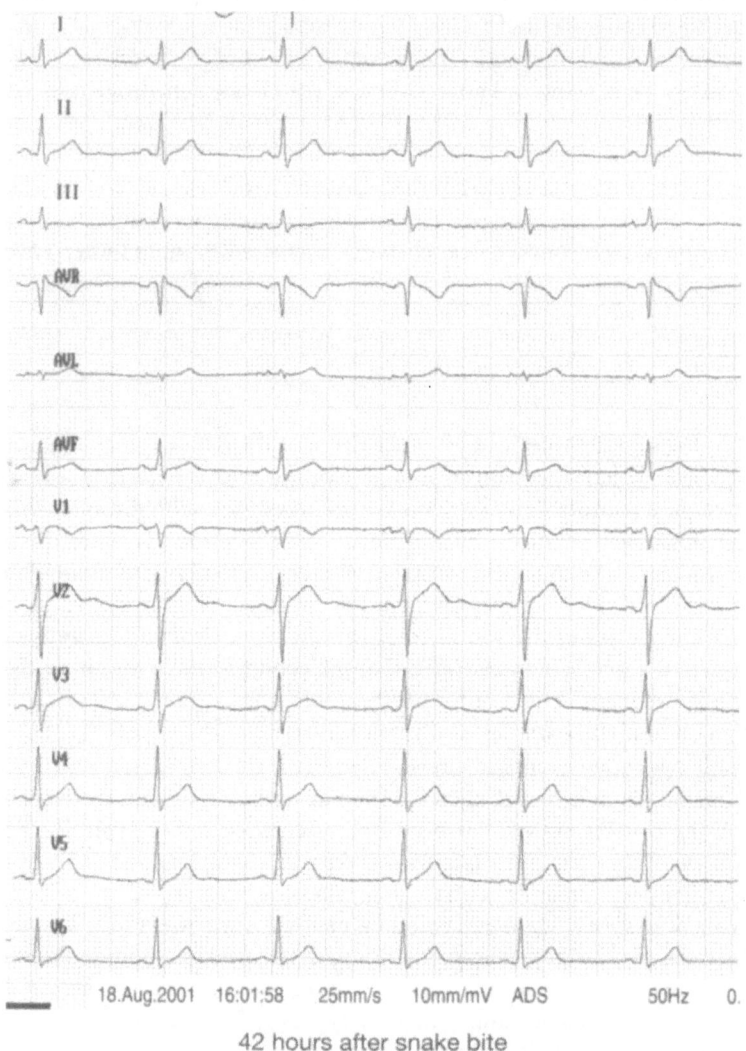

18.Aug.2001   16:01:58   25mm/s   10mm/mV   ADS   50Hz   0.

42 hours after snake bite

Fig. 2a. Electrocardiogram – normal

Summary

The toxin of the middle American pit viper Crotalus durissus dryinas caused a dys-fibrinogenemia in our patient, with minimal bleeding with immediate supportive therapy. A myotoxic effect was apparent as an incomplete right bundle branch block.
– The biological activity and the clinical manifestation of envenomation from Crotalus durissus varies greatly, dependent on the geographical origin of the species.

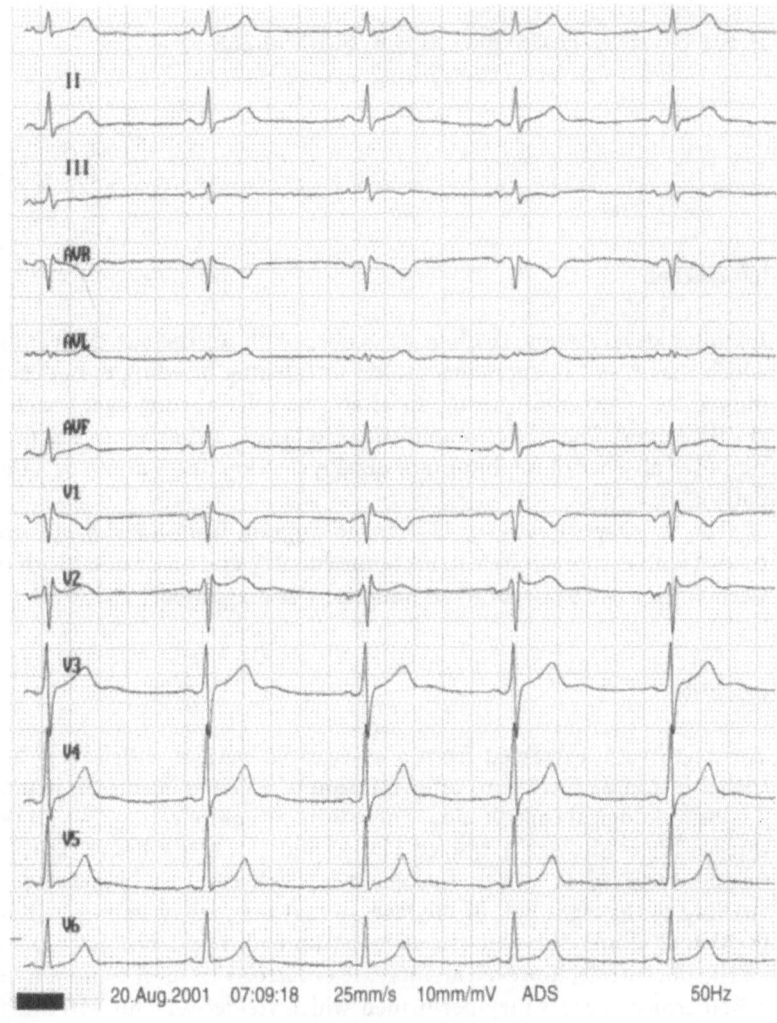

II

III

AVR

AVL

AVF

V1

V2

V3

V4

V5

V6

20.Aug.2001   07:09:18   25mm/s   10mm/mV   ADS   50Hz

82 hours after snake bite

Bleeding Complication following Tooth Extraction in a Hemophilia A Patient with Inhibitor – A Case Report

B. Eifrig, D.K. Hossfeld, and R. Schmelzle

Introduction

Inhibitor development is often associated with an increased bleeding tendency, which may result in spontaneous, life-threatening bleeding episodes and requires immediate intervention using an established therapeutic agent such as aPCC or rFVIIa. But even bleeding complications following a simple surgical procedure with supposed absence of inhibitor may quickly develop into a dramatic situation for the patient.

This is a report about a 49-year-old migrant from Kazakhstan who had been treated with cryoprecipitate in his home country, and on demand with Immunate in Germany for two years, until an inhibitor was diagnosed.

Casuistics

Two teeth were extracted from a 49-year-old patient with severe hemophilia A (distal intron 22 inversion) after infusion of FVIII concentrate, without previous hemostaseological consultation. There were no complications, and three days later, three more teeth were extracted (13, 47 and 48). A few hours later, hemorrhagic oozing occurred at empty alveolus 47, which resulted in massive and painful swelling of the right half of the face, so that the patient had to be hospitalized at the dental clinic. The hemostaseologist immediately administered 3000 units of FVIII concentrate; however, an increase of factor VIII level could not be measured. A Bethesda assay was then performed, which yielded a factor VIII inhibitor level of 120 BE. In addition, the patient reported that his response to the FVIII substitution therapy had started to be lower several weeks prior to the first tooth extraction.

Material and methods

IMMUNATE STIM plus Immuno is a plasma-derived FVIII concentrate highly purified by chromatography and virally inactivated through several steps. For its production, only plasma is used which has been PCR-tested for genomes of HIV-1/-2, HCV, HBV, HAV and Parvovirus B19.

I. Scharrer/W. Schramm (Ed.)
32nd Hemophilia Symposion Hamburg 2001
© Springer-Verlag Berlin Heidelberg 2003

FEIBA S-TIM 4 Immuno is an activated prothrombin complex concentrate which is also exclusively produced from plasmas tested for the above viruses using PCR.

Laboratory tests

Factor VIII determination:
Coagulation measurement using FVIII deficient plasma
Factor VIII inhibitor determination:
Nijmegen modification of the original Bethesda assay

Treatment of acute bleeding

The acute hemorrhagic oozing was treated with local hemostasis by means of mechanical compaction of the alveolar spongy bone. At the same time, 4000 units of FEIBA were infused every six hours, accompanied by administration of an antifibrinolytic agent – 0.5 g Anvitoff three times a day (Fig. 1).

When the bleeding had ceased, the treatment interval was extended to eight hours from day 2, and twelve hours from day 5. During hospitalization there were no bleedings during FEIBA administration, and the FVIII inhibitor titer fell to 19 BU.

The patient was discharged from the hospital on day 12.

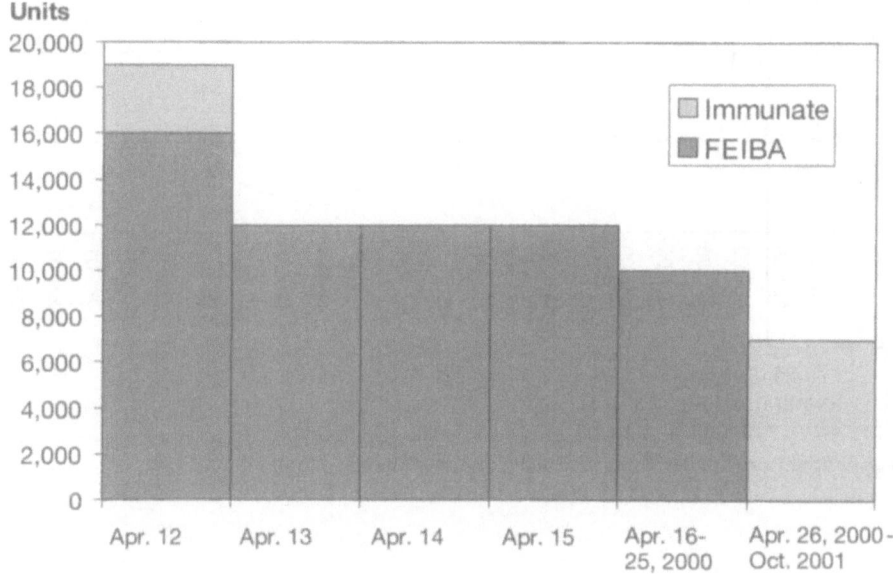

Fig. 1. Treatment of hemorrhagic oozing by means of FEIBA

Immune tolerance induction

On day 14 after initiating treatment of the hemorrhage, immune tolerance induction based on the well-established »Bonn Protocol« was started with 100 IU/kg body weight two times a day according to the »German recommendations« [1, 2]. There was an immediate increase of the inhibitor titer up to a level of 67 BU (Fig. 2). For organizational reasons, only 100 IU/kg body weight within 24 hours could be administered, as the patient had a very long journey to the hemophilia center.

After 18 months of immune tolerance induction (ITI), the inhibitor titer was 7 BE, FVIII activity was below 0.2 %, and aPPT was 120 seconds. There was only a short episode of macrohematuria, which occurred immediately after discharge from the hospital and had iatrogenic causes. It was controlled by a single dose of FEIBA (5000 U). There were no other bleeding complications.

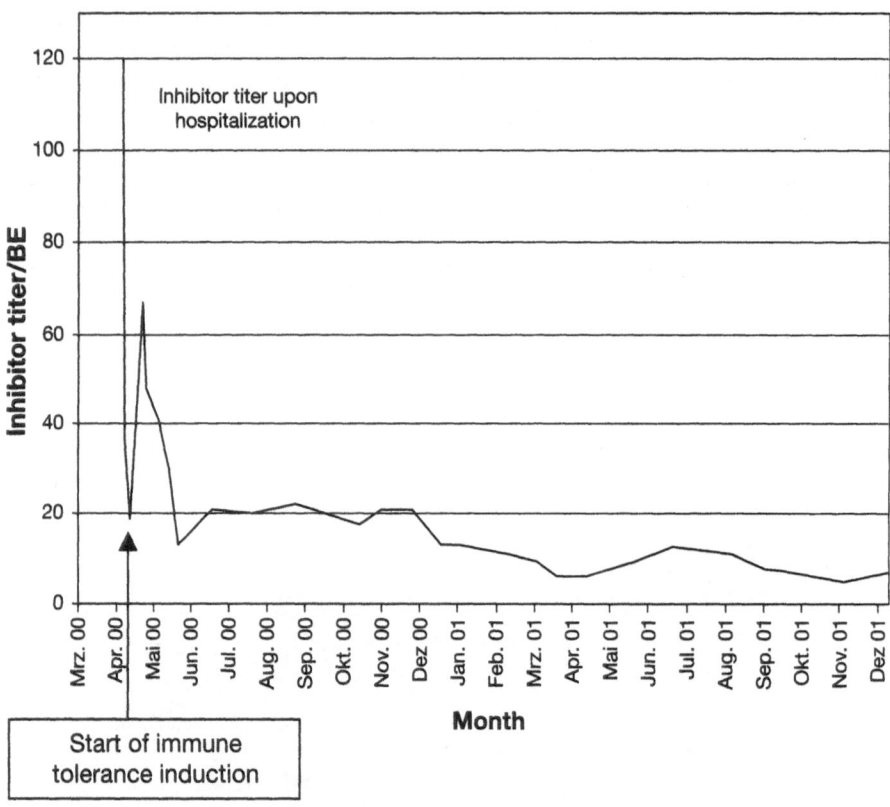

Fig. 2. Inhibitor titer development during immune tolerance induction

Discussion

Whereas the alveolar hemorrhagic oozing was successfully treated with FEIBA, daily administration of 100 IU Immunate/kg BW failed to eradicate the inhibitor even after 16 months, but only managed to reduce the titer to 5–7 BU. According to the literature about 10 % of inhibitors prove resistant to treatment in immune tolerance induction [3]. Whether the patient presented here falls into that category due to his individual disposition, or whether the fact that FVIII was only administered once a day is responsible for the long duration of treatment, remains an open question. To maximize the chances of success, compliance with the well-established »Bonn Protocol« would surely have been necessary. This shows the importance of the patient's cooperation and understanding as regards the daily puncture for administration of the concentrate, as well as the significance of the respective visit to the physician at the clinic.

In order to reach the goal of complete elimination of the inhibitor, continuation of the current treatment regimen for a period of 4–6 months has been recommended upon consultation with other experienced hemophilia physicians. The target will be to continually reduce the inhibitor level and to establish a normal 24-hour FVIII recovery.

References

1. Brackmann HH, Oldenburg J, Schwaab R (1994) Immune tolerance for the treatment of factor VIII inhibitors – twenty years 'bonn protocol'. Vox Sang 70 Suppl 1: 30–5
2. Brackmann HH, Lenk H, Scharrer I, Auerswald G, Kreuz S (1999) German recommendations for immune tolerance therapy in type A haemophiliacs with antibodies. Haemophilia 5(3): 203–6
3. Lenk H and the ITT study group (2000) ITT in haemophilia – 1999 update of the German registry. Haematologica 85 (Suppl): 45–47

Cerebral Sinus Thrombosis: Recanalization after intravenous Dalteparin Administration

H.-H. Wolf, C. Behrmann, O. Dorligschaw, and H.J. Schmoll

Cerebral sinus thrombosis is a serious, life threatening complication of infectious diseases or malignancy. Ascending thrombosis of the jugular veins or cerebral sinuses may occur in patients with thrombophilic diathesis following cerebral infection or trauma as well as in tumor patients.

Ascending venous thrombosis may occur in case of mediastinal tumor and vena caval compression or after placement of central venous access. Especially patients with acute lymphoblastic leukemia and L-asparaginase treatment undergo a high risk for thrombotic complications [1-3].

Usually, thrombotic material cannot be resected neurosurgically, and intravenous lysis cannot be performed in tumour patients [4] due to thrombocytopenia or disorders of plasmatic coagulation. In order to prevent intracerebral hemorrhages administration of thrombolytic therapy should be safe, efficacious and controlled without diagnostic difficulties.

Patients` characteristics and hemostaseologic parameters

We report two patients with thrombophilic diathesis and diffuse thrombosis of cerebral sinuses.

A 28 year old man with newly diagnosed acute T-lymphoblastic leukemia presented mediastinal lymphoma. Supraclavicular and cervical swelling were caused by partial thrombosis of the left subclavian vein, superior caval vein, and jugular veins, respectively. Central venous line had been placed via right subclavian vein. Chemotherapy with cyclophosphamide, high-dose steroids, doxorubicin and vincristine was performed day 1–15. Peg-asparaginase 1000 IE/m^2 was administered intravenously day 11. After asparaginase administration thrombosis of jugular veins as well as cerebral sinuses proceeded despite severe thrombocytopenia.

The patient presented severe granulocytopenia < 0.5 Gpt/l and thrombocytopenia < 20 Gpt/l day 11. Heparin had been administered for 7 days in order to adjust aPTT (80 seconds) but was stopped when platelet count was <50 Gpt/l. Despite heparin therapy there was a progress of thrombosis. Neither thrombectomy nor systemic lysis could be performed due to complex coagulation disorders.

The patient presented epileptic convulsion. Computed tomography revealed complete thrombosis of cavernosus sinus and all basal cerebral veins and profuse intracerebral hemorrhage frontotemporal reaching third and lateral ventricle.

I. Scharrer/W. Schramm (Ed.)
32nd Hemophilia Symposion Hamburg 2001
© Springer-Verlag Berlin Heidelberg 2003

There was no way to diminish cerebral compression other than multiple neuro-surgical interventions, partial resection of the calotte and implantation of a ventri-culo-peritoneal drainage.

Thrombophilic risk factors were heterozygotic factor V gene G1691A mutation and homozygotic C677T mutation of methylene-tetrahydrofolat-reductase-gene. APC-ratio was 1.4. Due to leukemic liver involvement and cytotoxic therapy low plasma concentrations of antithrombin III (51%), protein C (36%), protein S activity (40%) as well as F XII (70%) and fibrinogen (< 1g/l) were found. Hemorrhagic risk factors were thrombocytopenia IV and low plasma concentrations of almost all coagulation factors induced by chemotherapy.

The second patient was a 47 year old female presenting cerebral sinus thrombosis without any history of injury or surgery. Thrombosis occurred following viral infection and meningitis within a few days (Fig. 1).

Thrombophilic rsik factors were C 677 T mutation and low plasma concentrations of protein S. F V Leiden G1691A, MTHFR C677T or prothrombin G 20210A gene mutations were not found. As intracerebral pressure excessed despite anti-edematous medication, craniotomy had to be performed also in this patient.

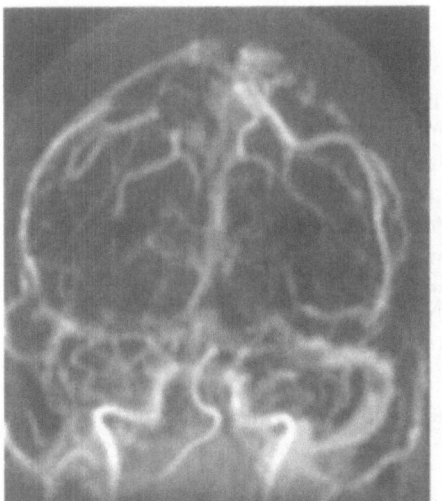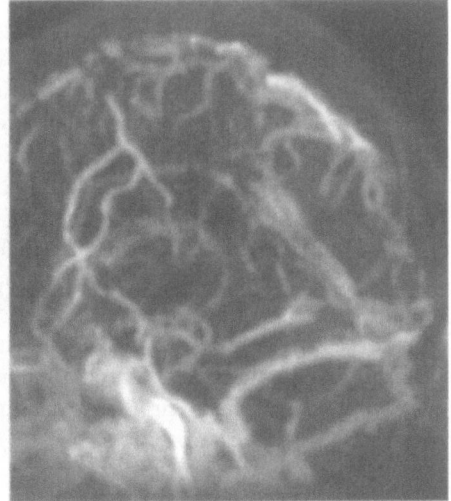

Fig. 1. Patient MN, 9.3.1954. Thrombosis of sinus sagittalis, sinus rectus, sinus cavernosus and sinus transversus (MR-angiography) 22/3/2001

Table 1. Patient MK, coagulation parameters during course of chemotherapy

	leuko-cytes Gpt/l	platelets Gpt/l	partial thromboplastin time %	aPTT sec	fibrinogen g/l	ATIII %	D-dimer mg/l
admission	23.2	132	89	23	3.3	114	
day 16	1.3	33	46	64	0.5	51	0.57

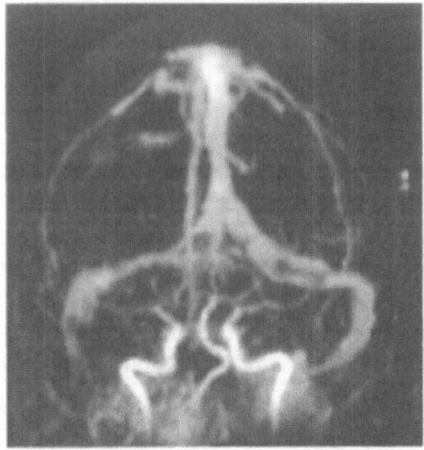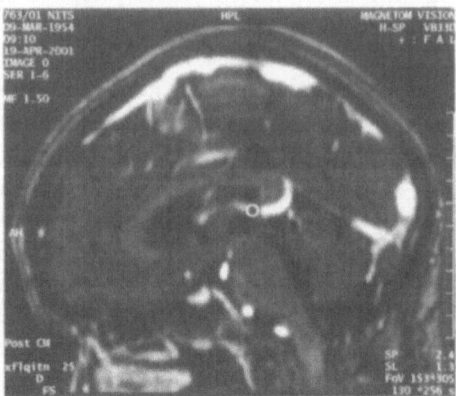

Fig. 2. Patient MN, 9.3.1954. Recanalization of cerebral sinus thrombosis after 4 weeks of dalteparin treatment (MR-angiography) 19/4/2001

Dalteparin therapy

After initial bolus injection (5 IU/kg body weight iv) we administered dalteparin 5 IU/kg body weight / hour as continuous intravenous infusion. Dosage was administered in order to adjust anti-Xa plasma concentrations to 0.4–0.6 IU/ml. Low molecular weight (LMW) heparin was administered because of its higher thrombolytic activity compared to non-fractionated heparin or cumarin [5]. In Germany dalteparin is the only LMW heparin approved for intravenous administration.

Continuous infusion was performed for 75 days in the leukemic patient and for 40 days in the female patient with meningeal infection, respectively. As recanalization progressed cumarin therapy could be administered to her for further 9 months after successful intravenous LMW heparin administration (Fig. 2).

In the leukemic patient subcutaneous administration of dalteparin was continued for 2 years as cumarin therapy did not seem to be applicable concerning seizures and possible trauma.

Results

In both patients almost complete recanalisation of cerebral sinus as well as jugular veins were seen without any hemorrhagic complications. Neurological symptoms improved significantly after two months of therapy.

In the leukemic patient (MK) intracerebral pressure normalized and ventriculoperitoneal drainage could be implanted after 6 weeks of dalteparin therapy. Thrombosis of sinus cavernosus, suclavian and cervical veins resolved slowly. Magnetic resonance (MR) angiography 6 months after onset of thrombosis presented recanalization of sinus rectus and almost complete lysis of thrombosis of the left sinus transversus.

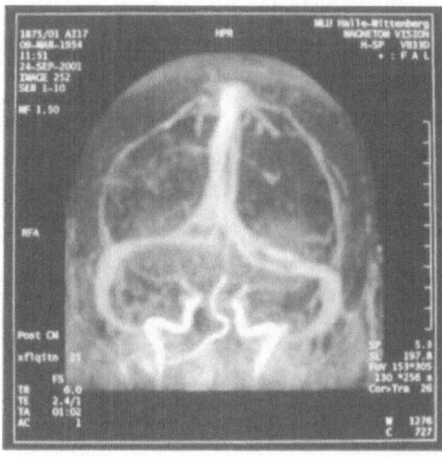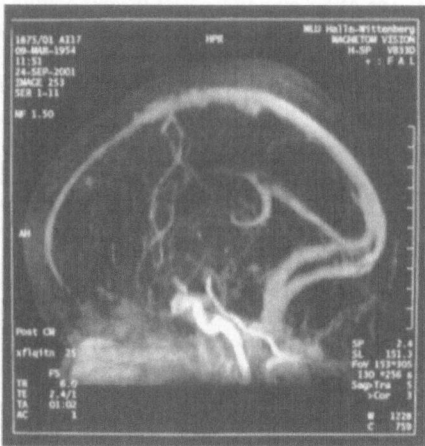

Fig. 3. Patient MN, 9.3.1954. Almost complete recanalization of cerebral sinus thrombosis after months of dalteparin treatment (MR-angiography) 23/9/2001

Finally, cerebral veins were recanalized. Neurologic residues are incomplete hemiparesis, motoric aphasia, and mental disorders as well as posttraumatic epilepsia.

In the female patient (MN) there are no significant neurologic residues after a 12 months therapy. MR angiography presented normal contrast of all cerebral veins (Fig. 3).

Conclusions

We conclude that continuous intravenous infusion of dalteparin provides high fibrinolytic activity and may be an adequat therapy of sinus thrombosis even in patients with high risk for cerebral bleeding. Plasma concentrations of dalteparin were adjusted to 0.4–0.6 IU/ml for at least 6 weeks. There were no difficulties in dosaging of anticoagulation.

Intravenous application of dalteparin seems to be safe and efficacious even in patients with high risks for hemorrhagic complications due to hematologic disorders and impaired plasmatic coagulation.

References

1. Alberts SR, Bretscher M, J.C. W, O'Niell BP, B. M, Witzig TE. Thrombosis related to the use of L-asparaginase in adults with acute lymphoblastic leukemia: a need to consider coagulation monitoring and clotting factor replacement. Leuk Lymphoma. 1999;32:489–496
2. Castaman G, F. R, Dini E. Thrombotic complications during L-asparaginase treatment for acute lymphocytic leukemia. Haemetologica. 1990;75:567–569
3. Feinberg WM, Swenson MR. Cerebrovascular complications of L-asparaginase therapy. Neurology. 1988;38:127–133

4. Lee AYY, Levine MN. The thrombophilic state induced by therapeutic agents in the cancer patient. Semin Thromb Haemostasis. 1999;25:137–145
5. Reddingius RE, Patte C, Couanet D, Kalifa C, Lemerle J. Dural sinus thrombosis in children with cancer. Med Pediatr Ocol. 1997;29:296–302
6. Parma M, Belotti D, Pgliani EM. Management of L-asparaginase induced prothrombotic state in acute lymphoblastic leukemia. Haematologica. 1996;81:191

VIb. *Hemophilia*
and Hemorrhagic Disorders

Treatment of FVIII-Autoantibodies by Protein A-based Immunoadsorption and Immunosuppression: A Regimen without FVIII Substitution

U. Geisen, R. Grossmann, B. Mansouri-Taleghani, C.M. Schambeck, M. Böck, and U. Walter

Introduction

There are two main goals in the treatment of acquired FVIII-inhibitors: first, to control acute bleeding episodes and second, to induce immune tolerance (IT). For the induction of IT mainly immunosuppressive drugs are given (e.g. cortico-steroids, cyclophosphamide). As part of the »Malmö treatment protocol« (MTP) and its modifications they are combined with immunoadsorptions (IA), intra-venous immunoglobulins (IVIG) and the causative antigen, i.e. FVIII. The appli-cation of FVIII in huge doses for immune modulation is associated with very high costs and therefore there is still an important question: *Is a FVIII substitution really mandatory?*

Patients and Methods

4 patients with FVIII-autoantibodies were treated (1 female, 3 males; age *63, 54, 27 and 67* years rsp.). The initial inhibitor titers were 128, 6, 222 and 3 BU/ml rsp. We used a therapeutic approach, which included a modified MTP with removal of FVIII inhibitors by extracorporeal protein-A-adsorptions (Immunosorba™, Excorim AB, Lund, Sweden), cyclophosphamide and/or corticosteroids/azathioprin (initially i.v., later on orally applied) and IVIG 0.4 g/kg (post IAs). A FVIII substitution was not part of this regimen.

Results

Treatment courses are shown in Figure 1–4. All patients achieved a complete, still ongoing remission. No FVIII concentrates were given. No bleeding complications were observed. One patient (described in Fig. 4) showed a herpes zoster infection. In all patients, IT was reached during intensified treatment periods comprising up to 4 serial (i.e. daily applied) IAs.

I. Scharrer/W. Schramm (Ed.)
32nd Hemophilia Symposion Hamburg 2001
© Springer-Verlag Berlin Heidelberg 2003

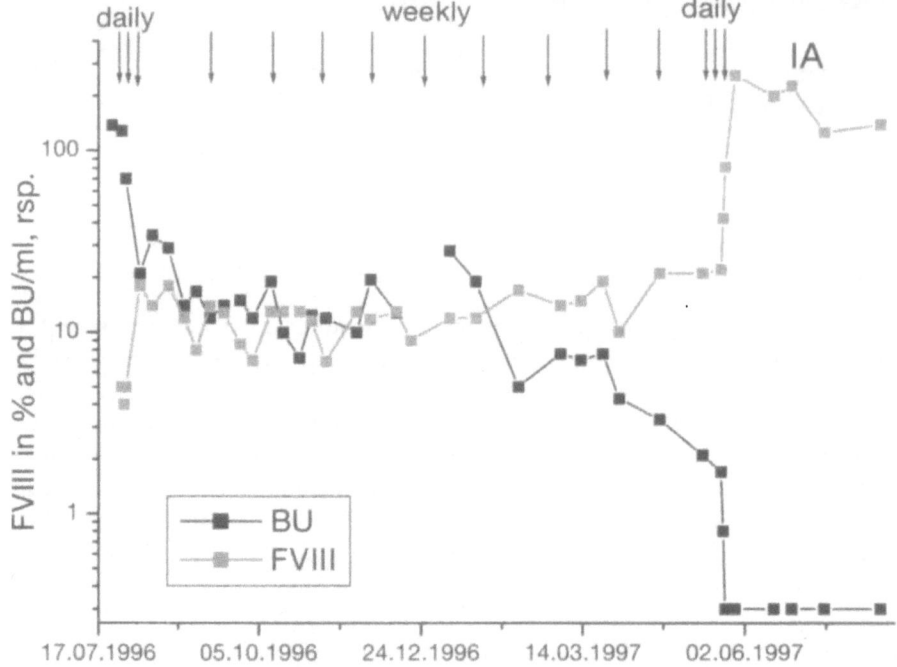

Fig. 1. 63 year old patient, 128 BU/ml.

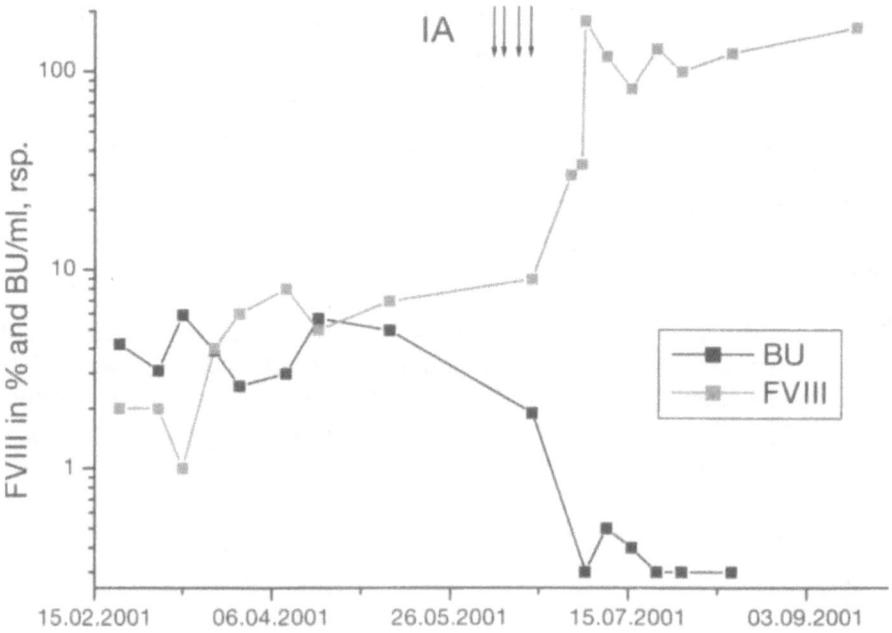

Fig. 2. 54 year old patient, 6 BU/ml.

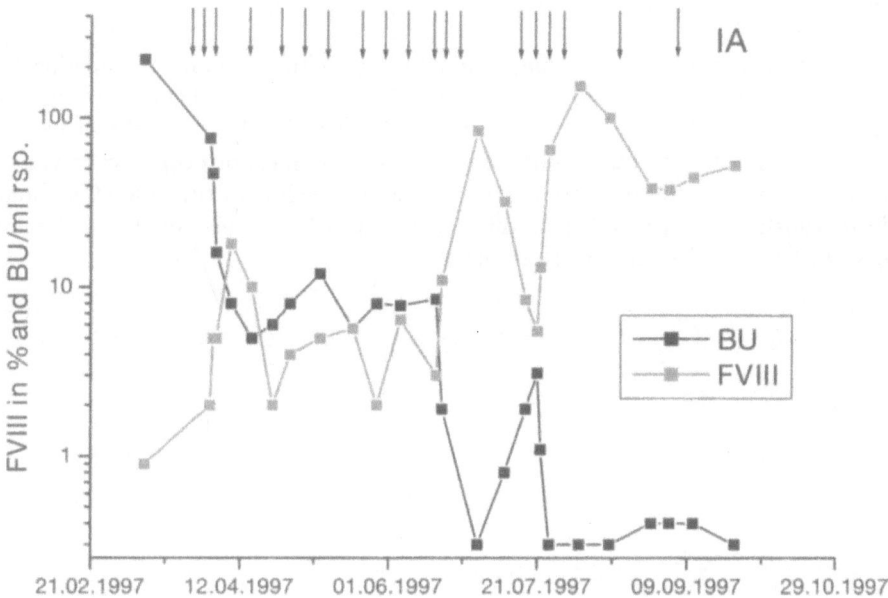

Fig. 3. 27 year old patient, 222 BU/ml.

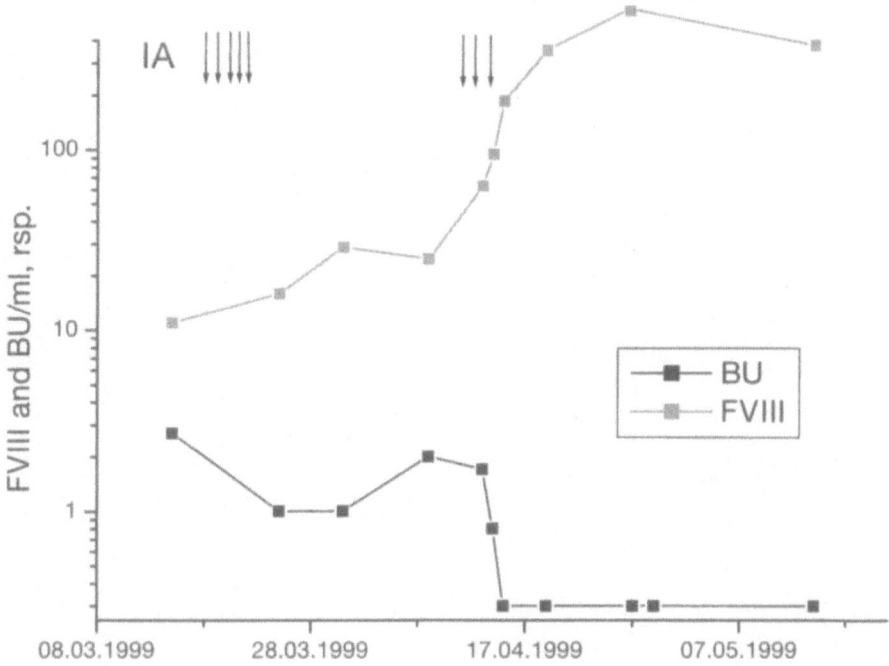

Fig. 4. 67 year old patient, 3 BU/ml.

Discussion

Immune tolerance could be achieved in all cases without immune modulation by FVIII substitution, leading to high cost-effectiveness. It seems, that a more aggressive treatment regimen, e.g. comprising several series of daily IAs, might lead more rapidly to IT. Nevertheless, one has to keep an eye on infectious complications due to a distinct immunosuppression and the risk of bleeding during a MTP without FVIII-substitution. The value of this regimen can be defined only in carefully designed, randomized multicenter-trials.

Factor XI Deficiency caused by a hitherto unknown Mutation in the Factor XI Gene

B. Maak, F. Bergmann, L. Kochhan, and Ch. Estel

Introduction

In 1953, Rosenthal et al. [14] described a new hemophilia-like bleeding disorder. In contrast to the true hemophilias, the newly detected coagulation defect was present in males and females. Moreover, in mixing experiments the observed defect could be corrected by blood specimens obtained from patients with both forms of hemophilia. The authors designated the presumably missing factor as „plasma thromboplastin antecedent" (PTA), which is today known as coagulation factor XI.

The factor XI deficiency is a rare defect in most populations worldwide, among the patients registered in the hemophilia treatment centers in the UK only 5% are factor XI deficient [4]. However, a very high prevalence rate of the factor XI deficiency exists in the population of the Ashkenazi Jews. Seligsohn [15] reported a frequency of 1 : 190 for the severe factor XI deficiency (homozygotes or compound-heterozygotes) and calculated a confidence limit for the heterozygous state of factor XI deficiency between 5.5 and 11%.

The disorder is inherited as an autosomal recessive trait [13]. The gene coding for the factor XI protein is located on the long arm of chromosome 4 (4 q 35) [6]. Up to now, more than 30 mutations are characterized [1, 2, 5, 7, 8, 11, 17, 19, 20] for the deficiency of factor XI among the Ashkenazi Jews only four different mutations are responsible [2, 12].

Spontaneous bleeding events are very uncommon, patients with a severe factor XI-deficiency exhibit bleedings in the most cases after surgical procedures or injuries [15]. Heterozygous individuals with factor XI-activities of more than 15 per

---

Abbreviations used:

PT	prothrombin time
aPTT	activated partial thromboplastin time
aPC	activated protein C
vWF:Ag	von-Willebrand factor antigen
vWF:RiCoF	von-Willebrand factor – ristocetin cofactor activity
vWF:CBA	von-Willebrand factor collagen binding activity

I. Scharrer/W. Schramm (Ed.)
32nd Hemophilia Symposion Hamburg 2001
© Springer-Verlag Berlin Heidelberg 2003

cent may have bleeding problems [3, 4]. In the family investigated by Litz et al. [9] there were bleeding patients with factor XI activities between 15 and 41% and nonbleeding individuals with practically the same range of activity (15 to 58%).

The reason for this different behaviour is not fully understood as yet. The type of mutation in the factor XI gene alone seems not to be responsible. The results of one study suggests the coexistence of factor XI deficiency and von-Willebrand's disease in bleeding patients [16]. In another study an increased frequency of von-Willebrand's disease among patients with factor XI deficiency could not be demonstrated but patients with bleeding symptoms tended to have lower values of von-Willebrand factor and also of factor VIII activity in comparison with patients without bleeding symptoms [4].

We describe here the results of our study of a symptomatic woman and her family members. The woman reported a life-long bleeding tendency and a mild factor XI deficiency (XI : C = 52 %) could be detected. As the cause of the factor XI deficiency we identified a hitherto unknown mutation in the factor XI gene. This mutation is located in exon 7 and responsible for an exchange of Arg 210 to Gln in the third apple domain of the factor XI molecule. In the family, individuals with a bleeding tendency exist. However, there are also members with the mutation and reduced factor XI activity who are asymptomatic.

Material and methods

Patient and family members

The patient, a 46 year old woman, blood group A, rhesus positive (II/2, Fig. 1) reported a life-long bleeding tendency. Only mild traumatic events are regularly followed by large cutaneous hematomas. Menstrual blood loss was strong during the day 1–6 and after an interval of three days oozing persists for several days. After dental extractions bleeding occurred after an interval of a few hours and persisted for the next 12 to 15 hours. Cholecystectomy and cesarean section were followed by massive intraabdominal blood losses with the consequence of surgical intervention. In the case of the cesarean section the bleeding occurred at the time of surgery and continued for more than two weeks.

The patients daughter (III/2, Fig. 1) reported easy bruising and a marked menstrual blood loss during day 1–6. After the introduction of an oral contraceptive treatment the menstrual blood loss decreased. The spontaneous vaginal delivery of her baby (IV/1, Fig. 1) was followed by an excessive bleeding. This child, a three year old girl, is in good health. However, her mother believes that a tendency to easy bruising may exist. The second child (III/1) of the patient was a victim of a traffic accident and therefore not available for investigation.

All other family members of the proposita reported no spontaneous bleedings or bleeding complications after dental or gynecological surgery (hysterectomy).

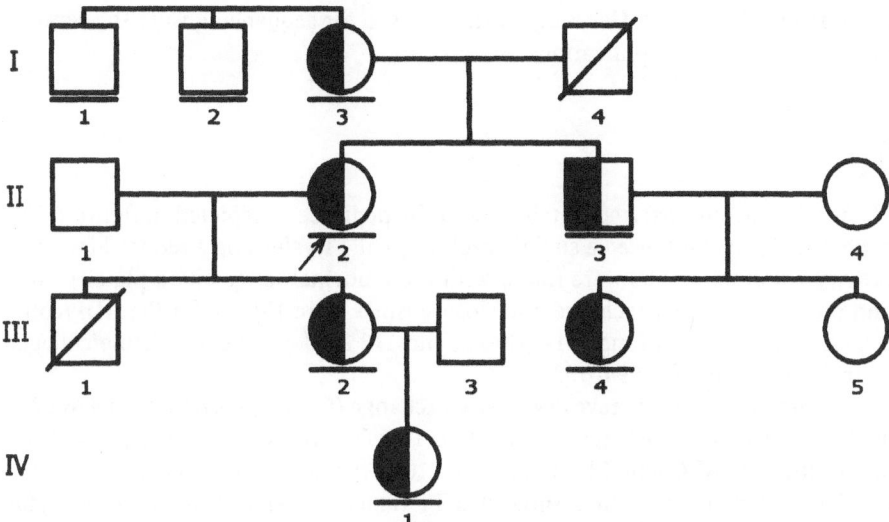

Fig. 1. Pedigree of the family. The arrow denotes the patient. Underlined symbols: Mutation analysis performed. Half-filled symbols indicate the heterozygous state for the mutation detected. Deceased individuals are characterized by a diagonal line through the boxes. Generations are indicated by roman numerals.

Coagulation tests

Blood was taken from an antecubital vein using a commercially available device (BD vacutainer). Nine parts of blood were carefully mixed with one part of 0.129 m trinatrium citrate solution. Thromboplastin time (PT, Quick value) and activated partial thromboplastin time (aPTT) were measured with an automated device. The fibrinogen content was determined as so-called derived fibrinogen during the PT assay. Coagulation factor assays were performed as clotting tests with specifically deficient plasmas according to the instructions given by the manufacturer. Antithrombin was estimated by a colorimetric assay. The APC-resistance was determined with an aPTT-based reagent kit. All reagents for the coagulation assays were purchased from IL. The concentration of von-Willebrand factor (vWF:Ag) was assayed by an ELISA kit (Bio-Merieux). Platelet function was tested with the PFA 100 device (Dade-Behring).

Genomic analysis

Total DNA of all patients was extracted from whole blood using micro spin columns (Quiagen, Hilden, Germany). Exons of the factor XI gene were amplified by polymerase chain reaction (PCR) using primers and conditions previously described [10]. Cycle sequencing was performed using the Big Dye Terminator Cycle Sequenzing kit (Perkin Elmer Applied Biosystems, Foster City, USA) and analyzed using an automated DNA sequenzer (ABI PRISM/377 DNA Sequencer, Applied

Biosystems, Weiterstadt, Germany). Primers used for sequencing were the same as those used for PCR amplification.

Results

The results are summarized in table 1 and the pedigree is depicted in figure 1. The patient (II/2, Fig. 1) showed a slightly prolonged aPTT value and a reduced factor XI activity. All other results were found within the normal range and a platelet function disorder was also excluded, the closure times were 101 sec for the ADP/collagen cartridge (normal range 71–118 sec) and 112 sec for the epinephrine/collagen cartridge (normal range 94–193 sec).

The genomic analysis revealed a base exchange (CGA → CAA) within exon 7 of the factor XI gene in the heterozygous state. This G → A transition is responsible for the substitution of Arg by Gln in position 210 of the factor XI molecule.

Five relatives of the patient showed aPTT values between 30 and 43 seconds, the factor XI activities of these persons ranged from 41 to 67 per cent and the same mutation in the factor XI gene was demonstrated. No further abnormal values of the coagulation system were present and the screening for antithrombotic factors (APC resistance, antithrombin activity) revealed normal results. Two uncles of the patient (I/1 and I/2, Fig. 1) showed normal aPTT values and factor XI activities of more than 100 % and the mutation in the factor XI gene was absent in both. The patient and her daughter showed bleeding symptoms, while in the case of the patients granddaughter a clear cut bleeding tendency can't be confirmed with certainty up to now. All family members with factor XI deficiency who bleed have von-Willebrand factor (vWF:Ag) values between 79 and 84 % in contrast to the nonbleeders with the factor XI mutation who have vWF:Ag values from 106 and 117 %.

Discussion

We present here the history and the results of coagulation studies and genomic analysis of a 46 year old woman with a lifelong bleeding tendency. Additionally, the results of the family investigation are demonstrated.

In the patient a mild factor XI deficiency exists. The analysis of her factor XI gene revealed a base exchange (CGA → CAA) within the exon 7. All other family members with a reduced factor XI activity exhibit the same genetic constellation, i.e. the heterozygous state of the above mentioned change in the factor XI gene. In contrast, in the persons with a normal factor XI activity this G → A transition is missing. Therefore we believe that the transition represents a mutation which is responsible for the reduced factor XI activity. Up to now, more than 30 different mutations in the factor XI gene are known (1, 2, 5, 7, 8, 11, 17, 19, 20). However, this type is not reported yet.

The amino acid exchange is located in the third apple domain of the factor XI molecule, a region which is needed for the binding of factor IX, the natural substrate

Table 1. Results of the coagulation studies and mutation analysis in the family with factor XI deficiency

	PT [%]	aPTT [sec]	XI:C [%]	Mutation factor XI-Gene	XII:C [%]	VII:C [%]	vWF-Ag [%]	APC ratio	AT III [%]	Fibrinogen [g/l]	Bleeding tendency
II/2	104	37	52	present	78	80	84	2.65	119	2.8	+
I/1	94	35	104	absent	125	78	81	2.30	102	2.9	–
I/2	96	34	103	absent	96	93	103	2.35	89	2.4	–
I/3	n.b.	35	47	present	n.d.	63	117	n.d.	n.d.	n.d.	–
II/3	n.b.	34	50	present	n.d.	87	106	n.d.	n.d.	n.d.	–
III/2	107	30	63	present	150	79	79	2.20	88	2.01	+
III/4	77	42	41	present	75	64	63	2.35	109	3.0	–
IV/1	113	43	67	present	102	89	80	2.55	112	3.9	(+)
Normal-values	70–120	25–35	70–150	absent	70–150	70–150	50–150	>2.0	75–120	1.8–4.5	

n.d. – not determined

of factor XI (18). Two further mutations in close vicinity to the amino acid exchange Arg 210 → Gln have been described: Gln → Arg exchange in position 226 [10] and a Trp 228 → Cys exchange [1]. Interestingly, the patient of Alhaq et al. [1], a 68 year old woman, presented with a cerebral thrombosis and had never demonstrated any bleeding signs.

In the family presented here there are bleeders and non-bleeders. The patient, her daughter and possibly also her granddaughter are bleeders. The vWF:Ag concentrations in these persons were estimated between 79 and 84 per cent and in the patient type 1 vWD was ruled out by multimeric analysis of vW factor. The patients mother and her brother who have never had bleeding episodes show vWF:Ag values of 117 and 106 per cent. This difference is in the same magnitude as the values reported by Bolton-Maggs et al. [4]. However, this behaviour of vWF:Ag is not sufficient to explain the missing bleeding tendency in the patient's niece (III/4, Fig. 1). We can speculate only that the young girl did not pass any risk situations (surgery, dental surgery) which might have challenged her coagulation system.

Another explanation for the different bleeding tendency within the family may be that the individuals without bleeding symptoms have normal amounts of platelet factor XI. However, investigations to test this hypothesis could not be performed.

It should be noted that the bleeding episodes of the patient were misdiagnosed in the past, for example as a platelet function defect. Repeatedly found mildly prolonged aPTT values were misinterpreted. Therefore, in such cases we recommend also factor XI estimations besides the testing of other coagulation factor activities. On the other hand, as can be seen from the summary of the results (Table 1), not all family members with proven factor XI deficiency show abnormal aPTT values. This finding is in agreement with the statement of Seligsohn [15] that the aPTT assay is not always suitable for the detection of patients with a heterozygous factor XI deficiency.

The factor XI activities in our heterozygous individuals ranged between 41 and 67 per cent. This observation confirms the results of Bolton-Maggs et al. [4] for heterozygous factor XI deficient patients, who pointed out that the lower limit of the normal range of the factor XI activity should be set at 70 per cent.

To predict any bleeding tendency in factor XI deficient individuals an extended coagulation analysis is necessary, including the components of the von-Willebrand complex, i.e. vWF:Ag, vWF:RiCoF, vWF:CBA and factor VIII activity should be tested. Low normal activities or concentrations of these components in patients with reduced factor XI activity point to an increased risk of bleeding complications after trauma or surgery, especially if tissues with a high fibrinolytic capacity are involved.

Summary

We report on a 46 year old woman with a lifelong bleeding tendency. A mildly prolonged aPTT value was explained as the result of a reduced factor XI activity. As the cause of the lowered factor XI activity we identified a CGA → CAA transition in exon 7 of the factor XI gene which results in an amino acid exchange Arg → Gln in position 210 of the factor XI molecule. In five family members with reduced factor XI activities between 41 and 67%, the mutation was also present. In two individuals from the same family the factor XI activity was normal (103 and 104%) and the above mentioned hitherto unknown mutation was not detectable.

The family members with reduced factor XI activity who bleed tend to have lower concentrations of vWF:Ag than the other individuals with reduced factor XI activity who are asymptomatic.

References

1. Alhaq A, Mitchel M, Sehti M, Rahman S, Flynn G, Boulton P, Caeno G, Smith M, Savidge G (1999) Identification of a novel mutation in a non-jewish factor XI deficient kindred. Brit J Haematol 104: 44–49
2. Asakai R, Chung D W, Ratnoff O D, Davie E W (1989) Factor XI (plasma thromboplastin antecedent) deficiency in Ashkenazi jews is a bleeding disorder that can result from three types of point mutations. Proc Natl Acad Sci USA 86: 7667–7671
3. Bolton-Maggs P H B, Young Wan-Yin B, Mc Craw A H, Slack J, Kernoff P B A (1988) Inheritance and bleeding in factor XI deficiency. Brit J Haematol 69: 521–528
4. Bolton-Maggs P H B, Patterson D A, Wensley R T, Tuddenham E G D (1995) Definition of the bleeding tendency in factor XI-deficient kindreds–clinical and laboratory study. Thromb Haemostas 73: 194–202
5. Gailani D, Bolton-Maggs P H B, Blinder M, Butler R, Mountford R, Heiny M, Dang T (2001) Amino acid substitutions in the factor XI catalytic domain associated with factor XI deficiency. Suppl Thromb Haemostas P 1112
6. Kato A, Asakai R, Davie E W, Aoki N (1989) Factor XI gene (F 11) is located on the distal end of the long arm of chromosome 4. Cytogenet Cell Genet 52: 77–78
7. Kraiijenhagen R A, Gerdes V E A, Vogels E W M, ten Cate H, Büller H R, Reitsma P H (2001) Factor XI gene analysis in thrombophilia and factor XI deficiency. Suppl Thromb Haemostas OC 167
8. Lex C, Kochhan L, Irsfeld H, Göbel U (2001): Identification of a novel mutation causing factor XI deficiency in a turkish family. Suppl Thromb Haemostas P 1144
9. Litz C E, Swaim W R, Dalmasso A P (1988) Factor XI deficiency: genetic and clinical studies of a single kindred. Am J Hematol 28: 8–12
10. Martincic D, Zimmerman S A, Ware R E, Sun M, Whitlock I A, Gailani D (1998) Identification of mutations and polymorphisms in the factor XI genes of an African-American family by dideoxyfingerprinting. Blood 92: 3309–3317 [Erratum (1999) Blood 93: 1786]
11. Mitchell M, Cutler J, Thompson S, Moore G, Jenkins Ap Rees E, Smith M, Savidge G, Alhaq A (1999) Heterozygous factor XI deficiency associated with three novel mutations. Brit J Haematol 107: 763–765
12. Peretz H, Zivelin A, Usher S, Seligsohn U (1996) A 14-bp deletion (codon 554 del AAGgtaacagagtg) at exon 14 / intron N junction of the coagulation factor XI gene disrupts splicing and causes severe factor XI deficiency. Human Mutation 8: 77–78.
13. Rapaport S I, Procter R R, Patch M J, Yetta M (1961) The mode of inheritance of PTA deficiency: evidence for the existence of major PTA deficiency and minor PTA deficiency. Blood 18: 149–165
14. Rosenthal R L, Dreskin O H, Rosenthal N (1953) New hemophilia-like disease caused by deficiency of a third plasma thromboplastin factor. Proc Soc Exp Biol Med 82: 171–174
15. Seligsohn U (1993) Factor XI deficiency. Thromb Haemostas 70: 68–71

16. Tavori S, Brenner B, Tatarsky I (1990) The effect of combined factor XI deficiency with von Willebrand factor abnormalities on haemorrhagic diathesis. Thromb Haemostas 63: 36–38.
17. Ventura C, Santos A I M, Tavares A, Gago T, Larinha J, Mc Vey J H, David D (2000) Molecular genetic analysis of factor XI deficiency: Identification of five novel gene alterations and the origin of type II mutation in Portuguese families. Thromb Haemostas 83: 833–840.
18. Walsh P N (1999) Platelets and factor XI bypass the contact system of blood coagulation. Thromb Haemostas 82: 234–242.
19. Zivelin A, Bauduer F, Yatuv R, Kornbrot N, Ifrah A, Peretz, H, Ducont L, Seligsohn U (2001) Cys 38 Arg substitution in the factor XI gene impairs secretion of factor XI and is the main mutation causing factor XI deficiency in Basques. Suppl Thromb Haemostas P 1110
20. Zivelin A, Yatuv R, Livnat T, Bulvik S, Peretz H, Salomon O, Seligsohn U (2001) Severe factor XI deficiency caused by a Gly 555 Glu mutation encodes for a cross reacting material positive factor XI. Suppl Thromb Haemostas P 1111

Polymorphisms in FV Gene associated with FV Deficiency – First Results

W. Schröder, and F.H. Herrmann

Introduction

Coagulation factor V plays an important role in maintaining the hemostatic balance in both the formation of thrombin in the procoagulant pathway as well as in the protein C anticoagulant pathway.

Coagulation factor V as well as FVIII do not possess catalytic activity per se. Once activated FVa is an essential cofactor for the serine protease F Xa. FXa, in presence of Ca^{2+} ions, combines with FVa on the membrane of activated platelets to form a macromolecular complex (prothrombinase) that converts prothrombin to thrombin.

Cloning and characterization of the human FV gene [1, 2] made it possible to infer the primary structure of the protein and to recognize its domain organization. The FV gene spans over 80kb and comprises 25 exons and 24 introns. The predicted native polypeptide encompasses 2224 AA, the first 28 representing a typical signal sequence. The structure is almost identical to that of the FVIII gene. Three A domains, one B domain, and two C domains are coded. Combining physical mapping data (southern hybridization to somatic cell hybrid DNA [3] and in situ hybridization: [4]) and linkage data McAlpine et al [5] concluded that F5 lies in the 1q23 band.

Factor V deficiency

FV deficiency firstly has been described by the Norwegian physician Owren in 1947 [6]. It is a rare bleeding disorder with variable phenotypic expression. About the molecular basis underlying this disease little is known. Zehnder et al. [7] pointed out that homozygous factor V deficiency (OMIM *227400) is rare, approximately 1 in 1 million. On this basis, heterozygotes should have a frequency of 1 in 1,000. It is characterized by reduced FV antigen and /or activity. A classification of different FV deficiencies has been proposed recently.

Classical factor V deficiency (Owren parahemophilia)

Classical factor V deficiency results in simultaneous prolongation of the prothrombin time (PT) and activated partial thromboplastin time (APPT). However, specific diagnosis relies on measurement of FV activity and antigen. Most FV deficient patients show a parallel reduction of FV:C and FV:Ag (type I). Some patients have a

I. Scharrer/W. Schramm (Ed.)
32nd Hemophilia Symposion Hamburg 2001
© Springer-Verlag Berlin Heidelberg 2003

FV:C level significantly lower than FV:Ag, suggesting a synthesis of dysfunctional FV molecule (Type II). Heterozygotes usually have plasma FV levels about 50%, homozygotes about 5%. Parahemophilia is inherited in an autosomal recessive trait within families. Heterozygous deficiency states are generally unrecognized because of a lack of significant clotting time prolongation or bleeding risk.

Platelet factor V deficiency (FV Quebec)

More rare is the autosomal dominant Platelet factor V deficiency (FV Quebec) with a mild thrombocytopenia and moderate reduction of the FV level (30–40%). Platelet FV has an very low activity (2–4%) in spite an normal antigen was detected. Up to now, FV Quebec has been described only in 2 non related French-Canadian families.

Combined FV-FVIII deficiency

In combined FV-FVIII deficiency FV and FVIII levels are reduced to 5–30% of normal, resulting in a bleeding tendency. This disease is inherited as an autosomal-recessive trait, the locus has been mapped at chromosome 18q21. The responsible gene has been detected and found to encode an transmembrane protein (ERGIC-53) involved in FV and FVIII trafficking from the ER to the Golgi apparatus.

Molecular variants in the FV gene

The molecular basis of classical FV deficiency is still largely unexplored as the condition is extremely rare and often asymptomatic. Since the first report only a few intragenic mutations have been described, mostly private. Because of the size of the gene a sequence analysis is expensive. Due to the lack of significant clotting time prolongation or bleeding risk it can be assumed that some mutations have no disadvantage for their carriers and therefore could have maintained in the population. Therefore we supposed that their polymorphisms in the factor V gene might have accumulated which modulate the activity or antigen level of the FV protein.

A correlation between the R2 allele of the FV HR2 haplotype and slightly reduced FV activity was reported by Lunghi et al. [8], de Visser et al. [9] and Hoekema et al. [10]. The factor V *haplotype HR2* described by Bernardi [11] is characterized by five polymorphic markers in exon 13 and one polymorphic marker in exon 16. All this polymorphisms are in a strong linkage disequilibrium. Thus the characterization of only one of them, the polymorphism FV 4070 A/G, predicting the replacement of His[1299] by Arg in the B-domain, is sufficient for the determination of this haplotype. The less frequent G-allele is called R2, the haplotype HR2 respectively. The allele frequency of this haplotype is about 7.3%–9.5% in the German population [12, 13].

Three further molecular variants which should be responsible for lowered FV activities/antigen levels have been described previously ([14] and pers. communication): the variant *R 712 stop* (*2308 C->T, exon 13*, B domain), *Glu 1608 Lys* (4996 G->A, exon 14, A3 domain) and *Tyr 1702 Cys* (5279 A->G, exon 15, A3 domain). Castoldi et al. [14] reported this variants several times in FV deficient patients from Italy with severe FV deficiency as well as with asymptomatic reduced FV levels.

We screened DNA probes of 14 FV deficient patients and 100 anonymous German blood donors for all four molecular variants in the FV gene. Additionally the FV Leiden mutation has been determined.

Material and methods

Patients

14 patients with factor V deficiency from different centers have been included in the study. Most of them but not all were of German origin. Seven of them had FV activities of about 50%, in one case an FV activity of about 20% was reported, 2 had an activity of about 10%. In 3 cases the activity was not known. Most of them were asymptomatic. Two patients with an FV residual activity of 50% had a thrombosis. Only in one case prolonged bleeding after tooth extraction was evident.

100 anonymous German blood donors were included in the study as a control group.

Methods

DNA from patients and controls was extracted from blood lymphocytes by standard method (salting out method [15]).

All polymorphisms and allelic variants – FV 4070 A/G (HR2), 2308 C/T, 4996 G/A, 5279 A/G and FV Leiden – have been detected by PCR and restriction analysis as described elsewhere [8,14, 16, Castoldi pers. communication].

Results and Discussion

The allele frequencies of the FV variants characterized in patients and controls are summarized in Table 1.

Arg 712 stop seems not to play a role in the German population studied. This variant was neither found in the patients nor in the control group. All Italian patients described came from the same region in Italy (Venetia) and had the same haplotype of exon 13 concerning 4 other polymorphisms in this exon. Although the patients were no relatives a common ancestor is discussed. Due to the missing clinical relevance this mutation could have spread in this population like a neutral variant.

An association of *HR2* and lower FV activity/level has been reported previously [8, 9]. In our patients group the allele frequency of the R2-allele is higher than in the control, but this difference it is not yet significant probably due to the low numbers of probands.

Tab. 1. Allele frequencies of the 4070 G (R2)-, 2308 T-, 4996 G-, 5279 G- and 1691 A-allele in patients with FV deficiency and controls

Variant	4070 A/G (ex 13)	2308 C/T (ex 13)	4996 G/A (ex 14)	5279 A/G (Ex 15)	FV Leiden
Mutant allele frequency	4070 G (R2)	2308 T	4996 G	5279 G	1691 A
Control (n=95)	0.076 (14/95)	0.00 (0/95)	0.001 (2/95)	0.021 (4/94)	0.031 (6/95)
Patients (n=14)	0.107 (3/14)	0.00 (0/14)	0.107 (3/14)	0.071 (2/14)	0.071 (2/14)
Controls Italy	0.075	0.00 (0/50)	no data	0.002 (1/252)	0.013
Patients Italy	0.308	0.04 (3/36)	no data	0.037 (5/66)	no data

One patient with an FV activity of 21% was homozygote for the R2 haplotype, another (FV:C 53%) was heterozygote. Therefore we assume the R2-allele as one reason of FV deficiency in this patients. However, a second mutation has to be expected.

The *Glu 1608 Lys* (4996 G->A) has a significant lower frequency in the German controls compared to the patients (χ^2=8.3; p=0.004). 3 out of 14 probands with reduced FV activity were heterozygous for this mutation. Determination of the FV activity in the carriers of the variant in the control group as well as genotype/phenotype still have to be done to confirm the role of that variant in FV deficiency.

Tyr 1702 Cys: The 5279 G allele was found to be more frequent among the patients with FV deficiency. Whereas in Italy the allele frequency of the G-allele was reported to be significantly higher in the patients group, it is not significant different in our study probably due to the low number of probands in both groups. 2 of 14 patients were heterozygote for this mutation and 4 of 94 controls.

Both, the Glu 1608 Lys as well as the Tyr 1702 Cys mutations are located in the A3 domain in a region which is involved in the anchoring of FV to the phospholipid membrane. Thus the stability of the prothrombinase complex could be influenced by that mutations. Further investigations have to confirm it.

The variants characterized in the FV gene influence with a high probability the FV activity as it is known e.g. in FVII and XII. Further phenotype/genotype analyses and expression studies have to be done to verify that assumption.

Acknowledgements. We thank Prof. Bernardi and Elisabetta Castoldi (Ferrara) who initiated the search for frequent functional variants in the FV gene, which correlate with reduced FV levels and who made available data from Italian patients and primer sequences.

We have to thank our clinical partners who recruited the patients for their cooperation: Dr. Boer, Erfurt; Dr. v. Depka and Dr. Eisert, Hanover; Dr. Eifrig, Hamburg; Dr. Grundeis, Chemnitz; Prof. Konrad, Rostock; Prof. Kunze, Berlin; OA Dr.Lenk, Leipzig; Dr. Schobeß, Halle; Prof. Trobisch, Duisburg, and Dr. Wendisch, Dresden.

References

1. Kane WH, Davie EW. Cloning of a cDNA coding for human factor V, a blood coagulation factor homologous to factor VIII and ceruloplasmin. Proc Natl Acad Sci 1986; 83:6800–6804

2. Jenny RJ, Pittmann DD, Toole JJ, Kritz RW, Aldape RA, Hewick RM, Kaufmann RJ., Mann KG. Complete cDNA and derived amino acid sequence of human Factor V. Proc. Nat Acad Sci 1987; 84: 4846–4850

3. Wang H, Riddell DC, Guinto ER, MacGillivray RTA, Hamerton JL. Localization of the gene encoding human factor V to chromosome 1q21-25. Genomics 1988; 2:324–328

4. Dahlbäck B, Hansson C, Islam MQ, Szpirer J, Szpirer C, Lundwall A., Levan G. Assignment of gene for coagulation factor V to chromosome 1 in man and to chromosome 13 in rat. Somat. Cell Molec. Genet 14:509–514: 1988

5. McAlpine PJ, Coopland G, Guy C, James S, Komarnicki L, MacDonald M, Stranc L, Lewis M, Philipps S, Coghlan G, Kaita H, Cox DW, Guinto ER, MacGillivray R. Mapping the genes for erythrocytic alpha-spectrin 1(SPTA1) and coagulation factor V (F5): Cytogenet Cell Genet 1989; 51:1042

6. Owren P. Parahaemophilia: haemorrhagic diathesis due to absence of a previously unknown clotting factor. Lancet 1947; I: 446–448

7. Zehnder JL, Hiraki DD, Jones CD, Gross N, Grumet FC. Familial coagulation factor V deficiency caused by a novel 4 base pair insertion in the FV gene: factor V Stanford. Thomb Haemos. 1999; 82:1097–1099

8. Lunghi B, Iacovello L, Gemmati D, Di Iasio MG, Castoldi E, Pinotti M, Castaman G, Redaelli R, Mariani G, Bernardi F. Detection od new polymorphic markers in the factor V gene: Association with factor V levels in plasma. Thromb Haemost 1996; 75: 45–48

9. De Visser MCH, Guasch JF, Kamphuisen PW, Vos HL, Rosendaal FR, Bertina RM. The HR2 haplotype of factor V: Effects on FV levels, normalized activated protein C sensitivity ratios and the risk of venous thrombosis. Thromb Haemost 2000, 83:577–582

10. Hoekema L, Castoldi E, Tans G, Girelli D, Gemmati D, Bernardi F, Rosing J. Functional properties of factor V and Va encoded by the R2-gene. Thromb. Haemost. 2001; 85:75–81

11. Bernardi F, Faioni EM, Castoldi E, Lunghi B, Castaman G, Sacci E, Mannucci PM. A factor V genetic component differing from factor V R506Q contributes to the activated protein C resistant phenotype. Blood 1997; 90:1552–1557

12. Herrmann FH, Salazar-Sanchez L, Wulff K, Grimm, R, Schuster G, Jimmez-Aru G, Chavez M, Schröder, W. Prevalence of common mutations and polymorphisms of the genes of FII, FV, FVII, FXIII, MTHFR and ACE – identified as risk factors for venous and arterial thrombosis – in Germany and different ethnic groups (Indians, Blacks) of Costa Rica. In: Scharrer I., Schramm W (eds). 30th Hemophilia Symposion Hamburg 1999, Springer Verlag Berlin, Heidelberg 2001; 241–260

13. Kostka H, Siegert G, Schwarz T, Gehrisch S, Kuhlisch E, Schellong S, Jaross W. Frequency of polymorphisms in the B domain of factor V gene in APC-resistant patients. Thromb Res 2000; 99:539–547

14. Castoldi E, Lunghi B, Mingozzi F, Muleo G, Redaelli R, Mariani G, Bernardi F. A missense mutation (Y1702C) in coagulation factor V gene is a cause of FV deficiency in the Italian population. Haematologica 2001; 86:629–633

15. Miller SA, Dykes DD, Polesky HF. A simple salting out procedure for extracting DNA from human nucleated cells. Nucleic Acids Res 1988: 16: 1215

16. Bertina RM, Koeleman BPC, Koster T, Rosendaal FR, Dirven RJ, de Ronde H, van der Velden PA, Reitsma PH. Mutation in blood coagulation factor V associated to activated protein C. Nature 1994; 369:64–67

Influence of Phospholipids of the Platelet Membrane of Newborns on the Thrombin Generation

M. Petritsch, G. Cvirn, B. Leschnik, M. Köstenberger, and W. Muntean

Introduction

Newborns have despite of low clotting factors and an in vitro poor platelet function a good functioning hemostasis. The reason for that is still not completely clear. Platelet counts of healthy neonates are similar to those of normal adults, but their platelets react hyporesponsively to a variety of physiological agonists, resulting in decreased platelet activation and aggregation [1–4].

Like most eukaryotic cells blood platelets have an asymmetrical distribution of phospholipids over their plasma membrane. The aminophospholipid phosphatidyl-serine is normally restricted to the inner leaflet of the plasma membrane. Cell activation, apoptosis and cell stress can induce redistribution of phospholipids and phosphatidylserine becomes rapidly exposed in the outer leaflet of the plasma membrane [5].

In our study we investigated, whether a difference exists between the support of the thrombin generation through the phospholipids of the platelet membrane of newborns and that of adults.

Materials and Methods

Blood Sampling

Blood was collected from umbilical vein of neonates (gestational age > 32 weeks) and from healthy adults. Nine parts of blood were collected into one part of 0.1 molar citrate.

Preparation of Platelet-Rich Plasma, Platelet-Poor Plasma, and Washed Platelets

Platelet-rich plasma (PRP) was obtained by centrifugation of whole blood at 200 g for 10 min at room temperature.

Platelet-poor plasma was prepared by centrifugation of whole blood at 2800 g for 10 min.

To obtain a platelet pellet PRP was recentrifuged for 20 min at 600 g. This pellet was resuspended in phosphate-buffered saline. Cells were washed and centrifuged three times at 300 g for 20 min.

I. Scharrer/W. Schramm (Ed.)
32nd Hemophilia Symposion Hamburg 2001
© Springer-Verlag Berlin Heidelberg 2003

Clotting times after recalcification were measured in 11 pairs of adult and new-born-PRP (250.000 platelets/µl), to that 5 µl A23187, a calcium-ionophor (Calbio-chem) which causes a higher expression of phosphatidylserine in the outer leaflet of the plasma membrane, or Tris-buffer was added.

Thrombin generation with 8 pairs of adult and newborn platelets in a purified prothrombinase complex was measured. To unstimulated or with 10 µl A23187 sti-mulated platelets (final concentration: 2.5×10^6, incubated for 6 min) 20 µl of factor Xa (f.c. 1.5 pmol), 20 µl of factor Va (f.c. 3 pmol) and 20 µl of calcium were added. 120 s later 40 µl of factor II (f.c. 4nmol) and 20 µl of calcium (f.c. 5 µmol) were added. Samples (25 µl) were taken from 180 s after addition of factor II and the thrombin generation was measured at 405 nm using the chromogenic substrate S2238.

Results

Stimulation of platelets with the calcium-ionophor A23187 shortened recalcificati-on time with newborn platelets as well as with adult platelets. Newborns stimulated with the ionophor had a reduction of $10 \pm 12.2\%$, adults had a reduction of $27 \pm 18.3\%$ (mean values).

The thrombin generation measured in a purified prothrombinase complex was increased by adding the ionophor, but there was no difference between stimulated newborn and adult platelets (Fig. 1–4).

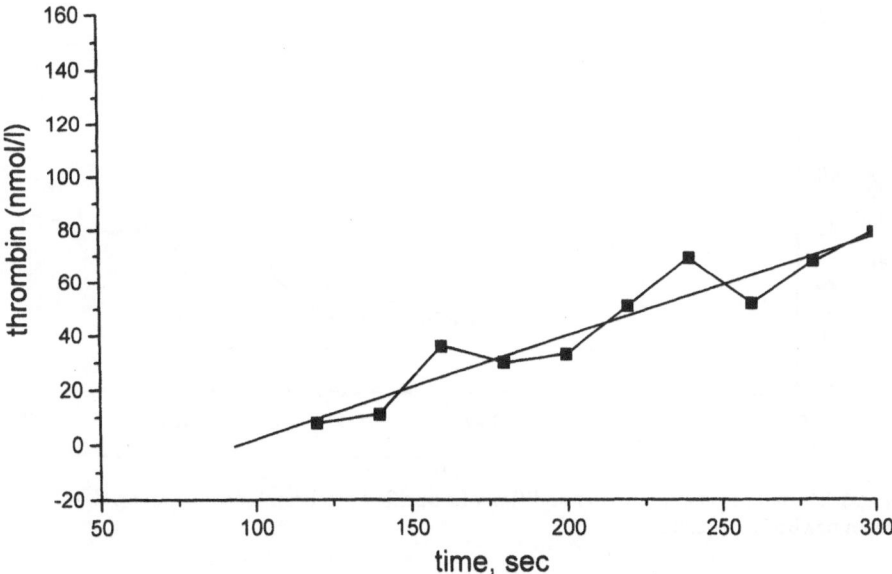

Fig. 1. Thrombin generation after addition of a purified prothrombinase complex to unstimu-lated adult platelets.

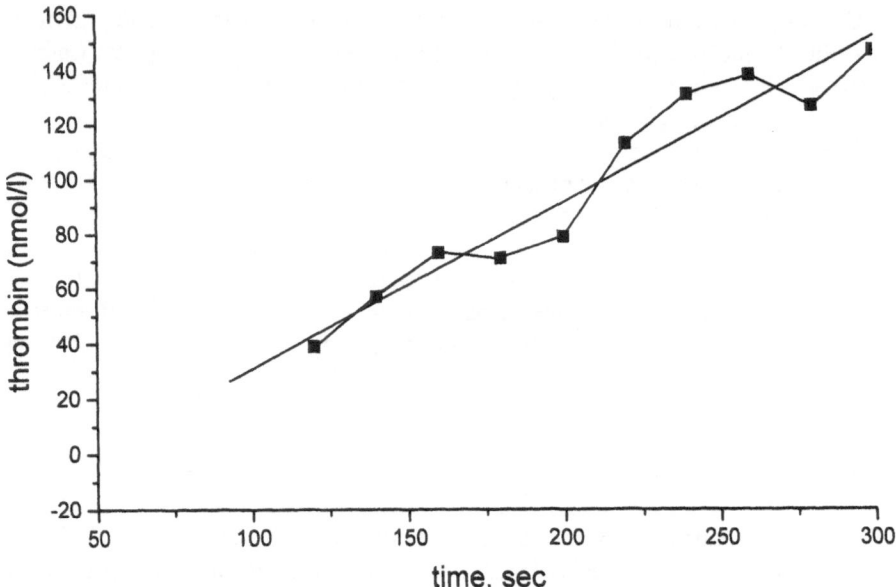

Fig. 2. Thrombin generation after addition of a purified prothrombinase complex to ionophor stimulated adult platelets.

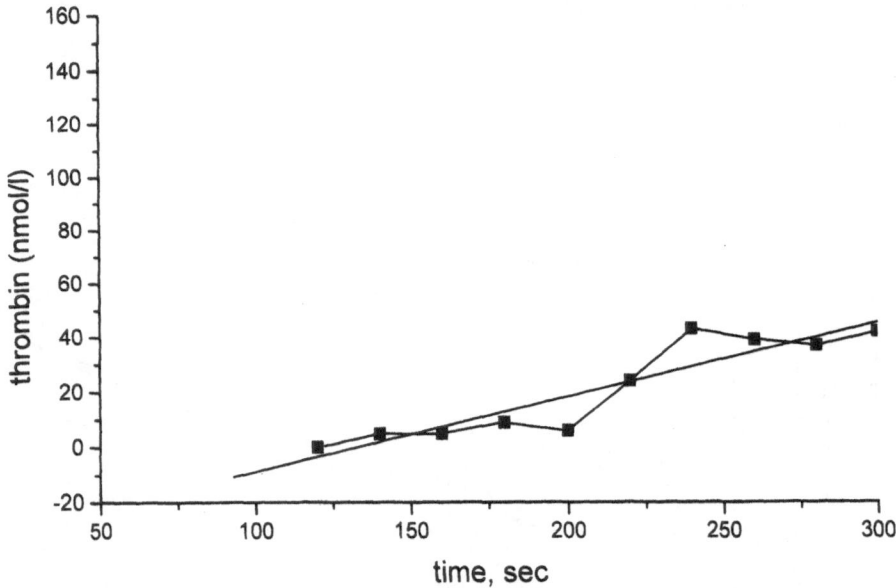

Fig. 3. Thrombin generation after addition of a purified prothrombinase complex to unstimulated newborn platelets.

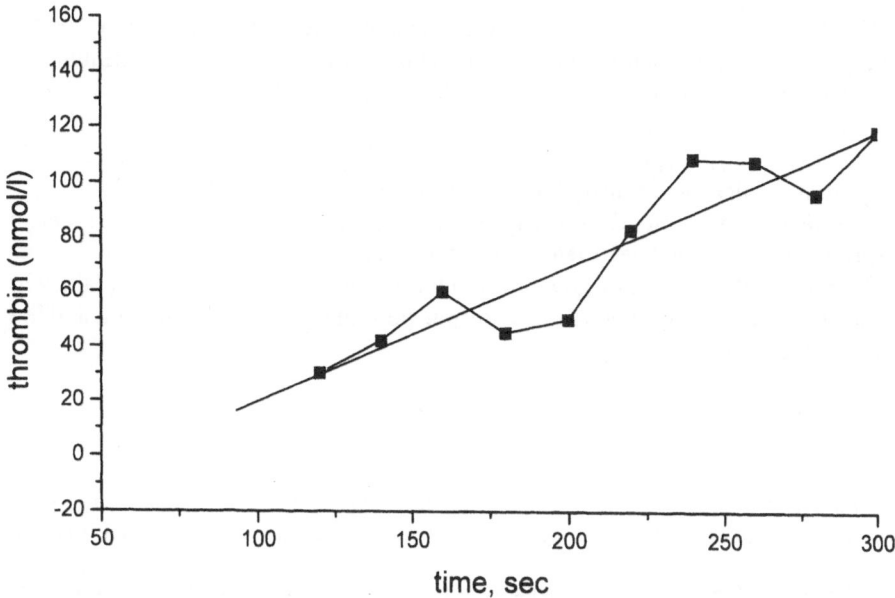

Fig. 4. Thrombin generation after addition of a prothrombinase complex to ionophor stimulated newborn platelets.

Discussion

Healthy newborns have a very low risk of thrombosis, due to lower plasma concentrations of vitamin K-dependent coagulation factors, i.e. prothrombin, and contact factors [1,6]. The bleeding time is, in good correlation to clinical experience and in contrast to poor in vitro platelet function, shorter in healthy neonates than in older children and adults [7]. The capacity of cord plasma to generate thrombin is decreased to 30–50 % of adult values [8].

Lines of evidence suggest that the hyporeactivity of neonatal platelets is the result of a defect intrinsic to them. Data suggest the possibility that the mechanism of the hyporeactivity is, at least in part, a relative defect in a shared signal transduction pathway [9]. Consistent with the hypothesis, it was reported that neonatal platelets have a relative impairment in their ability to mobilize calcium, an important mediator of many platelet functions [10].

It has been demonstrated that, compared with adult controls, neonatal platelets are hyporeactive to thrombin, a combination of adenosine diphosphate (ADP) and epinephrine, and U46619 (a stable thromboxane A2 analogue) in the physiological milieu of whole blood [9].

Phosphatidylserine in the plasma membrane of non activated human platelets is almost entirely located on the cytoplasmatic side. Stimulation with the calcium-ionophor A23187 or combined action of collagen plus thrombin results in a rapid loss of the asymmetric distribution of phosphatidylserine [11]. This alteration was much less apparent in platelets activated either by thrombin or collagen alone [12].

A23187 transports divalent cations across biologic membranes and increases the cytoplasmic level of calcium ions. This might be a critical factor linking stimulation to secretion through the platelet contractile mechanism [13-15].

In our study we investigated whether neonatal platelets have a different content or expression of phospholipids on the outer leaflet of the membrane which might have an influence on the thrombin generation and so on hemostasis.

However, our results do not suggest that a different phospholipid content or expression of the platelet membrane of newborns compared to adults has an influence on the thrombin generation. Our results do not help to explain why hemostasis works so well in neonates despite poor in vitro platelet function and low clotting factor plasma levels.

References

1. Andrew M., Paes B., Miller R., Johnston M., Mitchell L., Tollefsen DM., Powers P., Development of the human coagulation system in the full-term infant. Blood, 1987; 70: 165-72.
2. Corrigan JJ. (1989) Neonatal coagulation disorders. In: Alter BP (ed). Perinatal hematology. Churchill Livingstone, New York, pp 165-193.
3. Hathaway WE., (1987) Haemostatic disorders in the newborn. In: Bloom AL, Thomas DP., (eds) Haemostasis and thrombosis. Churchill Livingstone, Edinburgh, pp 554-569.
4. Israels SJ., Daniels M., McMillan EM. Deficient collagen-induced activation in the newborn platelet. Pediatr Res, 1990; 27: 337-43.
5. Stuart MCA., Bevers EM., Comfurius P., Zwaal RFA., Reutelingsperger CPM., Frederik PM. Ultrastructural detection of surface exposed phosphatidylserine on activated blood platelets. Thromb. Haemost, 1995, 74 (4): 1145-51.
6. Andrew M, Vegh P, Johnston M, Bowker J, Ofosu F, Mitchell L: Maturation of the hemostatic system during childhood. Blood, 1992; 8: 1998-2005.
7. Andrew M, Castle V, Mitchell L, Paes B. Modified bleeding time in the infant. Am J Haematol 1989; 30: 190-1.
8. Andrew M, Schmidt B, Mitchell L, Paes B, Ofosu F: Thrombin generation in newborn plasma is critically dependent on the concentration of prothrombin. Thromb Haemost 1990, 63: 27-30.
9. Rajasekhar D, Kestin AS, Bednarek FJ, et al. Neonatal platelets are less reactive than adult platelets to physiological agonists in whole blood. Thromb Haemost 1994; 72: 957-963.
10. Gelman B, Setty BNY, Chen D, Amin-Hanjani S, Stuart MJ. Impaired mobilization of intracellular calcium in neonatal platelets. Pediatr Res , 1996; 39: 692-696.
11. Bevers EM, Tilly RHJ, Senden JMG, Comfurius P, Zwaal RFA. Exposure of endogenous phosphatidylserine at the outer surface of stimulated platelets is reversed by restoration of aminophospholipid translocase activity. Biochemistry, 1989; 28: 2382-2387.
12. Bevers EM, Comfurius P, Van Rijn JLML, Hemker HC, Zwaal RFA. Eur. J. Biochem. 1982; 122: 429-436
13. Pressman BC: Properties of ionophores with broad range of cation selectivity. Fed Proc 32: 1698-1703, 1973
14. Hamill RL, Gorman M, Gale RM, Higgins CE, Hoehn MM. A23187, a new ionophor for divalent cations. I. Discovery, isolation and properties. Twelfth Interscience Conference on Antimicrobial Agents and Chemotherapy. 1972, p 32 (Abstr).
15. Reed PW, Lardy HA: A23187: a divalent cation ionophor. J Biol Chem. 1972; 247: 6970-6973.

Socio-economic Evaluation of Hemophilia Assistance

D. Mihailov, K. Schramm, W. Schramm, M. Şerban, and D. Lighezan

Introduction

The inadequate treatment, as well as the absence of prophylactic therapy of hemophiliacs in Romania lead to unfavorable long and short-term consequences (life-threatening and non-life threatening bleedings, chronic arthropathy, transfusion-transmitted diseases, etc.), affecting their life quality. The complications of the disease and those related to treatment are real problems for both the patients and the health care system.

Aim of the study

The aim of the present study was to perform a socio-economic evaluation of hemophilia patients.

Material and methods

Our study group included 46 hemophilia patients, registered and treated in the Center of Hemophilia Timisoara, 86.9% of them being hemophilia A patients, and the rest hemophilia B patients. The coagulopathy was severe in 76% of the cases, moderate in 11% of the cases and mild in 13% of the cases. None of these patients received prophylactic therapy.

We followed-up:
- sociodemographic data
- distance from home to hospital and the modality of transportation to hospital
- mean family income
- treatment compliance
- transfusion-transmitted diseases
- functional joint status (Petterson score)
- recovery mean time after severe bleeding episodes
- neuro-sensitive-sensorial sequelae
- average number of days off school or work
- symptomatic therapy

I. Scharrer/W. Schramm (Ed.)
32nd Hemophilia Symposion Hamburg 2001
© Springer-Verlag Berlin Heidelberg 2003

Results

The average age at the time of evaluation was 23.9 years (range: 7–35 years). The age-groups of the patients at admittance were: younger than 18 years old – 23.4% and older than 18 years old – 76.6%. In our study group, 15% of the patients were from Timisoara, 15% - from Timis county and 70% of them are from other counties.

The socio-professional status of the patients was: 24% of the hemophilia patients were schoolboys, 13% – university students, 13% – unemployed, 10% – employees, 40% of them being handicapped with social support.

Distribution of the hemophiliacs according to home-hospital distance revealed that 39% of them lived closer than 10 km from the hospital, in 41% cases the distance from their home and the hospital varied between 10–100 km, and 20% lived farther than 100 km from hospital.

The modality of transportation to hospital was as follows: 43% of the patients by car, 24% by train, 34% by bus, 13% by cab; the ambulance was used in 10% of the cases.

The mean family income in our study group is 80 USD/month (Fig. 1). 30% of the patients missed the hospitalization for bleeding episodes about 6 times a year because of financial reasons and 21 % of them came too late, on an average of 6 times a year.

Serological analysis were made to determine the type of transfusion-transmitted diseases (Fig. 2).

The assessment of functional joint status was performed according to Petterson score (Fig. 3). 71% of the patients attended joint functional recovery training on an average of 2 times a year. The recovery mean time after severe bleeding episodes was 35 days.

13% of the patients from our study group had neuro-sensitive-sensorial sequelae: epilepsia, lateral popliteal nerve paralysis, radial nerve paralysis and ambliopia. The average number of days off school or work is 57 a year (Fig. 4). 92%

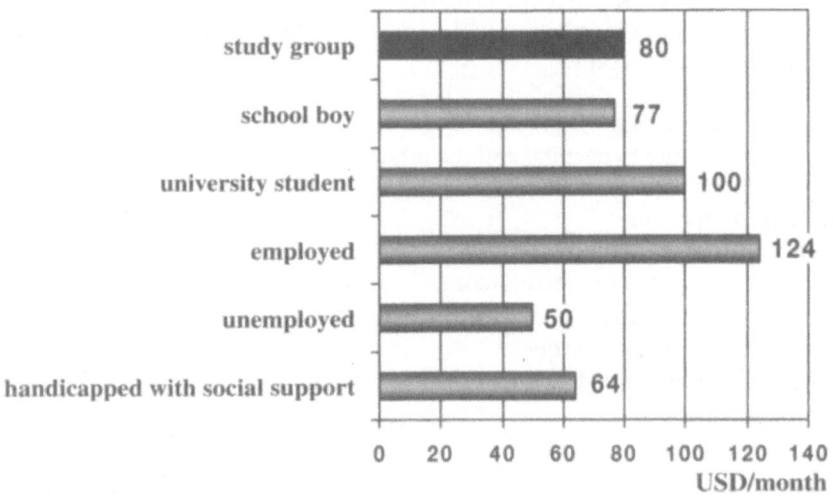

Fig. 1. Average family income in hemophilia patients

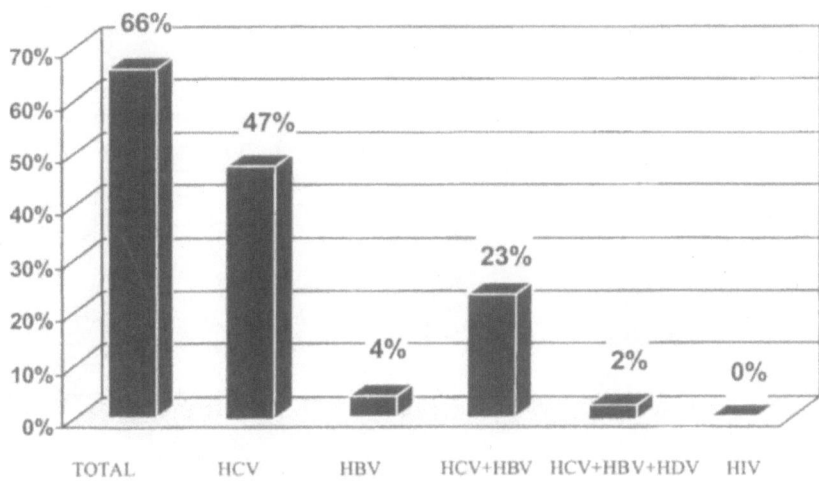

Fig. 2. Transfusion-transmitted diseases in hemophilia patients

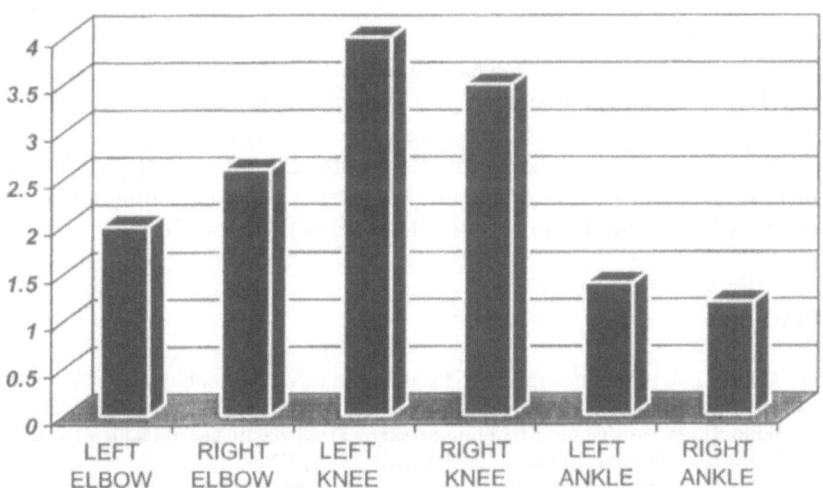

Fig. 3. Functional joint score in hemophilia patients

of the patients occasionally used symptomatic therapy (analgesic and anti-inflammatory drugs); 84% of them pay themselves for this treatment.

Conclusions

Our data suggest that the absence of the prophylactic therapy, as well as the use of inadequate doses and duration of the "on demand" therapy are responsible for consumption of other health care resources.

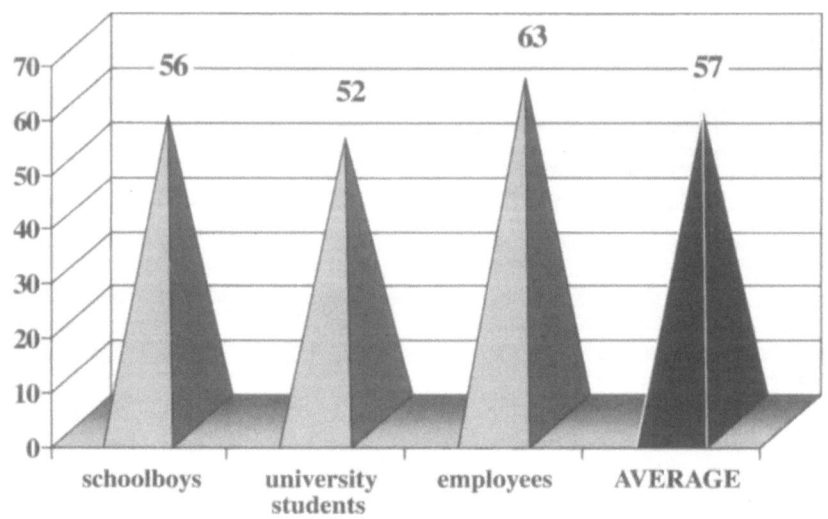

Fig. 4. Average number of days off school or work

Joint status, neuro-sensitive-sensorial sequelae and prolonged recovery time after bleeding episodes are responsible for the important number of days off school or work, affecting the integration in the social life of hemophilia patients.

The allocation of more appropriate health care resources to hemophilia treatment would decrease the number and the severity of complications and would allow these patients to be able to remain integrated in the social life.

References

1. Aledort LM. Economic aspects of haemophilia care, Haemophilia, 1999, Nov, 5 (6), 373
2. Aledort LM. Unsolved problems in haemophilia, Haemophilia, 4, 1998, 341–345
3. Bohn RL, Avorn J, Glynn RJ, Choodnovskiy I. Prophylactic use of factor VIII: an economic Evaluation, Thromb Haemost, 1998, May, 79 (5), 932–937
4. Bohn RL, Avorn J. Cost-Effectiveness – Can It Be Measured ?, Sem Hematol, 1993, 3 (Suppl 2) 20–23
5. Schramm W, Szucs TD. State-of-the-Art and Practices of Medical Economics, Haemophilia, 4, 1998, 491–497
6. Smith PS, Teutsch SM, Shaffer PA, Rolka H, Evatt B. Episodic Versus Prophylactic Infusions For Hemophilia A: A Cost-Effectiveness Analysis, J Pediatr, Sep, 129 (3), 424–431
7. Szucs TD, Offner A, Kroner B, Giangrande P, Berntrop E, Schramm W. Resource Utilization In Hemophiliacs Treated In Europe: Results From the European Study On Socioeconomic Aspects of Haemophilia Care, Haemophilia, 4, 1998, 498–501
8. Szucs TD, Schramm W. The economics of replacement therapy, Hämostaseologie, Dez 1996, 291–295
9. Szucs TD, Schramm W. Wirtschaftlichkeitsuntersuchungen von medizinischen Therapien-Methodologische Grundlagen, Zentralblatt für Chirurgie, 1995, 577–583
10. Schramm W, Öffner A, Szucs T. Sozioökonomische Untersuchungen zur hämostaseologischen Therapie und Antikoagulation, Zentralblatt für Chirurgie, 1995, 593–597

Aspects regarding Locomotor Rehabilitation of Hemophiliacs

M. Şerban, V. Şerban, H. Schuszler, D. Lighezan, D. Mihailov, V. Dumitraşcu, K. Schramm, and W. Schramm

Introduction

Progressive joint disease due to recurrent hemarthrosis and muscular bleedings or atrophy are the source of a significant morbidity and disability for hemophiliacs. They are common manifestations particularly in the severely affected patients, where bleeding can occur spontaneously or follow minimal stress.

In the absence of primary prophylaxis and of a correct early treatment of acute joint hemorrhages, in the situation of a very low availability of factor concentrates (<0.01IU/capita/year) and their imbalanced distribution through the country, more than 60% of our hemophilia patients are suffering from chronic arthropathy and more than 30% from muscular disabilities.

Objective

The study was conducted in order to evaluate the efficiency of a complex locomotor rehabilitation program on the joint status and its functional performances, achieved under minimal factor concentrate substitution and followed-up for 2–4 years. The crossectional study was carried out in the Clinical Rehabilitation Center Cristian Serban in Buzias between September 1997 and September 2001. None of the patients has ever been on primary prophylaxis.

Material and method

The studied cohort consisted of 130 patients with hemophilia and von Willebrand disease (Fig. 1), belonging to the age group of 3–30 years (Fig. 2), admitted in the Clinical Center Buzias. Most of them (88.5% of hemophilia A and 66.6% of hemophilia B) have manifested arthropathy (Fig. 3), 27.5% of them in more than four joints (Fig. 4) and 17.3% of them experiencing important (class III–IV) locomotor disability (Fig. 5).

The aims of the therapy were:
- improving range of motion and control of joint neutral
- global muscle strengthening and stabilizing of joints

I. Scharrer/W. Schramm (Ed.)
32nd Hemophilia Symposion Hamburg 2001
© Springer-Verlag Berlin Heidelberg 2003

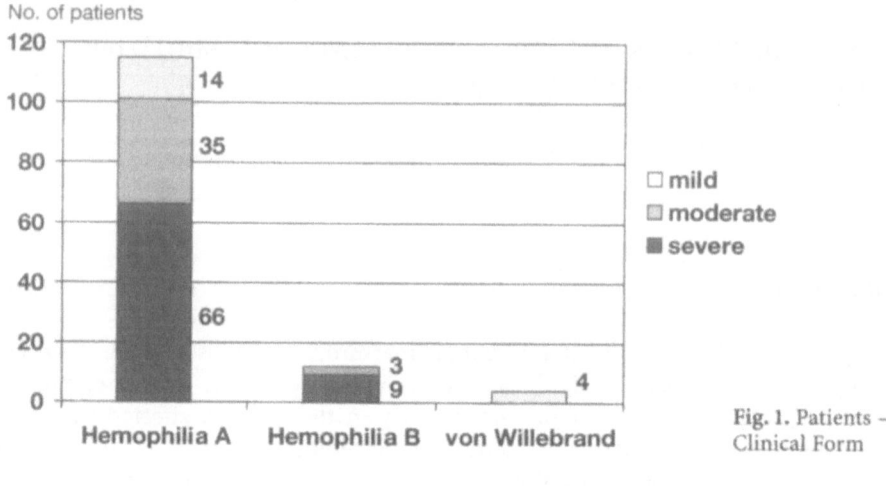

Fig. 1. Patients – Clinical Form

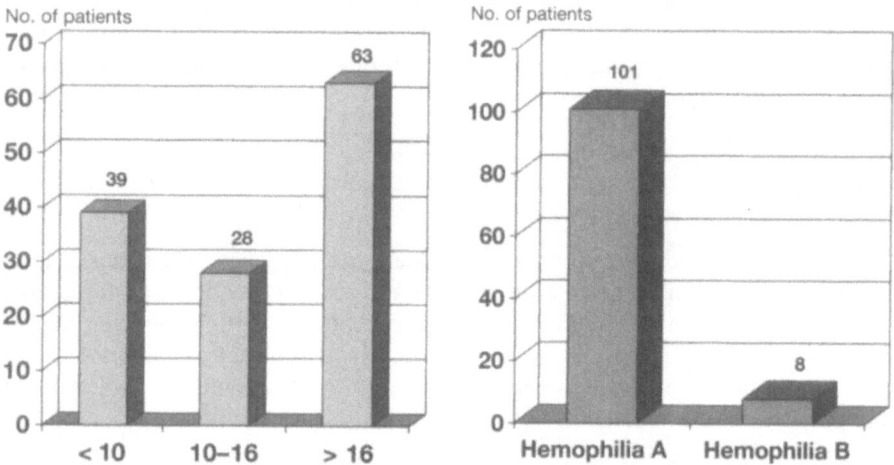

Fig. 2. Patients – Age distribution

Fig. 3. Patients – with chronic artropathy

- stretching and lengthening of global mobilizier muscles
- regaining dynamic control of stabilizing muscles
- integration into normal life.

The rehabilitation activity consisted of:
- hydrotherapy
- physical exercise
- therapeutical ultrasound
- pulsed electro-magnetotherapy
- pulsed short wave diathermy
- massage
- local ointment application or medical bath with arnica

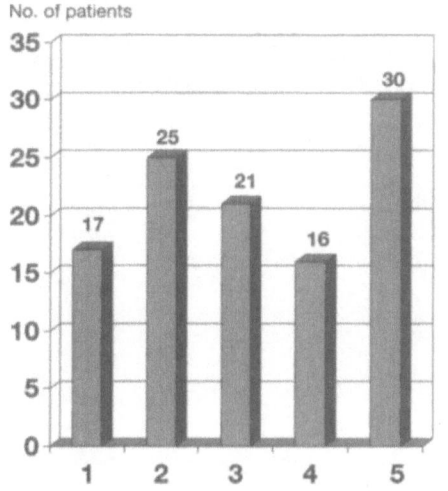

Fig. 4. Patients – Number of target joints

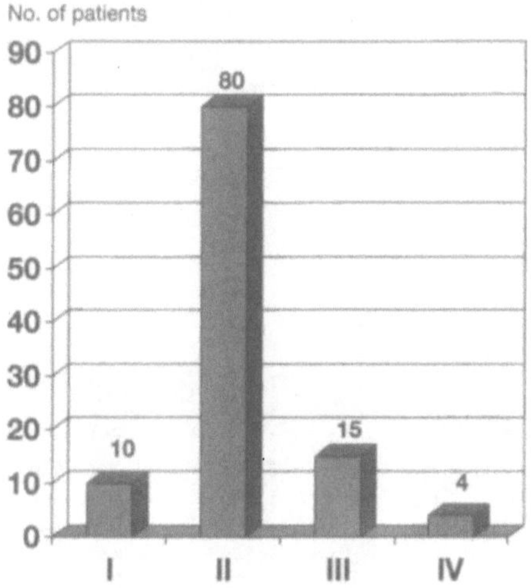

Fig. 5. Patients – Functional class of artropathy

It was part of a complex therapeutical approach:
- educational program, daily performed, regarding lifestyle in the situation of unavailability to appropriate factor concentrate substitution and regarding the attitude in bleeding emergencies; it also was aimed at early recognition and care of bleeding episodes, with simple and effective measures in order to control hemorrhages and to restore muscle and joint function
- psychological assistance particularly important for those with class III–IV locomotor handicap and for those missing integration in school and social life
- factor (VIII or IX) concentrate substitution was performed »on demand« promptly (10–20 IU/kg) for any joint or muscle complains and prophylaxis only in particular severe cases (10 IU/kg – 2–3 times/week)
- assessment of joint status was performed by the same doctor according to WFH and Petterson score at the start and the end of the therapy
- average number of therapy cycles (14–18 days) was 3.37/patient.

Results

The number of the affected joints was reduced after therapy (Fig. 6, 7), in both, hemophilia A and B patients. Despite of this fact, the changes of the average clinical joint scores and of the radiological scores (Fig. 8, 9) were not significant. But it was evident the improvement of the locomotor status in the handicapped patients with class III–IV disability (Fig. 10).

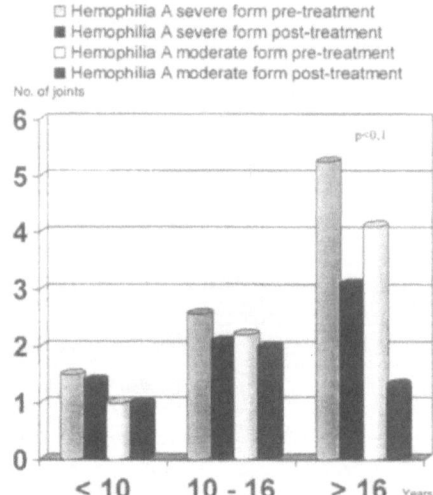

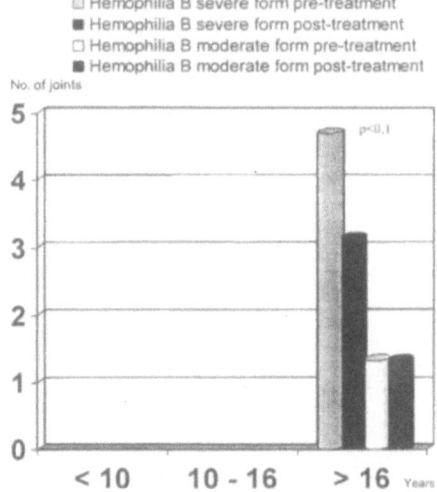

Fig. 6. Evolution of the average number of affected joints in hemophilia A patients

Fig. 7. Evolution of the average number of affected joints in hemophilia B patients

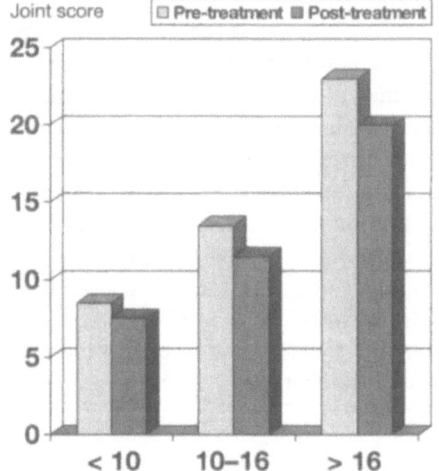

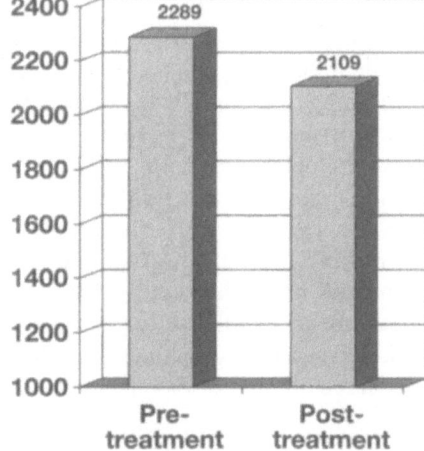

Fig. 8. Evolution of the average WFH joint score/patient

Fig. 9. Evolution of the average Petterson score

Discussions and conclusions

As expression of the limits and deficiencies in the medical treatment of hemophiliacs, chronic arthropathy and muscle atrophy, with pain, deformity, loss of range of movement and decreased function are sad realities for more than 80% of our young patients.

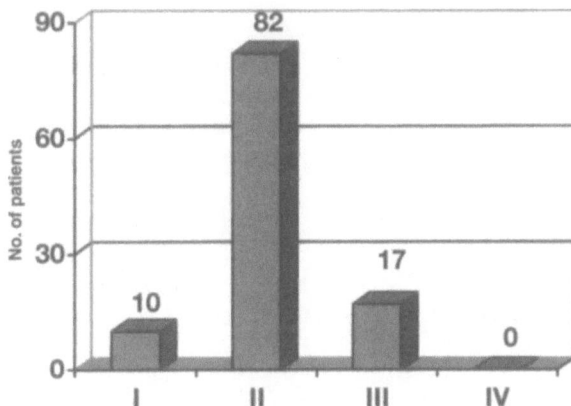

Fig. 10. Functional class of
arthropathy after treatment

In these conditions, physiotherapy as part of a comprehensive care, must and can assist the patient in restoring or improving musculo-skeletal function.

In 82.5 % of cases, depending on the severity of arthropathy, but also on the duration and discipline in performing the physiotherapy program, we could assess improving of the locomotor condition. The positive changes in the functional disability classes and the rehabilitation of those belonging to class IV are impressive and motivating for the patient and also for the whole involved team (physicians, physiotherapist, psychologist).

Decisive conditions for the evolution were the duration of the therapy (best results have been experienced by those with more than 8 cycles of treatment and those who have continued with home treatment) and the compliance of patients.

Thus, the seriously impaired life quality and physical performance ability of persons suffering from hemophilia justify the rehabilitation as a main challenge for the present and future Romanian medical assistance.

References

1. Buzzard Brenda, Beeton Karen: »Physiotherapy, Management of Haemophilia«, Blackwell Science, Oxford, 2000
2. Sohail Muhammed Tareg, Heijnen Lily: »Comprehensive haemophilia care in developing countries«, Ferzoans, Lahora, 2001
3. Schramm Wolfgang, Serban Margit: »Hemostazeologie clinica«, Brumar, Timisoara, 2001
4. Rizzo Battistella L: »Rehabilitation in Haemophilia- options in the developing world«, Haemophilia, 1998, 4, 486–490
5. Rodriguez-Merehan EC: »Therapeutic options in the management of articular contractures in haemophiliacs«, Haemophilia, 1995, 5 (suppl.1), 5–9

VIc. Thrombophilic Disorders

Prothrombin and Factor VII Genotypes and Phenotypes in healthy Individuals – Results from the Lugen Study

T. Landmann, H. Haubelt, J. Bach, and P. Hellstern

Introduction

Elevated plasma levels of prothrombin (PT) and coagulation factor VII (FVII) are discussed to be associated with an increased risk of venous thromboembolism or coronary heart disease [1, 3, 6, 8]. Activities of PT and FVII are influenced by genetic and environmental factors: In addition to polymorphisms of the PT gene (G20210A) and the FVII gene (R353Q, HVR4), smoking habits, use of oral contraceptives or postmenopausal hormone replacement therapy may also influence PT and FVII activities [1–4, 7, 12].

Aim of the study

The aims of the study were:

- to analyze prevalences of PT and FVII gene polymorphisms in a cohort of well-characterized healthy individuals
- to examine the influence of gene polymorphisms on the activity of the corresponding coagulation factor
- to demonstrate the association of different endogenous and exogenous factors with the corresponding coagulation factor level
- to analyze the association of coagulation factor II and VII activities with an activated hemostasis

Materials, methods and basic data

Study design and study population

We examined 488 healthy individuals (267 men, 221 women) from Southwest Germany, whose parents and grandparents had also been born in Central Europe (basic data Table 1). Women in pregnancy or nursing period and individuals with acute inflammatory or any other chronic disease were excluded. The medical history including risk factors for cardiovascular and thromboembolic disease was obtained.

I. Scharrer/W. Schramm (Ed.)
32nd Hemophilia Symposion Hamburg 2001
© Springer-Verlag Berlin Heidelberg 2003

Table 1. Basic data of the LUGEN study population

	men	women
n	267	221
age, yr (range)	48.2 ± 12.9 (14–74)	41.0 ± 14.1 (17–68)
BMI, kg/m² (range)	26.0 ± 3.1 (16.1–35.7)	24.4 ± 4.0 (16.4–40.8)
smokers, n (%)	133 (49.8%)	83 (37.6%)
pack/years	18.3	8.5
menopause, n (%)		75 (33.9%)
postmenopausal hormone replacement therapy, n (%)		36 (48.0%)
oral contraceptiva users, n (%)		54 (37.0%)

Determination of clotting factors and polymorphisms

PT activity was determined by a one-stage clotting assay [STA Neoplastin plus, Roche Diagnostics, Mannheim and factor II deficiency plasma, Progen, Heidelberg], FVII activity (FVII:C) by a chromogenic assay [Immunochrom FVII:C, Progen, Heidelberg]. We determined activated FVII (FVIIa) by a clotting assay [Staclot VIIa-rTF, Diagnostica Stago, Mannheim] and prothrombin fragments 1+2 (F1+2) and β-thromboglobulin (β-TG) by ELISAs [F(1+2): Enzygnost, Behring, Marburg and β-TG: Asserchrom, Roche Diagnostics, Mannheim].

Polymorphisms (PT G20210A, FVII R353Q and FVII HVR4) were analyzed by PCR. *PT G20210A:* (primer sense: 5′ TCT AGA AAC AGT TGC CTG GC 3′; primer antisense: 5′ ATA GCA CTG GGA GCA TTG AAG C 3′; PCR: 3 min 94°C, 30 cycles: 60 sec 94°C, 60 sec 57°C, 90 sec 72°C; 5 min 72°C). Hind III digestion products were separated on 6% polyacrylamide gels and visualized by staining with ethidium bromide [10].
FVII R353Q: (primer sense: 5′ GGG AGA CTC CCC AAA TAT CA 3′; primer antisense: 5′ ACG CAG CCT TGG CTT TCT CTC 3′; PCR: 3 min 94°C, 30 cycles: 60 sec 94°C, 60 sec 60°C, 90 sec 72°C; 5 min 72°C). Msp I digestion products were separeted on 2% agarose gels and visualizid by staining with ethidium bromide [5].
FVII HVR4: (primer sense: 5′ AATGTGACTTCCACACCTCC 3′; primer antisense: 5′ GATGTCTGTCTGTCTGTGGA 3′; PCR: 3 min 94°C, 32 cycles: 60 sec 94°C, 6 sec 57°C, 60 sec 72°C; 150 sec 72°C). PCR-products were separated on 6% polyacrylamide gels and visualized by staining with ethidium bromide [9].

Table 2. Prevalences of PT G20210A in LUGEN

	G20210G wildtype n (%)	G20210A heterozygote n (%)	A20210A homozygote n (%)
men n =267	256 (95.9)	11 (4.1)	0 (0.0)
women n =221	214 (96.8)	7 (3.2)	0 (0.0)
all n = 488	470 (96.3)	18 (3.7)	0 (0.0)

Results

Prevalences of PT G20210A and PT levels:

Prevalence of the PT A20210 mutation in total study population was 3,7%. No differences between men and women were observed (p= 0.578, Table 2).

Heterozygotes of G20210A polymorphism had significantly higher plasma levels of PT and F(1+2) when compared to wildtypes (p < 0.001 and p< 0.05, respectively, Fig. 1).

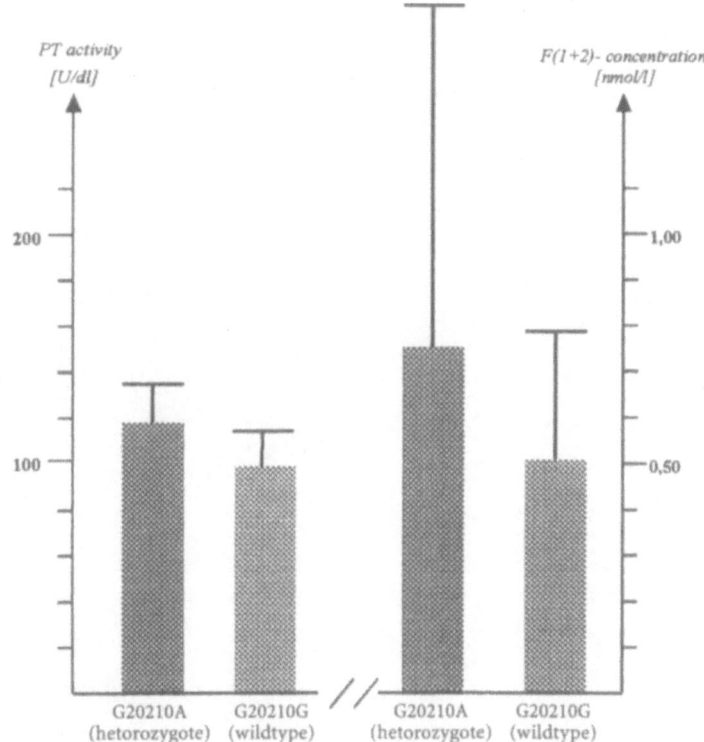

Fig. 1. Influence of PT G20210A on PT activity and F(1+2)

Women (< 50 yr) had significantly higher PT and F(1+2) levels when compared to men (< 50 yr): PT 106 ± 17.6 U/dl vs 101 ± 14.5 U/dl, p = 0.025; F(1+2) 0.48 ± 0.24 nmol/l vs 0.38 ± 0.14, p < 0.001). Oral contraceptive (OC) users had significantly higher PT and F(1+2) levels than OC nonusers (p = 0.001 and 0.006, repectively). In contrast, PT levels were not altered by menopause (p = 0.316), smoking (p = 0.758) or postmenopausal hormone replacement therapy (p = 0.220).

Prevalences of FVII R353Q and FVII levels

Prevalences of FVII R353Q polymorphism are shown in Table 3. Again, we found no differences in the prevalences of factor VII polymorphisms between men and women (p = 0.117).

We observed significant differences in FVII:C and FVIIa with respect to FVII R353Q genotype (R353R > R353Q > Q353Q; p < 0.001) (Fig. 2 and 3).

Table 3. Prevalence of FVII R353Q in LUGEN

	R353R wildtype n (%)	R353Q heterozygote n (%)	Q353Q homozygote n (%)
men n =267	199 (74.5)	62 (23.2)	6 (2.3)
women n =221	178 (80.5)	42 (19.0)	1 (0.5)
all n = 488	377 (77.3)	104 (21.3)	7 (1.4)

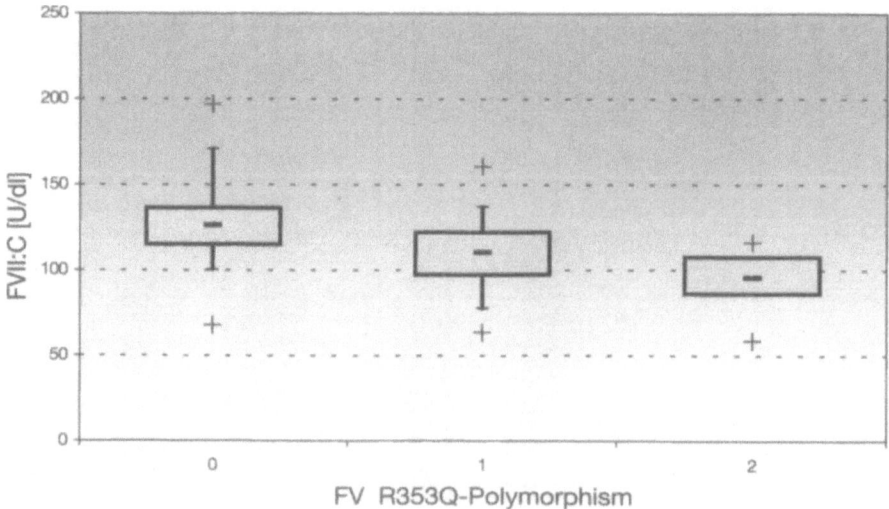

Fig. 2. Influence of FVII R353Q on FVII:C

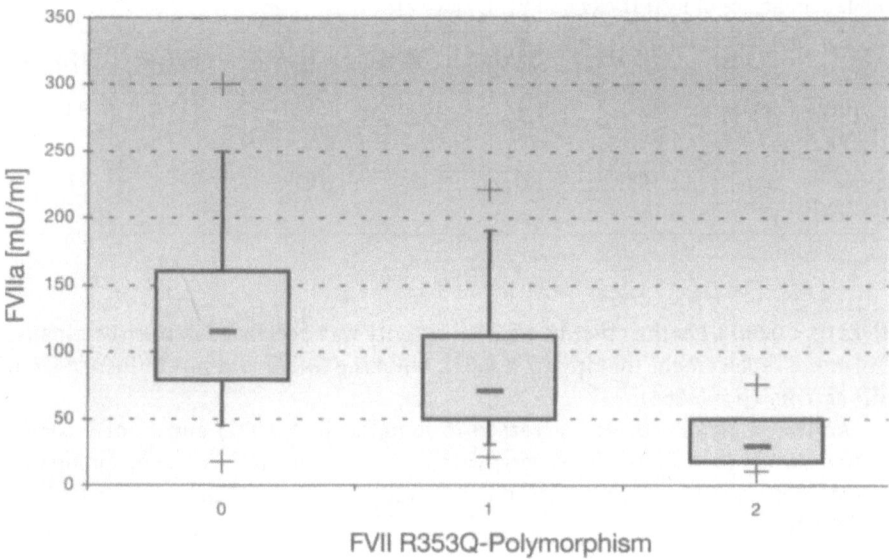

Fig. 3. Influence of FVII R353Q on FVIIa

Prevalence of FVII HVR4 and FVII levels:

Prevalences of HVR4 are shown in Table 4. No differences between men and women were observed ($p = 0.635$).

FVII HVR4 polymorphism was significantly associated with factor VII activity and FVIIa. Highest levels of FVII:C and FVIIa were observed in the H5/H6 genotypes (Table 5).

Additional factors influencing FVII levels:

Elevated levels of FVII:C were significantly associated with female gender ($p = 0.001$), older age ($p < 0.01$), postmenopause ($p < 0.01$) and use of oral contracep-

Table 4. Prevalences of FVII HVR4 in LUGEN

	H5/H6 n (%)	H5/H7 n (%)	H6/H6 n (%)	H6/H7 n (%)	H6/H8 n (%)	H7/H7 n (%)	H7/H8 n (%)
men n = 267	5 (1.9)	5 (1.9)	125 (46.8)	107 (40.0)	2 (0.8)	23 (8.6)	0 (0.0)
women n = 221	6 (2.7)	2 (0.9)	109 (49.3)	81 (36.6)	1 (0.5)	20 (9.1)	2 (0.9)
all n = 488	11 (2.3)	7 (1.4)	234 (48.0)	188 (38.5)	3 (0.6)	43 (8.8)	2 (0.4)

Table 5. Influence of FVII HVR4 on FVII:C and FVIIA

	H5/H6	H5/H7	H6/H6	H6/H7	H6/H8	H7/H7	H7/H8
FVII:C [U/dl]	137	122	126	120	126	122	92
FVIIa [mU/ml]	166	108	127	105	96	97	71

tives (p < 0.001). On the other hand, FVII activity was decreased in postmenopausal hormone replacement therapy (p < 0.05). Smoking habits did not influence factor VII activity (p = 0.684).

Activated factor VII was increased in females (p < 0.001) and in oral contraceptives users (p < 0.001). However, FVIIa was not associated with age, menopause, postmenopausal hormone replacement therapy or smoking habits (p > 0.05, respectively).

β-TG in LUGEN

β-TG was not associated with any of the polymorphisms or other analysed parameters in the study.

Conclusion

Prevalences of PT G20210A, FVII R353Q and FVII HVR4 were comparable to those observed in control groups of published case-control studies [3, 11]. From our data we conclude, that multiple endogenous (e.g. genotypes, age, gender) and exogenous (e.g. sexual hormons) factors alter plasma levels of PT and FVII. None of the polymorphisms caused a significant alteration of ß-TG levels. In contrast to prothrombin G20210A, none of the factor VII polymorphisms altered plasma levels of F(1+2). These differences clearly demonstrate that PT G20210A, but not the FVII polymorphisms, promotes intravascular thrombin formation. The LUGEN Study presents a well-characterized cohort of healthy individuals for forthcoming case-control studies.

References

1. Bernardi F, Marchetti G, Pinotti M, Arcieri P, Baroncini C, Papacchini M, Zepponi E, Ursicino N, Chiarotti F, Mariani G. Factor VII gene polymorphisms contribute about one third of the factor VII level variation in plasma. Arterioscler Thromb Vasc Biol 1996 Jan;16(1):72–6
2. Bernardi F, Arcieri P, Bertina RM, Chiarotti F, Corral J, Pinotti M, Prydz H, Samama M, Sandset PM, Strom R, Garcia VV, Mariani G. Contribution of factor VII genotype to activa-

ted FVII levels. Differences in genotype frequencies between northern and southern European populations. Arterioscler Thromb Vasc Biol 1997 Nov;17(11):2548–53

3. Bertina RM. The prothrombin 20210 G to A variation and thrombosis. Curr Opin Hematol 1998 Sep;5(5):339–42

4. Di Castelnuovo A, D'Orazio A, Amore C, Falanga A, Kluft C, Donati MB, Iacoviello L. Genetic modulation of coagulation factor VII plasma levels: contribution of different polymorphisms and gender-related effects. Thromb Haemost 1998 Oct;80(4):592–7

5. Green F, Kelleher C, Wilkes H, Temple A, Meade T, Humphries S. A common genetic polymorphism associated with lower coagulation factor VII levels in healthy individuals. Arterioscler Thromb 1991 May-Jun;11(3):540–6

6. Hellstern P, Bach J, Haubelt H, Preiss A, Winkelmann BR, Senges J. Gene polymorphisms of hemostasis and coronary risk. Med Klin 2001 Apr 15;96(4):217–27

7. Humphries SE, Lane A, Dawson S, Green FR. The study of gene-environment interactions that influence thrombosis and fibrinolysis. Genetic variation at the loci for factor VII and plasminogen activator inhibitor-1. Arch Pathol Lab Med 1992 Dec;116(12):1322–9

8. Lane DA, Grant PJ. Role of hemostatic gene polymorphisms in venous and arterial thrombotic disease. Blood 2000 Mar 1;95(5):1517–32

9. Marchetti G, Gemmati D, Patracchini P, Pinotti M, Bernardi F. PCR detection of a repeat polymorphism within the F7 gene. Nucleic Acids Res 1991 Aug 25;19(16):4570

10. Poort SR, Rosendaal FR, Reitsma PH, Bertina RM. A common genetic variation in the 3'-untranslated region of the prothrombin gene is associated with elevated plasma prothrombin levels and an increase in venous thrombosis. Blood 1996 Nov 15;88(10): 3698–703

11. Rosendaal FR, Doggen CJ, Zivelin A, Arruda VR, Aiach M, Siscovick DS, Hillarp A, Watzke HH, Bernardi F, Cumming AM, Preston FE, Reitsma PH. Geographic distribution of the 20210 G to A prothrombin variant. Thromb Haemost 1998 Apr;79(4):706–8

12. von Ahsen N, Lewczuk P, Schutz E, Oellerich M, Ehrenreich H. Prothrombin activity and concentration in healthy subjects with and without the prothrombin G20210A mutation. Thromb Res 2000 Sep 15;99(6):549–56

Factor V Leiden and other thrombotic risk factors in CHD and myocardial Infarction

W. Schröder, R. Grimm, G. Schuster, M. Brüser, K. Wulff,
M. Rieger, H. Völzke, U. John, and F.H. Herrmann

Introduction

Hemostatic imbalance might be an etiological factor in the transition of coronary heart disease (CHD) to myocardial infarction (MI). Several polymorphisms in genes regulating coagulation and hemostasis have been described as risk factors for venous thrombosis. However, their contribution to the development of arterial thrombosis is still unresolved. There are many reports in literature dealing with the role of specific coagulation factors in MI, ischemic stroke or peripheral arterial occlusion (for references see [1]), but for none of them a clear association to CHD or MI was finally accepted.

The aims of the present study were

1. to determine the exact prevalences of mutations and polymorphisms in the genes for FV (FV Leiden mutation Arg506Gln and haplotype FV HR2, His1299Arg), MTHFR (677C>T), FII (20210G>A), FVII (Arg353Gln), FXIII (Val34Leu) and ACE (insertion/deletion polymorphism in intron 16), known to be risk factors or discussed as protective factors (FVII, FXIII) for venous thrombosis, in a group of angiographically confirmed CHD patients,
2. to determine an association between individual genetic markers and/or combinations of them and CHD and
3. to characterize the relationship of genetic marker frequency and the degree of coronary artery stenosis.

Subjects and Methods

Subjects

We have analyzed 132 (102 male, 30 female) angiographically characterized patients with CHD, admitted to the Clinic for Internal Medicine at University Hospital Greifswald, North-Eastern Germany. 89 of them had a history of non-fatal MI. With regard to the number of stenoses 38 of them had a single vessel disease, 39 a double vessel disease and 53 a triple vessel disease. In two cases no result of angiography was available. As a control group we investigated 155 (72 male, 83 female) participants of a population-based cross-sectional epidemiological study of the same region (Study of Health in Pomerania SHIP [2]), having no sign of CHD (i.e. persons with history of deep vein thrombosis, MI or stroke were excluded).

I. Scharrer/W. Schramm (Ed.)
32nd Hemophilia Symposion Hamburg 2001
© Springer-Verlag Berlin Heidelberg 2003

Moleculargenetic methods for detection of sequence variants

For the DNA analysis of the variants of FV, FII, MTHFR and ACE blood samples were soaked onto filterpaper cards and used for PCR as described previously [3].

The detection of the molecular markers has been performed by standard methods by PCR and restriction analysis (FV Leiden: [4]; FII: (5); MTHFR: [6]). For the analysis of the newly described FV haplotype HR2 we detected the mutation 4070 A(R1)/G(R2) (His1299Arg) in exon 13 of FV as described by Lunghi et al. [7]. The analysis of the I/D polymorphism in intron 16 of the ACE gene was performed according to the protocols described by Rigat et al. [8] and for control of mistyping the D/D genotype by Odawara et al. [9]. For the other mutations/polymorphisms genomic DNA was extracted from blood samples by standard methods. The Arg353Gln polymorphism in exon 8 of FVII [10] was analyzed by PCR amplification and digestion with Msp I. Primer were designed from the FVII sequence [11]. The FXIII Val34Leu polymorphism was analyzed by PCR amplification and heteroduplex analysis [12].

Statistics

For statistical analysis allele frequencies were calculated by counting genes from the observed genotypes. Differences in allele frequencies and categorical variables like sex, history of hypertonia or diabetes between groups were tested for heterogeneity by χ^2 test. T-Test for two independent samples was used to compare means of age, body mass index (BMI) and plasma levels of triglycerides, total cholesterol and fibrinogen between groups. Adjusting for classical cardiovascular risk factors was performed by bivariate logistic regression. All analyses were performed using SPSS version 10.07 for Windows (SPSS GmbH Software München, Germany).

Results

Table 1 shows the clinical characteristics of patients and controls and the distribution of classical cardiovascular risk factors in these groups. As expected, some of these factors were more common in patients than in controls. As expected significantly more males than females had an CHD. In all CHD patients there were more persons with a history of diabetes mellitus (p<0.0011) than in controls. However, in this specific group of patients we found significantly lower plasma levels of total cholesterol (p=0.005) and a lower BMI (p=0.021). In patients with MI, sex distribution (p<0.0001), BMI (p=0.016), total cholesterol (p=0.006), fibrinogen levels (p=0.001) and diabetes frequency (p=0.0005) were significantly different to controls. Patients with single-vessel disease were significantly younger than our controls (p=0.004), had lower plasma levels of total cholesterol (p=0.007). In tendency there were less persons with hypertonia (p=0.0558), and again more men present in that group (p=0.0027) than in the control group. No data were available for current smoking status or use of hormones in patients.

Table 1. Clinical characteristics of patients and controls

	all CHD patients n = 133	patients with MI n = 89	single vessel n = 38	controls n = 155
age (years)	64.9 ± 10.0	66.8 ± 8.2	61.1 ± 10.8	66.9 ± 10.8
sex (% male/female)	77.3 / 22.7	82.0 / 18.0	73.7 / 26.3	46.5 / 53.5
BMI (kg/m²)	27.1 ± 3.4	26.9 ± 3.0	27.4 ± 3.5	28.2 ± 4.6
triglycerides (mmol/l)	2.1 ± 1.1	2.2 ± 1.3	1.9 ± 1.0	2.1 ± 1.3
total cholesterol (mmol/l)	6.0 ± 1.3	6.0 ± 1.3	5.8 ± 1.2	6.5 ± 1.5
fibrinogen (g/l)	3.3 ± 1.1	3.1 ± 0.9	3.3 ± 1.3	3.5 ± 0.8
hypertension	46.2%	47.2%	36.8%	54.2%
diabetes mellitus	31.8%	34.8%	13.2%	15.5%

Results concerning prevalences of the genetic markers investigated in different groups of patients and controls are summarized in Table 2. Frequencies of all mutations/polymorphism in all groups were exactly as expected when a distribution according to Hardy-Weinberg was assumed. The heterozygous FVL genotype was detected more often in patients than in controls: 16 (12.1%) CHD patients (p=0.0591), 12 (13.5%) MI-survivors (p=0.04), 7 (18.4%) patients with single-vessel disease (p=0.0117), but only 9 (5.8%) controls.

There was no other significant difference in mutation frequency detectable between the groups. We were not able to find the expected lower number of patients with the potentially protective polymorphisms Gln 353 of FVII or Leu 34 FXIII gene. Although there was a slight enhancement in frequency of homozygous MTHFR genotype or ACE D/D compared to controls, this was not significant and the allele frequencies did not differ at all. Frequencies of FII and FV R2 allele were even lower in all patient groups than in controls.

Table 2. Prevalences of genetic markers in patients and controls

		all CHD patients n = 132	patients with MI n = 89	single vessel n = 38	controls n = 155
FVL	% hz	12.1	13.5	18.4	5.8
MTHFR	% hz	40.2	34.8	47.4	40.0
	% ho	11.4	13.5	13.2	9.0
FII	% hz	0.8	1.2	0	1.3
FVHR2	% hz	10.6	10.1	10.5	15.5
ACE	% I/I	18.9	24.7	23.7	18.1
	% I/D	48.5	43.8	44.7	52.9
	% D/D	32.6	31.5	31.6	29.0
FXIII	% hz	39.7	50.0	39.5	40.0
	% ho	5.3	5.7	2.6	6.5
FVII	% hz	18.9	17.1	21.1	19.9
	% ho	2.3	1.6	2.6	1.3

Table 3. FVL in patients and controls

	FVL % hz	p (χ^2)	p (log.Regr.)	OR (95 % CI)
all CHD patients	12.1	0.059	0.097	2.26 (0.86–5.93)
male (n=102)	10.8	0.227	0.368	1.76 (0.51–6.04)
female (n= 30)	16.7	0.079	0.047	4.69 (1.02–21.62)
patients with MI	13.5	0.04	0.158	2.19 (0.74–6.47)
male (n=73)	12.3	0.155	0.454	1.65 (0.44–6.12)
female (n=16)	18.8	0.089	0.034	7.71 (1.16–51.0)
controls	5.8			
male (n=72)	5.6			
female (n=83)	6.0			

When adjusted for all major classical cardiovascular risk factors we had information about (see Table 1) it appears, that FVL mutation is not a significant risk factor in all CHD patients (p=0.097) or all MI-survivors (p=0.158). However, stratified by gender we could show, that FVL is an independent significant risk factor for CHD and MI only in female patients (Table 3). The presence of the FVL allele in women only seems to enhance the risk for CHD more than fourfold and for MI more than 7-fold.

Given the prevalence of the FVL mutation in the control population of North-Eastern Germany of 5.8 % and in the female population of 5.6% it reveals, that the population based attributable risk PAR is 7.46% for CHD and 7.12% for MI, i.e. more than 7% of CHD or MI cases in the general population are due to the presence of the FVL allele, which could be diagnosed in advance. For women the PAR for CHD or MI is even higher (17.1% and 28.12%, resp.).

When analyzed by number of stenosed main coronary arteries by angiography, it appears that FVL mutation is only significantly more often present in patients with single-vessel disease, not in two- or multi-vessel-disease (Table 4).

In patients with lower grade of coronary stenosis (single-vessel disease) is the FVL mutation only significantly more present in women compared to control women, not in men. However, the absolute figure of affected women is very small; conclusions in this regard can only be drawn preliminary.

When adjusted for age, sex, hypertension, diabetes, BMI, triglycerides, total cholesterol and fibrinogen we found, that the risk getting CHD for patients with single-vessel disease is enhanced more than sixfold by the presence of the FVL allele. There is no risk elevation by FVL in patients with higher grades of coronary stenosis.

Note, that single-vessel disease and multi-vessel disease did not have the same distribution of conventional risk factors for CHD. For example, patients with multi-vessel disease were significantly older than patients with single-vessel disease (68.02 years vs. 61.13 years, p=0.001) and they had significantly more often a history of diabetes mellitus (43.4% vs. 13.2%, p=0.0022, OR 5.06, CI 1.77-14.47). In tendency, although not statistically significant, they had more often hypertonia (56.6% vs.

Table 4. FVL in different groups of coronary stenosis

	FVL % hz	p (χ^2)	p (log.Regr.)	OR (95 % CI)
patients with single-vessel disease	18.4	0.012	0.004	6.11 (1.78–20.88)
male (n=28)	10.7	0.366	0.315	2.35 (0.44–12.44)
female (n=10)	40.0	0.0006	0.007	43.06 (2.80–662.24)
patients with two-vessel disease	5.1	0.870	0.740	0.74 (0.12–4.37)
male (n=30)	6.7	0.828	0.813	1.26 (0.19–8.24)
female (n= 9)	–	–	–	–
patients with multi vessel disease	13.2	0.082	0.457	1.58 (0.47–5.34)
male (n=42)	14.3	0.114	0.402	1.85 (0.44–7.83)
female (n=11)	9.1	0.697	0.871	1.25 (0.08–19.06)

36.8%, p=0.064, OR 2.24, CI 0.97-5.17), there were more male patients present (79.2% vs. 73.7% p=0.5) and they had slightly higher plasma levels of total cholesterol (6.19 vs. 5.8 mmol/l), triglycerides 2.19 vs. 1.92 mmol/l) and fibrinogen (3.4 vs. 3.28 g/l). These findings might be the reason for the higher prevalence of MI in patients with multi-vessel disease compared to single-vessel disease. In our study 40 out of 53 (75.5%) patients with multi-vessel disease had a history of non-fatal MI, but only 22 out of 38 (57.9%) patients with single-vessel disease (p=0.077, OR 2.24, CI 0.93-5.4). Nevertheless, the presence of the FVL mutation does not further enhance the risk in this high risk-group of patients, as was shown in Table 4.

Discussion

In the present study the FVL mutation was found more often in patients with CHD and in patients with MI compared to healthy controls, the effect was mostly pronounced in women. It was shown, that presence of FVL enhances the risk for CHD and MI in female patients significantly. Furthermore, FVL seems to be of special importance in patient groups with low degree of coronary stenosis.

FVL is the most common genetic factor associated with risk of venous thromboembolism. The role of the FVL mutation in arterial thrombosis, CHD and MI has been investigated in many studies with varying results. Holm et al. [13] found a high prevalence of the mutation amongst 101 Swedish MI patients (18%), especially among men. In a later study at 295 patients with acute coronary syndrome [14] it was reported that FVL enhances the risk of infarction or death in smokers threefold. Rosendaal et al. [15] found FVL more often in young women with MI (10%), the risk was increased fourfold when adjusted for major cardiovascular risk factors and was particularly high among smokers. Doggen et al. [16] also reported an increased risk of MI due to carriership of FVL that was most pronounced in men with other classical risk factors. In a study performed by Middendorf et al. [17]in Bavaria, southern

Germany, also a significantly enhanced prevalence of FVL (9.1%) was found in patients with myocardial infarction. However, most subsequent studies have failed to show an association between FVL and coronary disease or non-fatal MI (for references see [1]). In contrast to the studies showing an importance of FVL in patient groups with higher risk we found FVL more significant in groups with lower risk for MI (single-vessel disease, women). Van de Water et al. [18] has shown that FVL is increased in frequency (14.6%) among young MI patients (<50 years) with normal or near normal coronary arteries (no stenosis >50%) and also in all MI-patients with no stenosis, irrespective of age (11.7%). This is comparable to our results found in patients with single-vessel disease.

As with FVL many controversial results are published for the role of FV HR2, FII, MTHFR, ACE, FXIII and FVII in arterial thrombosis. Gardemann et al. [19] reported an importance of FII 20210G>A gene variation for CHD restricted to cases with major cardiovascular risk factors. In contrast, Morita et al. [20] found a significantly enhanced prevalence of MTHFR and ACE D/D only in MI patients which had a conventionally low risk. These authors also have strengthened the hypothesis, that genetic factors have to be taken in account especially in conventionally low-risk groups of patients.

However, in our study we couldn't find any hint for the hypothesis that FII, MTHFR, ACE D/D, FV HR2 are risk factors or FVII and FXIII are protective factors for CHD or myocardial infarction.

Conclusions

We conclude that the prothrombotic mutation FVL is increased in frequency in groups of CHD patients being at conventionally low risk (lower degree of coronary artery stenosis/woman). The relatively weak contribution of one genetic susceptibility marker (FVL) to the transition of CHD to an arterial thrombotic event (MI) might become obvious only in groups, where other conventional risk factors, hiding this influence, are less frequent. FVL in these groups seems to be associated with an increased risk for CHD and myocardial infarction. Our results did not demonstrate any importance of genetic markers like FII, FV HR2, FVII, FXIII, MTHFR or ACE I/D polymorphism for arterial thrombosis. However, due to the relatively small number of patients, results have to be confirmed in larger studies.

References

1. Reiner AP, Siscovick DS, Rosendaal FR. Hemostatic risk factors and arterial thrombotic disease. Thromb Haemost 2001; 85:584–595
2. John U, Greiner B, Hensel E, Lüdemann J, Pieck M, Sauer S, Adam C, Born G, Alte D, Greiser E, Haertel U, Hense H-W, Haerting J, Willich S, Kessler C. Study of Health in Pomerania (SHIP): a health examination survey in an east German region: objectives and design. Soz. Präventivmed 2001; 46:186-194
3. Schröder W, Koeslimg M, Wulff K, Wehnert M, Herrmann FH. Large-scale screening for Factor V leiden mutation in a north-eastern population. Haemostasis 1996; 26: 233-236

4. Bertina RM, Koeleman BC, Koster T, Rosendaal RF, Dirven RJ, Ronde de H, Velden van der PA, Reitsma PH. Mutation in blood coagulation factor V associated with resistance to activated protein C. Nature 1994; 369: 64–7

5. Poort SR, Rosendaal FR, Reitsma PH, Bertina RM. A common genetic variation in the 3'-untranslated region of the prothrombin gene is associated with elevated plasma prothrombin levels and an increase in venous thrombosis. Blood 1996; 88: 3698–3703

6. Frosst P, Blom HJ, Milos R, Goyette P, Sheppard CA, Matthews RG, Boers GJ, den Heijer M, Kluijtmans LAJ, van den Heuvel LP, Rozen R. A candidate genetic risk factor for vascular diseases: a common mutation in methylenetetrahydrofolate reductase. Nat Genet 1995; 10: 111-113

7. Lunghi B, Iacoviello L, Gemmati D, DiIasio MG, Castoldi E, Pinotti M, Castaman G, Redaelli R, Mariani G, Marchetti G, Bernardi F. Detection of new polymorphic markers in the factor V gene: Association with factor V levels in plasma. Thromb Haemost 1996; 75:45–48

8. Rigat B, Hubert C, Corvol P, Soubrier F. PCR detection of the insertion/deletion polymorphism of the human angiotensin converting enzyme gene (DCP 1) (dipeptidyl carboxypepetidase1). Nucl Acids Res 1992; 20:1433

9. Odawara M, Matsunuma A, Yamashita K. Mistyping frequency of the angiotensin-converting enzyme gene polymorphism and an improved method for its avoidance. Hum Genet 1997; 100 163-166

10. Green F, Kelleher C, Wilkes H, Temple A, Meade T, Humphries SA. A common genetic polymorphism associated with lower coagulation factor VII level in healthy individuals. Arterioscler Thromb 1991; 11:540–546

11. Wulff K, Herrmann FH. Twenty two novel mutations of the factor VII gene in factor VII deficiency. Human Mutation 2000; 15:489–496

12. Wulff K, Ebener U, Wehnert C-S, Ward PA, Reuner U, Hiebsch W, Herrmann FH, Wehnert M. Direct molecular genetic diagnosis and heterozygote identification in X-linked Emery-Dreyfuss muscular dystrophy by heteroduplex analysis. Disease Markers 1997; 13:77–86

13. Holm J, Hillarp A, Zöller B, Erhardt L, Berntorp E, Dahlbäck B. Factor V Q506 (resistance to activated protein C) and prognosis after acute coronary syndrome. Thromb Haemostas 1999; 81(6):857–60

14. Holm J, Zöller B, Berntorp E, Erhardt L, Dahlbäck B. Prevalence of factor V gene mutation amongst myocardial infarction patients and healthy controls is higher in Sweden than in other countries. J Intern Med 1996; 239(3):221–6

15. Rosendaal FR, Siscovick DS, Schwartz SM., Beverly RK, Psaty BM, Longstreth WT, Raghunathan TE, Koepsell TD, Reitsma PH. Factor V Leiden (resistance to avctivated protein C) increases the risk of myocardial infarction in young women. Blood 1997; 89(8):2817–21

16. Doggen CJ, Cats VM, Bertina RM, Rosendaal FR. Interaction of coagulation defects and cardiovascular risk factors: increased risk of myocardial infarction associated with factor V Leiden or prothrombin G20210A. Circulation 1998; 97(11):1037–41

17. Middendorf K., Nikol S. Prevalence of resistance against activated protein C resulting from FV Leiden is significantly increased in myocardial infarction: investigation of 519 patients with myocardial infarction and meta-analysis of previous publications. 45. Jahrestagung der Gesellschaft für Thrombose- und Hämostaseforschung e.V. 14.-17.2.2001 Düsseldorf; 2001

18. Van de Water NS, French JK, Lund M, Hyde TA, White HD, Browett PJ. Factor V Leiden and prothrombin variant G20210A are associated with myocardial infarction in patients aged <50 years with no angiographic stenosis. XVIIth Congress of the International Society of Thrombosis and Haemostasis, Washington; 1999

19. Gardemann A, Arsic T, Katz N, Tillmanns H, Hehrlein FW, Haberbosch W. The factor II G20210A and factor V G1691A gene transitions and coronary heart disease. Thromb Haemost 1999; 81(2):208–213

20. Morita H, Kurihara H, Imai Y, Yazaki Y, Nagai R. Genetic coronary risk factors in conventionally low-risk patients. Thromb Haemost 2000; 84:137

In vitro Effects of combined Administration of Eptifibatide and Anticoagulants on Thrombin induced Platelet Aggregation after high versus low Coagulant Activation of Platelet Rich Plasma

M. Köstenberger, S. Gallistl, G. Cvirn, M. Petritsch, B. Leschnik, and W. Muntean

Abstract

Aim of our study was to compare effects of eptifibatide and anticoagulants on platelet aggregation and thrombin generation under low versus high coagulant challenge in tissue factor-activated platelet rich plasma. We used a model allowing simultaneous determination of the time course of platelet aggregation and thrombin generation in the presence of eptifibatide and anticoagulants after extrinsic activation of plasma. Eptifibatide exerted a dose dependent anti-aggregating effect which reached its maximum at 1000 ng/ml. Under low coagulant challenge the anti-aggregating effect was significantly higher compared to results obtained under high coagulant challenge, but also reached its maximum at 1000 ng/ml. Addition of eptifibatide revealed no influence after both high and low coagulant challenge on thrombin generation under our experimental conditions. Eptifibatide prolonged dose dependently the lag phase until the onset of platelet aggregation under low coagulant but not under high coagulant challenge. Under both high and low coagulant challenge UH, LMWH, and rH dose dependently decreased thrombin generation, but had no influence on platelet aggregation. Combination of eptifibatide and anticoagulants resulted in significant additive prolongation of the lag phase, more pronounced under low coagulant challenge. Combination of eptifibatide and anticoagulants under high coagulant challenge had a significant synergistic inhibitory effect on platelet aggregation. In contrast, under low coagulant challenge addition of anticoagulants to plasma that contained eptifibatide did not add to inhibition of platelet aggregation. Combined addition of eptifibatide and anticoagulants to plasma did not significantly add to the decrease of thrombin generation at high coagulant challenge. Interestingly, under low coagulant challenge combination of eptifibatide and LMWH resulted in significantly reduced thrombin generation compared to measurements in the absence of eptifibatide. Combined administration of eptifibatide with rH, or UH under low coagulant challenge did not result in reduced thrombin generation.

Our in vitro experiments support the notion that combined application of eptifibatide and anticoagulants might be beneficial in atherosclerotic disease to palliate the high thrombogenic challenge of ruptured atherosclerotic plaques.

I. Scharrer/W. Schramm (Ed.)
32nd Hemophilia Symposion Hamburg 2001

Introduction

Eptifibatide (Integrilin), a highly specific competitive inhibitor of the glycoprotein IIb/IIIa complex, has been shown to inhibit platelet aggregation in a dose dependent manner. Eptifibatide functions by blocking the binding of fibrinogen and von-Willebrand factor to glycoprotein IIb/IIIa on the surface of activated platelets [1]. It is further characterized by a short pharmacokinetic and pharmacodynamic half life, and the rate of eptifibatide elimination from circulation is rapid [2,3]. Eptifibatide is known to inhibit platelet aggregation but not to prevent platelet activation. Unfractionated heparin (UH), low molecular weight heparin (LMWH), and recombinant hirudin (rH) have been demonstrated to inhibit thrombin generation dose dependently after intrinsic or extrinsic activation of plasma [4-6]. Anticoagulants have been shown to delay thrombin induced platelet activation [5-7]. Clinical studies dealing with PTCA and acute coronary syndromes [8-9] demonstrated the effectiveness of combined application of a glycoprotein IIb/IIIa receptor antagonist and UH and supported the necessity of an anticoagulant therapy even in the presence of eptifibatide to reduce thrombin activity [9].

In vitro studies with eptifibatide done in whole blood [10] or washed platelets [11] suggested an anticoagulant effect of the drug that became more obvious in combination with UH or LMWH in activation with low concentrations of tissue factor. On the other hand, no influence on thrombin generation was observed in clinical [12] or baboon trials [13]. In vitro experiments performed with low tissue factor concentrations probably come closest to the physiological situation but should be complemented with experiments performed under strong activation to demonstrate the respective specific and additive effects of the drugs under conditions that might exist especially by rupture of lipid-rich plaques.

To our knowledge, until now no in vitro data are available about the combined effect of eptifibatide and anticoagulants on platelet aggregation and thrombin generation induced by endogenously generated thrombin under high and low coagulant challenge. We, therefore, used a previously described model allowing simultaneous determination of the time course of platelet aggregation and thrombin generation [5,7] in the presence of eptifibatide and anticoagulants after extrinsic activation of platelet rich plasma. For high coagulant challenge clotting was triggered using tissue factor (TF) concentrations that resulted in fibrinogen polymerization independent of platelets. For low coagulant activation we used tissue factor concentrations that did not eliminate the responsiveness of the system to variations of drug concentrations.

Materials and methods

Preparation and activation of platelet rich plasma (PRP)

Nine parts of blood from healthy volunteers were collected into one part of 0.1 molar citrate using a two syringe technique. The blood was centrifuged at room temperature for 10 min at 200 x g. The platelet count was adjusted to 250,000/µl with platelet poor plasma (PPP) prepared from the PRP. 400 µl of PRP were incubated with 1.3 mg/ml of the fibrinogen polymerization inhibitor PRP for 1 min at 37°C. Subsequently plasma samples were incubated with 10 µl buffer A containing different amounts of eptifibatide for 10 min at 37°C followed by administration of 20 µl buffer A containing rH, LMWH, or UH at desired concentrations for 2 min at 37°C in flat-bottom plastic tubes while stirring.

Clotting of plasma under »high coagulant challenge« was induced by administration of 48 µl activating solution containing Thromborel S (940 pg/ml = 26.9 nM final tissue factor concentration) and $CaCl_2$ (2mM final concentration). The activating solution to induce clotting under »low coagulant challenge« contained TF/FVIIa (5 pM final concentration) and $CaCl_2$ (2mM final concentration).

Determination of thrombin generation

The PRP was activated as described above. At timed intervals 10 µl aliquots were withdrawn and subsampled into 490 µl buffer B containing 255 µM S-2238™. The reagents were prewarmed to 37°C. Amidolysis of S-2238™ was stopped after 6 minutes by addition of 250 µl 50% acetic acid. The amount of thrombin generated was quantified by measuring the absorbency by double wave length (405–690 nm) in the Anthos microplate-reader 2001, from Anthos Labtec Instruments GmbH, Salzburg, Austria. The amidolytic activity measured is caused by the simultaneous activity of free thrombin and α2-macroglobulin-thrombin complex. The amount of free thrombin was calculated using a method developed by Hemker et al. [14–15].

Platelet aggregation

Platelet rich plasma (PRP) was obtained by centrifuging citrated blood at room temperature for 10 min at 200 x g. Platelet poor plasma (PPP) was obtained by centrifuging citrated blood for 10 min at 2800 x g. The PRP was diluted prior to testing by PPP to a final platelet count of 250,000/µl plasma. Platelet aggregation studies were done using a standard turbidimetric technique in an aggregometer (Bio/Data Corporation, Horsham, PA, USA). PRP was added to an aggregometer cuvette containing a stir bar. The cuvette was placed in the aggregometer prewarmed to 37°C. PPP was used as the blank. Platelet aggregation was induced by endogenously generated thrombin [5,7]. The anti-aggregating activity of the drugs was expressed as percent inhibition related to aggregation measured in the absence of inhibitors.

Determination of prothrombin fragment 1+2 (F 1+2)

Plasmas were prepared and activated as described above. At timed intervals 10 µl aliquots were withdrawn from the plasma and subsampled into 490 µl stopping solution. After subsequent 1:10-dilution in stopping solution, the amount of F 1+2 generated was quantified by using an immuno enzymatic kit.

Statistical analysis

The effects of different concentrations of eptifibatide, UH, LMWH, and rH on platelet aggregation, thrombin generation, lag phase until the onset of platelet aggregation, and F 1+2 activation were analyzed using paired t-test. For comparison of platelet aggregation, thrombin generation, lag phase until the onset of platelet aggregation, and F 1+2 measurements after activation of plasma at high and low coagulant challenge Mann Whitney U test was performed. The significant level of p-values was set at $p<0.05$.

Results

The anti-aggregating action of eptifibatide and anticoagulants was expressed as percent inhibition by relating the endlevels of the aggregation curves in the presence to that in the absence of drugs.

To assess thrombin generation (TG) curves samples were removed from activated plasma at timed intervals and assayed for thrombin potential (TP). Results are expressed as means (± SD) of six experiments.

Activation of PRP in the absence of eptifibatide, UH, LMWH, or rH under *high* coagulant challenge resulted in a sudden onset of thrombin generation after a lag time of 22.5 ± 1.6 seconds. The peak amount of thrombin concentration was about 150 nM and the calculated thrombin potential was 302 ± 9.4 nM.minute. To demonstrate that platelets had no influence on TP under high coagulant challenge PPP was activated as described above. The peak amount of thrombin concentration and the calculated TP were not different in PPP compared to PRP.

Under *low* coagulant challenge activation of PRP in the absence of eptifibatide, UH, LMWH, or rH revealed a calculated TP of 254 ± 9.3 nM.minute. In contrast to measurements under high coagulant challenge lack of platelets (PPP) decreased TP to 41 ± 8.2 nM.minute. The lag phase until the onset of platelet aggregation was 75 ± 6.5 seconds in the absence of inhibitors. As shown previously [8,9], onset of platelet aggregation and free thrombin generation occurred simultaneously under our experimental conditions.

Effects of eptifibatide and anticoagulants on platelet aggregation

Under *high* and *low* coagulant challenge increasing eptifibatide concentrations up to 1000 ng/ml resulted in dose dependent inhibition of platelet aggregation compared to measurements in absence of eptifibatide (Fig. 1). The anti-aggregating effect was significantly higher under low coagulant challenge in all experiments. Higher concentrations of eptifibatide did not result in significant further inhibition of platelet aggregation. Under *high* and *low* coagulant challenge different amounts of UH, LMWH, or rH had no anti-aggregating effect compared to not anticoagulated plasma.

Under *high* coagulant challenge combination of eptifibatide and anticoagulants resulted in significant additive inhibition of platelet aggregation compared to mea-

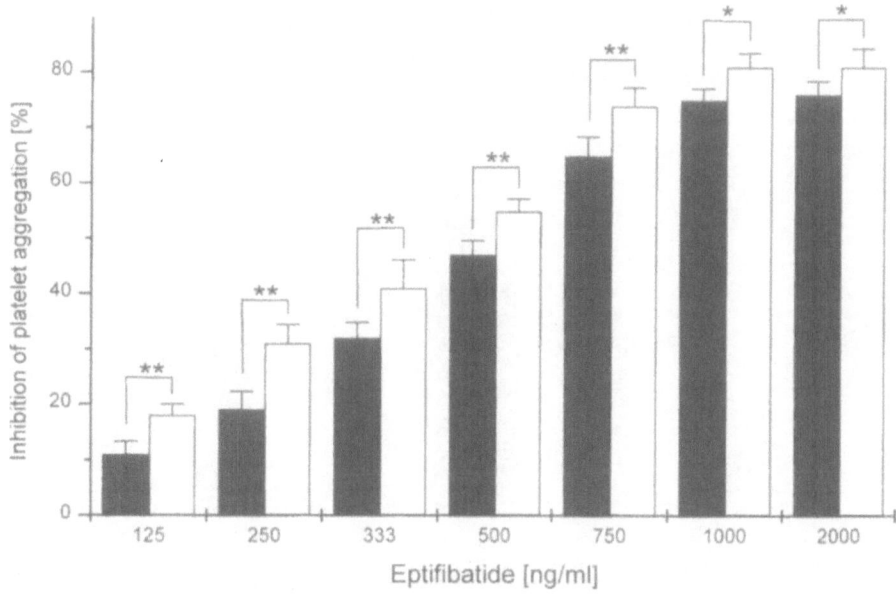

Fig. 1. Per cent inhibition of platelet aggregation with increasing concentrations of eptifibatide after high and low coagulant activation of PRP. *Black columns*: eptifibatide; high coagulant challenge (cc). *White columns*: eptifibatide; low cc. ★ = p<0.05; ★★ = p<0.01.

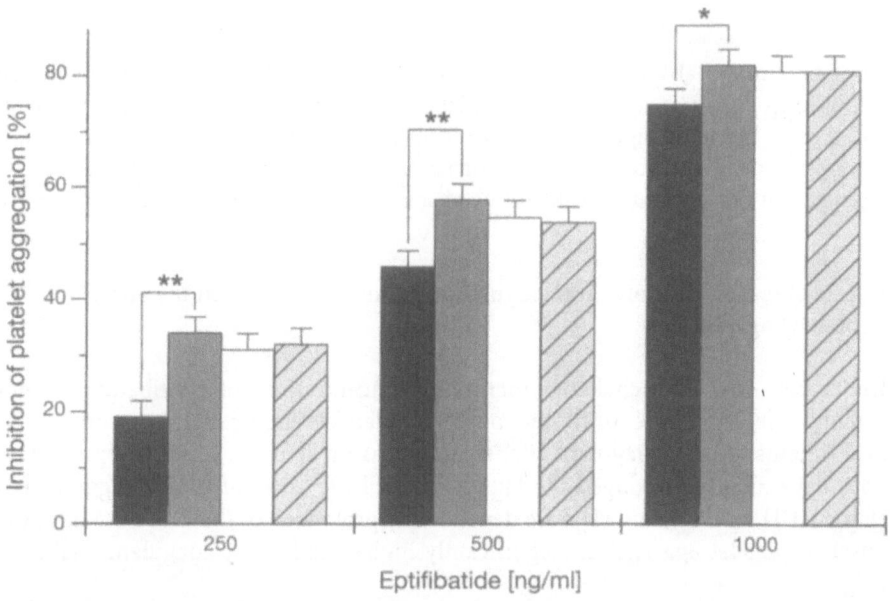

Fig. 2. Per cent inhibition of platelet aggregation at 250, 500, and 1000 ng/ml eptifibatide with or without addition of rH after high and low coagulant activation of PRP. *Black columns*: Eptifibatide; high cc. *Grey columns*: Eptifibatide and rH; high cc. *White columns*: Eptifibatide; low cc. *Striped columns*: Eptifibatide and rH; low cc. ★ = p<0.01; ★★ = p<0.001.

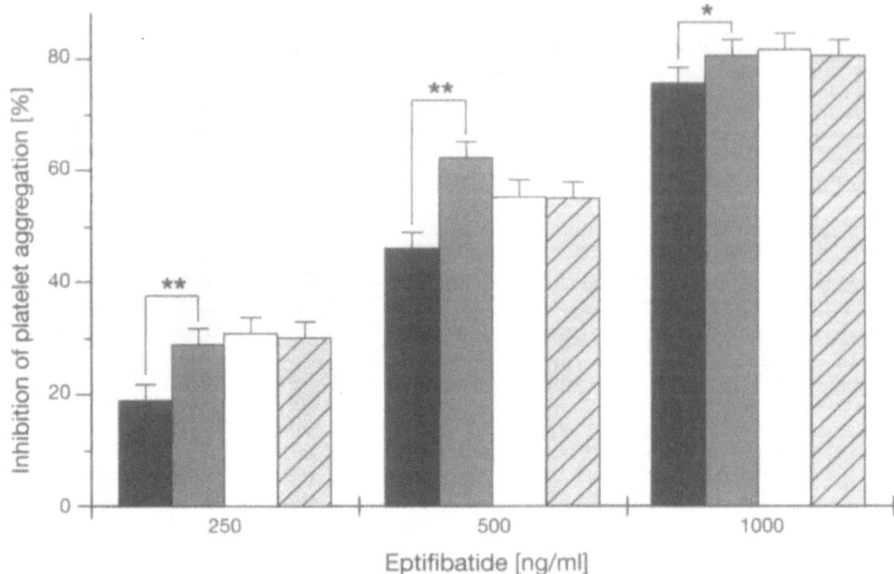

Fig. 3. Per cent inhibition of platelet aggregation at 250, 500, and 1000 ng/ml eptifibatide with or without addition of LMWH after high and low coagulant activation of PRP. *Black columns:* Eptifibatide; high cc. *Grey columns:* Eptifibatide and LMWH; high cc. *White columns:* Eptifibatide; low cc. *Striped columns:* Eptifibatide and LMWH; low cc. ★ = p<0.05; ★★ = p<0.001.

surements in the absence of anticoagulants (Fig. 2–4). Effect of anticoagulants on inhibition of platelet aggregation in plasma that contained eptifibatide was irrespective of the anticoagulant concentration used. Under *low* coagulant challenge combination of eptifibatide and anticoagulants did not further inhibit platelet aggregation compared to results in the absence of anticoagulants (Fig. 2–4).

Effects of eptifibatide and anticoagulants on the lag phase until the onset of platelet aggregation

Under *high* coagulant challenge increasing concentrations of eptifibatide did not prolong the lag phase until the onset of platelet aggregation. In contrast to experiments at high coagulant challenge increasing concentrations of eptifibatide dose dependently prolonged the lag phase until the onset of platelet aggregation (Fig. 5). UH, LMWH, and rH dose dependently prolonged of the lag phase until the onset of platelet aggregation, significantly higher under low coagulant challenge (Fig. 5).

Prolongation of the lag phase until the onset of platelet aggregation after addition of eptifibatide to anticoagulated plasmas is shown as percentage prolongation compared to lag phases of anticoagulated plasmas in the absence of eptifibatide. Combination of eptifibatide and anticoagulants significantly prolonged the lag

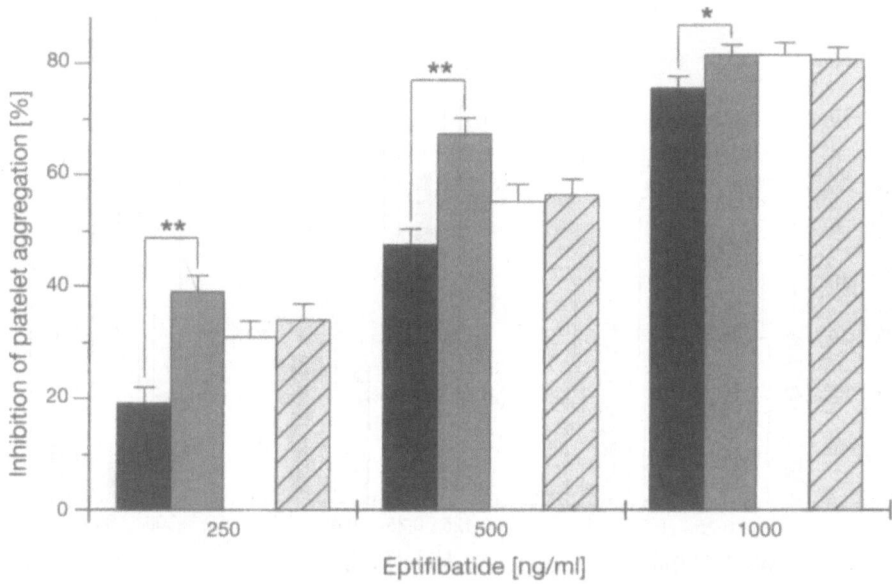

Fig. 4. Per cent inhibition of platelet aggregation at 250, 500, and 1000 ng/ml eptifibatide with or without addition of UH after high and low coagulant activation of PRP. *Black columns*: Eptifibatide; high cc. *Grey columns*: Eptifibatide and UH; high cc. *White columns*: Eptifibatide; low cc. *Striped columns*: Eptifibatide and UH; low cc. ★ = p<0.01; ★★ = p<0.001.

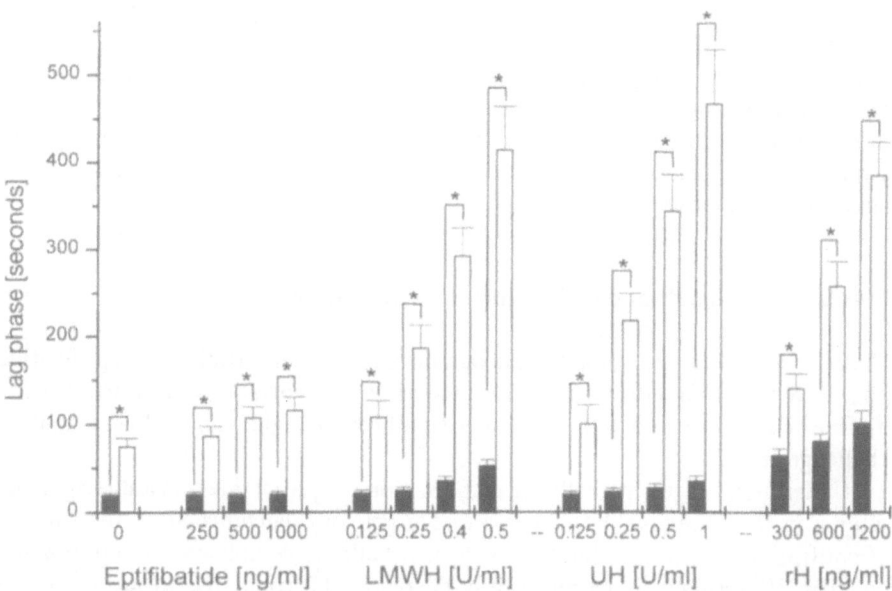

Fig. 5. Lag phase until the onset of platelet aggregation in PRP that contained eptifibatide, UH, LMWH, or rH after high and low coagulant activation of PRP. *Black columns*: High cc. *White columns*: low cc. ★ = p<0.0001.

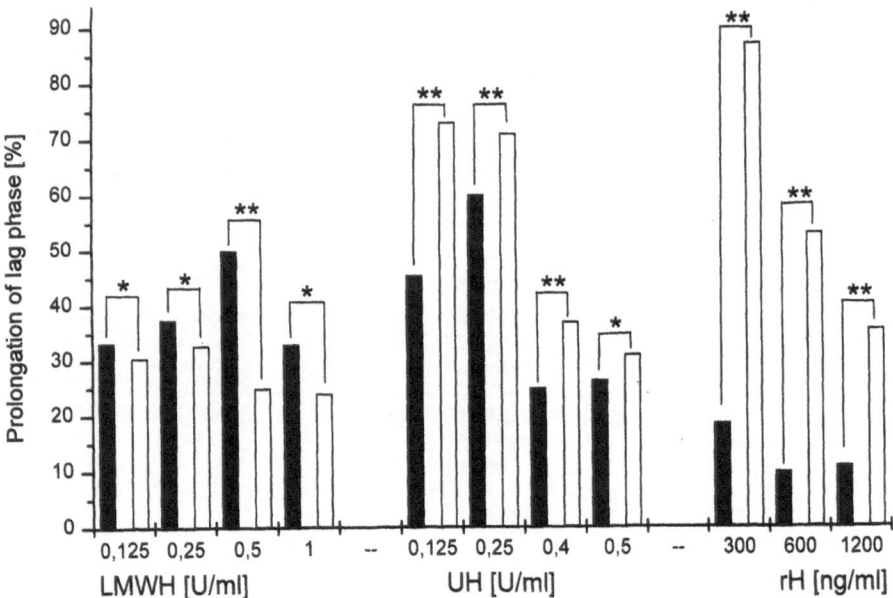

Fig. 6. Prolongation of the lag phase until the onset of platelet aggregation after addition of eptifibatide to LMWH, UH, or rH plasmas after high and low coagulant activation of PRP. Data shown as percentage prolongation compared to lag phases of LMWH, UH, or rH plasmas in the absence of eptifibatide. *Black columns*: Eptifibatide and Anticoagulants; high cc. *White columns*: Eptifibatide and Anticoagulants; low cc. ⋆ = p<0.001; ⋆⋆ = p<0.0001 compared to lag phases obtained in LMWH, UH, or rH plasmas in the absence of eptifibatide.

phase until the onset of platelet aggregation under *high* and *low* coagulant challenge, independent of the eptifibatide concentration used. In contrast to combination of eptifibatide with UH, and rH, combination of eptifibatide and LMWH demonstrated a minor per cent prolongation of the lag phase until the onset of platelet aggregation under *low* than under *high* coagulant challenge (Fig. 6).

Effects of eptifibatide and anticoagulants on the thrombin potential (TP)

Under *high* and *low* coagulant challenge increasing concentrations of eptifibatide had no diminishing effect on the TP. Increasing concentrations of anticoagulants diminished the TP, and this effect was significantly higher under low coagulant challenge (Fig. 7).

Under *high* coagulant challenge combination of eptifibatide and anticoagulants did not further diminish the TP compared to anticoagulated plasma in the absence of eptifibatide (Fig. 8). Under *low* coagulant challenge combination of eptifibatide and LMWH resulted in a significantly decreased TP compared to results in the absence of eptifibatide (Fig. 8). Only trace amounts of thrombin were detected testing 1 U/ml LMWH in the absence or presence of eptifibatide. No combined effects of eptifibatide and UH, and rH regarding the TP were observed.

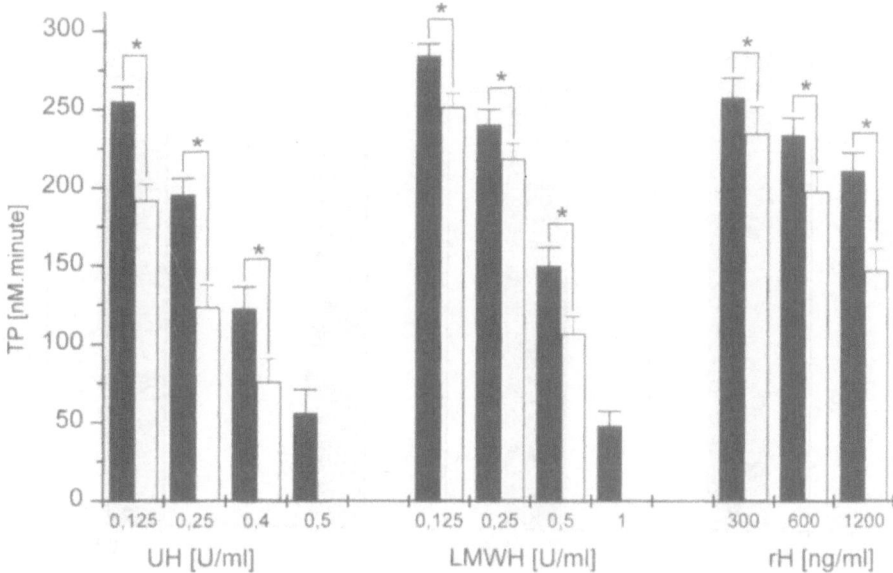

Fig. 7. Thrombin potential (TP) in the presence of UH, LMWH, or rH after high and low coagulant activation of PRP. *Black columns*: high cc. *White columns*: low cc. ★ = p<0.001.

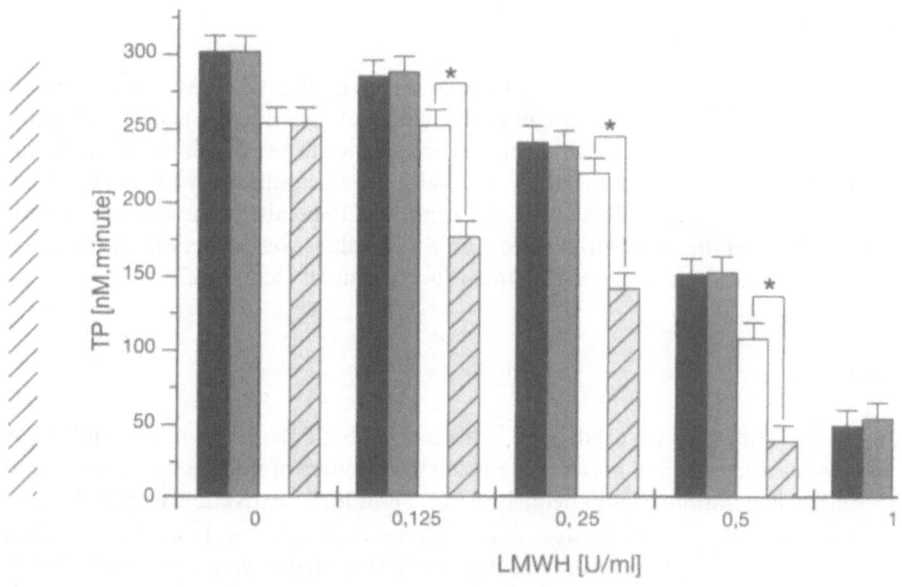

Fig. 8. Thrombin potential (TP) with or without addition of eptifibatide to plasma that contained LMWH after high and low coagulant activation of PRP. *Black columns*: LMWH, high cc. *Grey columns*: LMWH and Eptifibatide; high cc. *White columns*: LMWH; low cc. *Striped columns*: LMWH and Eptifibatide; low cc. ★ = p<0.001.

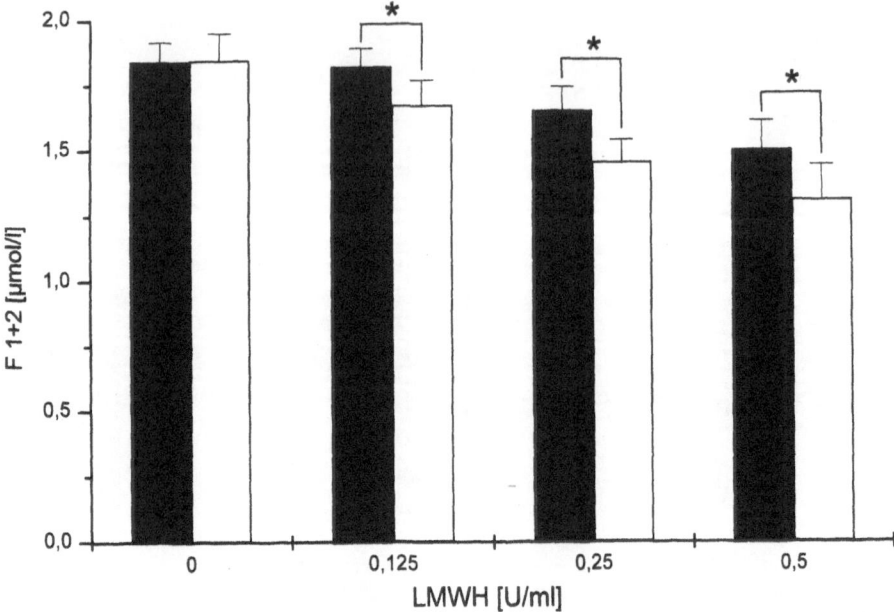

Fig. 9. F 1+2 values after low coagulant activation of PRP. Combination of eptifibatide and LMWH significantly reduced the F 1+2 values compared to results in the absence of eptifibatide. *Black columns*: LMWH. *White columns*: LMWH and Eptifibatide. ⋆ = p<0.01.

F 1+2 values

Under *high* coagulant challenge combination of eptifibatide and anticoagulants resulted in similar F 1+2 values compared to data obtained in the absence of eptifibatide. Under *low* coagulant challenge, in accordance to results obtained in thrombin generation measurements, the F 1+2 values were significantly lower (Fig. 9) in combination of eptifibatide and LMWH compared to results in the absence of eptifibatide. No significant additive effects on F 1+2 values were observed in combination of eptifibatide with rH or UH under low coagulant challenge.

Discussion

In the present study we used an in vitro model that enabled us to determine the effect of eptifibatide and anticoagulants on time course of platelet aggregation and thrombin generation simultaneously. After TF-induced activation of platelet rich plasma eptifibatide exerted a dose dependent anti-aggregating effect which reached its maximum of 75 per cent inhibition of platelet aggregation at a concentration of 1000 ng/ml. Under low coagulant challenge the anti-aggregating effect was significantly higher compared to results obtained under high coagulant challenge, and reached its maximum at 81 per cent inhibition of platelet aggregation also at a concentration of 1000 ng/ml. In the absence of drugs free thrombin generation was significantly lower under low than under high coagulant challenge. Addition of eptifibatide showed no influence on thrombin generation under high and low coagulant challenge. Prothrombin fragment 1+2 values were not lower in plasma containing eptifibatide compared to control. Eptifibatide addition to PRP prolonged dose dependently the lag phase until the onset of platelet aggregation under low coagulant but had no influence on the lag phase under high coagulant challenge. This results are in agreement with Butenas et al. [10], who found no effect of eptifibatide on clotting time at high but significant prolongation of the clotting time at low TF concentration activation. Our results might be explained by the both action of eptifibatide and tissue factor pathway inhibitor (TFPI). TFPI, a reversible, active site-directed inhibitor of factor Xa is a major inhibitor of thrombin generation, extends the lag time of thrombin formation, and reduces the rate of thrombin formation [16–17]. It has been shown that TFPI under low but not under high coagulant challenge [16] is able to inhibit the initiation of the coagulation cascade after tissue factor activation. We, therefore, suggest that under low coagulant challenge eptifibatide supports the anticoagulant action of TFPI.

The combination of eptifibatide and anticoagulants resulted in significant additive prolongation of the lag phase, which was significantly more pronounced under low coagulant challenge. Combination of eptifibatide and anticoagulants under high coagulant challenge revealed a significant synergistic decreasing effect on platelet aggregation. This observation might be explained by the ability of anticoagulants to affect binding of thrombin to GP Ib on the platelet surface. The binding site for thrombin on GP Ib has been demonstrated to play a key role in exposure of phospholipids on platelet surface and thrombin generation in response to thrombin, that also requires GP IIb/IIIa and platelet-platelet contact [18]. In its capacity as a receptor for vWF, GPIb promotes adhesion of inactivated platelets at sites of vascular injury. Surprisingly, under our low coagulant challenge addition of anticoagulants to plasma containing eptifibatide did not alter inhibition of platelet aggregation.

Addition of eptifibatide to UH, LMWH, and rH anticoagulated plasma did not further diminish the TG neither at high nor at low coagulant challenge with one exception. Under low coagulant challenge combination of eptifibatide and LMWH resulted in significantly reduced TG compared to measurements in the absence of eptifibatide. This observation might be due to the anti-Xa activity of LMWH. We speculate that the higher anti-Xa ratio of LMWH and the ability of TFPI at low TF/FVIIa concentrations to reduce thrombin formation might be the reasons for the additional decreasing effect of LMWH and eptifibatide on thrombin generation at low coagulant challenge.

Eptifibatide, although being a highly specific inhibitor of the glycoprotein IIb/IIIa receptor function, has been suggested to inhibit thrombin generation. Butenas et al. [10] demonstrated that the disruption of the GP IIb/IIIa-ligand interaction not only effects platelet aggregation but also decreases the role of TF-initiated thrombin generation in whole blood, suggesting a potent antithrombotic effect superimposed on the aggregation characteristics. On the other hand it was seen in a baboon study [13] that thrombin formation and activity were not significantly reduced in the eptifibatide group compared to control. In addition, Kleiman et al.

[12] demonstrated that levels of fibrinopeptide A (FPA), thrombin-antithrombin complexes, and prothrombin fragment 1+2 (F1+2) were not lower in patients treated with eptifibatide than in the control group in patients undergoing thrombolysis, suggesting that treatment with inhibitors of thrombin generation and activity may be required even when eptifibatide is used. The necessity for an antithrombin therapy even in the presence of GP IIb/IIIa blockade to reduce thrombin activity was further suggested by Ohman et al. [9].

GP IIb/IIIa inhibition when combined with heparin [8-9,19], or LMWH [20], has been demonstrated to be effective in PCTA and acute coronary syndromes. Anticoagulants such as UH, LMWH, and rH have been shown to reduce thrombin generation under low and high coagulant challenge [5,7] and have been demonstrated to be effective in treatment of arterial thrombosis [21-22]. In clinical studies combination of eptifibatide with UH has proven effective in PTCA, thrombolysis after myocardial infarction, and acute coronary syndromes [8-9].

Based on our experiments the anticoagulant effect of eptifibatide depends on the coagulant challenge, which is hardly to estimate in clinical situations. Results derived from our in vitro investigations support the notion that combination of eptifibatide and anticoagulants might improve the clinical outcome in atherosclerotic disease.

Acknowledgements. We would like to thank Prof. H.C. Hemker for kindly providing the method to calculate free thrombin generation from the amidolytic activity curve.

References

1. Scarborough RM. Development of eptifibatide. Am Heart J 1999;138:1093–104.
2. Phillips DR, Scarborough RM. Clinical pharmacology of eptifibatide. Am J Cardiol 1997;80:11B–20B.
3. Scarborough RM. Eptifibatide. Drugs future 1998;23:1–6.
4. Gallistl S, Muntean W. Thrombin-hirudin complex formation, thrombin-antithrombin III complex formation, and thrombin generation after intrinsic activation of plasma. Thromb Haemost 1994;72:387–92.
5. Gallistl S, Muntean W, Leis HJ. Effects of heparin and hirudin on thrombin generation and platelet aggregation after intrinsic activation of platelet rich plasma. Thromb Haemost 1995;74:1163–68.
6. Pieters J, Lindhout T. The limited importance of factor Xa inhibition to the anticoagulant property of heparin in thromboplastin-activated plasma. Blood 1988;72:2048–52.
7. Koestenberger M, Gallistl S, Cvirn G, Roschitz B, Muntean W. Effects of the glycoprotein IIb/IIIa receptor antagonist c7E3 Fab and anticoagulants on platelet aggregation and thrombin potential under high coagulant challenge in vitro. Blood Coagul Fibrinolysis 2000;11:425–32.
8. The IMPACT-II investigators. Randomized placebo-controlled trial of effect of eptifibatide on complications of percutaneous coronary intervention: IMPACT II. Lancet 1997;349:1422–28.
9. Ohman EM, Kleiman NS, Gacioch G, Worley SJ, Navetta FI, Talley JD, Anderson HV, Ellis SG, Cohen MD, Sriggs D, Miller M, Kereiakes D, Yakubov S, Kitt MM, Sigmon KN, Califf RM, Krucoff MW, Topol EJ. Combined accelerated tissue-plasminogen activator and platelet glycoprotein IIb/IIIa integrin receptor blockade with integrilin in acute myocardial infarction. Circulation 1997;95:846–54.

10. Butenas S, Cawthern KM, van't Veer C, DiLorenzo ME, Lock JB, Mann KG. Antiplatelet agents in tissue factor-induced blood coagulation. Blood 2001;97:2314–22.
11. Li Y, Spencer FA, Ball S, Becker RC. Inhibition of platelet-dependent prothrombinase activity and thrombin generation by glycoprotein IIb/IIIa receptor-directed antagonists: Potential contributing mechanism of benefit in acute coronary syndromes. J Thromb Thrombolysis 2000;10:69–76.
12. Kleiman NS, Tracy RP, Talley JD, Sigmon K, Joseph D, Topol EJ, Califf RM, Kitt M, Ohman EM. Inhibition of platelet aggregation with a glycoprotein IIb-IIIa antagonist does not prevent thrombin generation in patients undergoing thrombolysis for acute myocardial infarction. J Thromb Thrombolysis 2000;9:5–12.
13. Suzuki YS, Hillyer P, Miyamoto S, Niewiaroski S, Sun L, Rao AK, Hollenbach S, Edmunds LH. Integrilin prevents prolonged bleeding times after cardiopulmonary bypass. Ann Thorac Surg 1998;66:373–81.
14. Hemker HC, Beguin S. Thrombin generation in plasma: Its assessment via the endogenous thrombin potential. Thromb Haemost 1995;74:134–38.
15. Hemker HC, Wielders S, Kessels H, Beguin S. Continuous registration of thrombin generation in plasma, its use for the determination of the thrombin potential. Thromb Haemost 1993;70:617–24.
16. Van't Veer C, Mann KG. Regulation of tissue factor initiated thrombin generation by the stoichiometric inhibitors tissue factor pathway inhibitor, antithrombin-III and heparin cofactor-II. J Biol Chem 1997;272:4367–77.
17. Rapaport SI. The extrinsic pathway inhibitor: a regulator of tissue factor-dependent blood coagulation. Thromb Haemost 1991;66(1):6–15.
18. Dörmann D, Clemetson KJ, Kehrel BE. The GPIb thrombin-binding site is essential for thrombin-induced platelet procoagulant activity. Blood 2000;96:2469–78.
19. Storey RF, Wilcox RG, Heptinstall S. Differential effects of glycoprotein IIb/IIIa antagonists on platelet microaggregate and macroaggregate formation and effect of anticoagulant on antagonist potency. Circulation 1998;98:1616–21.
20. Cohen M, Theroux P, Weber S, Lavamee P, Huynh T, Borzak S, Diodati JG, Squire IB, Deckelbaum LI, Thornton AR, Harris KE, Sax FL, Lo MW, White HD. Combination therapy with tirofiban and enoxaparin in acute coronary syndromes. Int J Cardiol 1999;71:273–81
21. Weitz JI. Activation of blood coagulation by plaque rupture: mechanisms and prevention. Am J Cardiol 1995;75:18B–22B.
22. Turpie AG. Clinical potential of antithrombotic drugs in coronary syndromes. Am J Cardiol 1998;82:11L–14L.

Cardiac and cerebral Manifestations
of the Antiphospholipid Syndrome

W. Miesbach, F. Jung, Th. Vigh, and I. Scharrer

Arterial or venous thrombosis, fetal loss and thrombocytopenia characterize the clinical trias of the antiphospholipid syndrome (APS) [1]. It has been reported that a history of thrombosis is present in approximately 40–50% of the patients with antiphospholipid (aPL) antibodies and that 70% of the events are venous and 30% are arterial [2]. Deep vein thrombosis and pulmonary embolism are the most common venous events whereas the cerebral and cardiac system is most commonly affected on the arterial site [3].

Whereas the secondary APS is usually associated with other systemic diseases, with infections, certain drugs or systemic lupus erythematodes, the primary APS is a separate clinical entity.

The APS is characterized by the presence of a family of immunoglobulins that react with phospholipids or with phospholipid-protein complexes.

Lupus anticoagulants inhibit in vitro phospholipid-dependent coagulation tests while anticardiolipin (aCL) antibodies are assayed by ELISAs.

The mechanism of procoagulant activity of these antibodies is not yet completely understood, although inhibition of ß2-glycoprotein or the interference with the protein C or protein S pathway seems to be most likely [4]. Moreover, the formation of bivalent complexes of antiphospholipids with ß2-glycoprotein on the phospholipid membrane may interfere with the function of annexin-V, shielding phospholipids from the availability for any coagulation reactions [5].

Although there is still controversy about cardiovascular involvement in patients with APS, it recently has become more evident, that patients with APS have a higher prevalence of cardiac complications [6]. It has been reported APS patients with acute coronary syndrome and thrombotic occlusion of coronary arteries, as well as the presence of intracavitary thrombi [7]. Moreover valvular abnormalities have been described in 5–38 % of patients with APS [8,9], which mostly consist of superficial or intravalvular fibrin deposits subsequently leading to vascular proliferation, fibroblast influx and calcification [10].

Also cerebrovascular involvement has been described in patients with APS. In a study by Kenet et al. the presence of aPL antibodies was associated with a 6-fold increased risk for stroke [12]. Any neurological presentation can occur in these patients, of which ischemic stroke seems to be the major event [11,13]. Other symptoms such as migraines, seizures, chorea, symptoms of multiple sclerosis, transverse myelitis, optic nerve pathology or cerebral venous thrombosis have been reported [14]. The prevalence of aPL antibodies in patients with cerebral venous thrombosis

I. Scharrer/W. Schramm (Ed.)
32nd Hemophilia Symposion Hamburg 2001
© Springer-Verlag Berlin Heidelberg 2003

is about 22.6% compared to 3.2 % of controls [15]. Although neurological presentation of patients with APS may vary, many patients have striking similarities, such as memory loss, aphasia, cognitive disorders with progressive cerebral deterioration and even dementia [14].

The most feared manifestation in aPL-positive patients is the catastrophic APS presenting with thrombocytopenia, acute respiratory distress syndrome, disseminated intravascular coagulation, coma, multiorgan failure and, in most cases, with death [16]. The trigger is unknown, though infection is the prime suspect.

Patients

27 patients with APS were admitted to the university hospital Frankfurt/Main between 1998 and 2001 for cardiac or cerebral complications. Patients were between 29 and 79 years old and already known to have an APS or newly diagnosed. All patients fulfilled the proposed classification criteria for the APS according to the SSC of the ISTH [17] with positive lupus anticoagulant tests or with elevated levels of IgG and IgM anticardiolipin antibodies >5PL by an ELISA method.

Four patients had secondary APS with clinical and autoimmune markers (Fig. 1). Three patients died and had an autopsy.

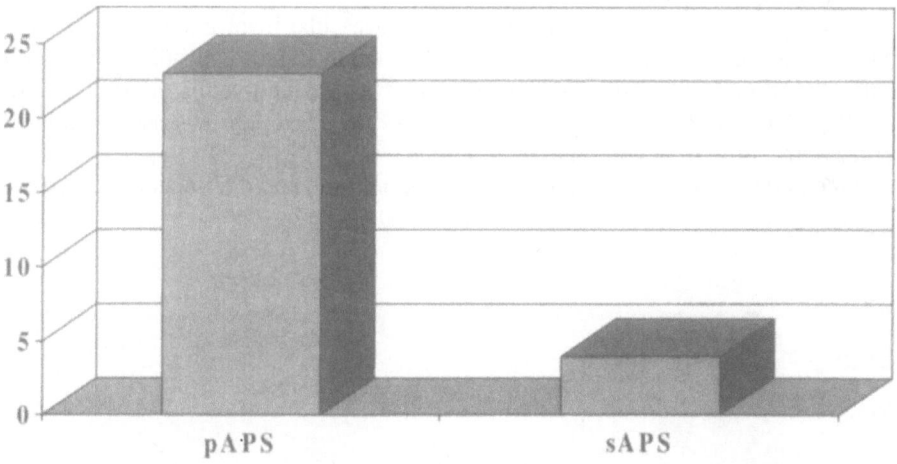

Fig. 1. Primary or secondary APS

Results

18 of the 27 patients had coronary artery disease with either thrombotic coronary occlusions, high grade stenosis, or complete vessel occlusion. In three patients the left main artery was involved. 10 patients had involvement of the left anterior descending artery (LAD), 6 patients of the circumflex artery (RCX) and 5 patients had

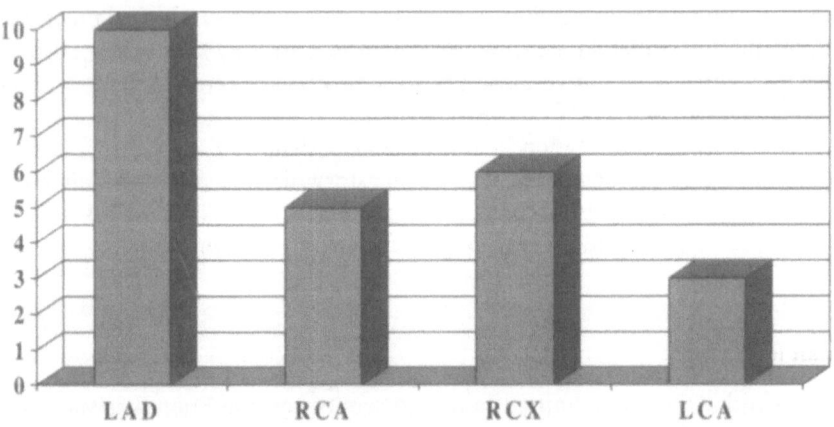

Fig. 2. Stenosis or vessel occlusion in coronary artery disease

involvement of the right coronary artery (RCA) (Fig. 2). In 3 patients there was thrombotic coronary occlusion without any signs of coronary artery disease.

As valvular lesions have been described in association with APS it has to be noted that in 16 cases there was mitral and/or aortic valva disease and in 3 cases tricuspid valve disease (Fig 3). Four patients underwent mitral- and/or aortic- and/or tricuspid valve replacement.

Seven patients presented a history of cerebrovascular involvement. Five of these patients had cerebral infarction, one patient recurrent cerebral bleeding under oral anticoagulation and another patient presented with cognitive disorders. Three of the 7 patients had a prior history of myocardial infarction, whereas 3 patients underwent mitral or aortic valve replacement.

One patient had an occlusion of artery spinalis ant. and developed paraplegia.

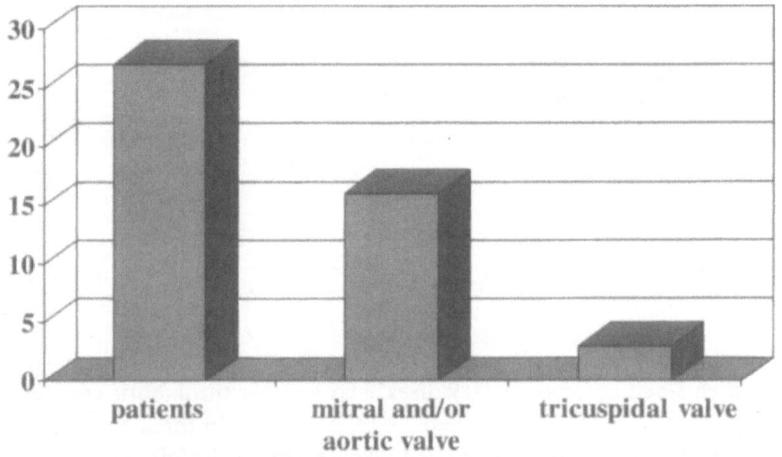

Fig. 3. Valvular lesions

Another patient with catastrophic APS was suffering from hand and leg ulcera due to arterial microembolism.

24 of the 27 patients survived, whereas one patient died from cardiogenic shock after massive myocardial infarction from acute thrombotic occlusion of the left coronary artery, one patient died of septicemia and endocarditis and another patient died of lung cancer.

Discussion

There is increasing body of evidence that the disease process in APS is systemic rather than localized with disturbance of endothelial integrity and procoagulability. This may explain the vascular manifestations of the disease with cardiovascular and cerebral involvement.

Especially in young patients under the age of 45 years, elevated titers of aPL antibodies seem to be associated with the incidence of acute myocardial infarction as well as higher incidence of subsequent cardiovascular events [17].

Similarly, patients who are aPL-positive have a higher risk of myocardial infarction: Varaala et al. postulated in a prospective study of 4081 men that elevated ACL titer is a risk factor of myocardial infarction or artery coronary disease, independent of age of the patient and other frequent risk factors [18].

The mechanism leading to an acute coronary syndrome is not entirely clear. Thrombotic vessel occlusion or myocardial vasculopathy, in the absence of vasculitis, may be the most likely [19]. Predominant localization of occlusion of coronary vessel pathology has not been studied extensively. It is striking that in our patients 18 of the 27 patients had coronary artery disease with either thrombotic coronary occlusions, high grade stenosis or complete vessel occlusion.

In three patients the left main artery was involved. 10 patients had involvement of the left anterior descending artery (LAD), 6 patients of the circumflex artery (RCX) and 5 patients had involvement of the right coronary artery (RCA). In 3 patients there was thrombotic coronary occlusion without any signs of coronary artery disease. There is more evidence for the involvement of the left coronary system, but the reason for this is not yet clear.

It is well known that the presence of aPL antibodies can be associated with valvular heart disease [20]. For example Galve et al. have described that patients with lupus and valvular involvement had aPL antibodies in 89 % [21]. Moreover valvular abnormalities have been described in 5–38 % of patients with APS, which mostly consist of superficial or intravalvular fibrin deposits subsequently leading to vascular proliferation, fibroblast influx, fibrosis and calcification [8]. The type of vascular lesions found in lupus disease mostly consists of noninfectious vegetations, which is different from those seen in APS, where irregular thickening of the valves is found [22]. Both stenotic and regurgitant lesions are found in patients with lupus erythematodes, whereas patients with APS predominantly present with left sided regurgitant lesions [22, 23]. As valvular lesions have been described in association with APS, the mitral valve is involved in 22–26 % of APS patients and the aortic valve in 6–10% [23].

Our study presents 16 cases with mitral and/or aortic valva disease and 3 cases with tricuspid valve disease. Four patients underwent mitral- and/or aortic- and/or tricuspid valve replacement after endocarditis and cardiomyopathie with diastolic dysfunction.

Association of APS with cerebrovascular events have been described already 1984 by Harris et al [24]. Barbut et al. reported that 86% of patients with ischemic cerebral strokes and aPL antibodies also had left sided vascular lesions compared to only 43% of patients with strokes, who did not have antibodies [25]. Cerebral ischemic events are the most frequent neurological manifestations, although migraine, epilepsy, recurrent TIAs, amaurosis fugax or transverse myelopathy, as well as progressive dementia have been described [13]. Although the neurological presentation of patients with APS may vary, many patients have striking similarities, such as initial memory loss, aphasia, cognitive disorders with progressive cerebral deterioration and even dementia [11,13]. In our study 7 patients presented with a history of cerebrovascular involvement. Five of these patients had cerebral infarction, one patient recurrent cerebral bleeding under oral anticoagulation and another patient was presented with cognitive disorders.

The hypothesis is appealing that the brain has a higher content of phospholipids, which may promote procoagulant activity or that aPL antibodies may have direct antineural properties [11]. Levine et al. suggested a correlation of antibody titers with the prognosis for recurrent stroke events. They stated that a titer > 40 GPL was associated with a higher risk of recurrent stroke [11,13].

Further research in this field will be of greatest interest. At present the prevention of recurrent thrombosis by anticoagulants and/or antiplatelet agents and the observation of asymptomatic patients with APS are essential tools in the care of APS patients.

References

1. Schmidt R, Scheuermann RH, Viertel A, Geiger H, Scharrer I. Antiphospholipid antibody syndrome. Med Klin 1999; 94:93–100.
2. Mc Neil HP, Chestermann CN, Krilis SA. Immunology and clinical importance of antiphospholipid antibodies. Adv Immunol 1991; 49:193–280.
3. Laraki R, Bletry O, Wechsler B, Piette JC, de Zuttere D, Godeau P. The heart and antiphospholipid antibodies. Rev Med Interne 1996; 17:46–57.
4. Ames PR, Tommasino R, Iannaccone L, Brillante M, Cimino R, Brancaccio V. Coagulation activation and fibrinolytic imbalance in subjects with idiopathic antiphospholipid antibodies – a crucial role for acquired free protein S deficiency. Thromb Haemost 1996; 76:190–4.
5. Rand JH, Wu XX. Antibody mediated disruption of the annexin V antithrombotic shield: a new mechanism for thrombosis in the antiphospholipid syndrome. Thromb haemost 1999; 82:649–55.
6. Ducceschi V, Sarubbi B, Iacono A. Primary antiphospholipid syndrome and cardiovascular disease. Eur Heart J 1995; 16:441–5.
7. Takeuchi, Obayashi T, Toyama J. Primary antiphospholipid syndrome with acute myocardial infarction recanalized by PTCA. Heart 1998; 79:96–8.
8. Asherson RA, Khamashta MA, Ordi-Ros J, Derksen RH, Machin SJ, Barquinero J, Outt HH, Harris EN, Vilardell-Torres M, Hughes GR. The »primary« antiphospholipid syndrome: major clinical and serological features. Medicine (Baltimore) 1989; 68:366–74.

9. Galve E, Ordi J, Barquinero J, Evangelista A, Vilardell M, Soler-Soler J. Valvular heart disease in the primary antiphospholipid syndrome. Ann Intern Med 1992; 116: 293–8.

10. Garcia-Torres R, Amigo MC, de la Rosa A, Moron A, Reyes PA. Valvular heart disease in primary antiphospholipid syndrome: clinical and morphological findings. Lupus 1996; 5: 56–61.

11. Levine SR, Brey RL. Neurological aspects of antiphospholipid antibody syndrome. Lupus 1996; 5: 347–53.

12. Kenet G, Sadetzki S, Murad H, Martinowitz U, Rosenberg N, Gitel S, Rechavi G, Inbal A. Factor V Leiden and antiphospholipid antibodies are significant risk factors for ischemic stroke in children. Stroke 2000; 31: 1283–8.

13. Levine SR, Brey RL, Sawaya KL, Salowich-Palm L, Kokkinos J, Kostrzema B, Perry M, Havstad S, Carey J. Recurrent stroke and thrombo-occlusive events in the antiphospholipid syndrome. Ann Neurol 1995; 38: 119–24.

14. Asherson RA, Mercey D, Phillips G, Sheehan N, Gharavi AE, Harris EN, Hughes GR. Recurrent stroke and multi-infarct dementia in systemic lupus erythematosus: association with antiphospholipid antibodies. Ann Rheum Dis 1987; 46: 605–11.

15. Christopher R, Nagaraja D, Dixit NS, Narayanan CP. Anticardiolipin antibodies : a study in cerebral vein thrombosis. Acta Neurol Scand 1999; 99: 121–4.

16. Asherson RA, Piette JC. The catastrophic antiphospholipid syndrome: acute multiorgan failure associated with antiphospholipid antibodies: a review of 31 patients. Lupus 1996; 5 : 414–7.

17. Brandt JT, Triplett DA, Alving B, Scharrer I. Criteria for the diagnosis of lupus anticoagulans: an update. On behalf of the Subcommittee on Lupus Anticoagulant/Antiphospholipid Antibody of the Scientific and Standardization Committee of the ISTH. Thromb Haemost. 1995; 74:1185–90.

18. Hamsten A, Norberg R, Bjorholm M, de Faire U, Holm G. Antibodies to cardiolipin in young survivors of myocardial infarction: an association with recurrent cardiovascular events. Lancet 1986; 1:113–6.

19. Vaarala O, Manttari M, Manninen V, Tenkanen L, Puurunen M, Aho K, Palpsuo T. Anti-cardiolipin antibodies and risk of myocardial infarction in a prospective cohort of middle-aged men. Circulation 1995; 91:23–7.

20. Kattwinkel N, Villanueva AG, Labib SB, Aretz HT, Walek JW, Burns DL, Klenz JT. Myocardial infarction caused by cardiac microvasculopathy in a patient with the primary antiphospholipid syndrome. Ann Intern Med 1992; 116:974–6.

21. Nihoyannopoulos P, Gomez PM, Joshi J, Loizou S, Walport MJ, Oakley CM. Cardiac abnormalities in systemic lupus erythematosus. Association with raised anticardiolipin antibodies Circulation 1990; 82:369–75.

22. Galve E, Candell-Riera J, Permanyer-Miralda G, Vilardell M, Soler-Soler J. Valvular heart disease in systemic lupus erythematosus. N Engl J Med 1989; 320: K739–41.

23. Galve E OJ, Candell-Riera J, Piegrau C, Permanyer-Miralda G, Garcia-Del-Castillo H, Soler-Soler J. Prevalence, morphological types and evolution of cardiac valvular disease in systemic lupus erythematosus. N Engl J Med 1988; 319:817–23.

24. Nesher G, Ilany J, Rosenmann D, Abraham AS. Valvular dysfunction in antiphospholipid syndrome: prevalence, clinical features and treatment. Semin Arthritis Rheum 1997; 27:27–53.

25. Harris EN, Gharavi AE, Asherson RA, Boey ML, Hughes GR. Cerebral infarction in systemic lupus: association with anticardiolipin antibodies. Clin Exp Rheumatol 1984; 2:47–51.

26. Barbut D, Borer JS, Wallerson D, Ameisen O, Lockshin M. Anticardiolipin antibody and stroke: possible relation of valvular heart disease and embolic events. Cardiology 1991; 79:99–109.

VId. Diagnosis

Inactivation of Animal Factor VIII by human Factor VIII Inhibitors: Special Methodological Features in Performing the Factor VIII Assay and the Bethesda Assay

G. Lutze (Jr.), V. Aumann, G. Lutze (Sen.), K. Kutschmann, and M. Schröpel

Introduction

Coagulation testing is currently gaining increasing importance in veterinary medicine. This applies particularly to coagulation factor VIII and its associated diseases [1, 2, 5, 6, 9, 10]. It therefore appeared necessary to examine the methods currently used for the determination of factor VIII activity with regard to their comparability and suitability for use in animals. The coagulometric and chromogenic assay methods established for the determination of factor VIII activity in human medicine were used.

The allo- and autoantibodies that occur in hemophilia A patients with inhibitors and in patients with acquired hemophilia A are currently of particular interest from both the clinical and the theoretical point of view. With the exception of porcine factor VIII, there have been practically no studies of the effects of human factor VIII antibodies on animal factor VIII [8].

The objectives of our investigations were

A. to determine special methodological features of determining factor VIII activity in animal plasma using the coagulometric and the chromogenic method

B. to examine the suitability of the Bethesda method for quantitation of factor VIII inhibitors using animal plasmas as source of factor VIII.

Methods

Plasma tested

In addition to human plasma, plasma from healthy individuals of the following species was tested: pig (Sus scrofa f. domestica), cattle (Bos primigenius f. taurus), dog (Canis lupus f. familiaris), cat (Felis silvestris f. catus), zebra (Equus grevyi), llama (Lama guanicoe f. glama), snow leopard (Panthera uncia), greater kudu (Tragelaphus strepsiceros) and mink (Mustela lutreola f. vison).

Platelet-free citrated plasma was obtained from human and animal citrated blood samples by centrifugation (30 minutes at 2500g). The plasma was aliquoted and stored in liquid nitrogen at –196°C.

I. Scharrer/W. Schramm (Ed.)
32nd Hemophilia Symposion Hamburg 2001
© Springer-Verlag Berlin Heidelberg 2003

Determination of factor VIII activity

The assays were performed on the Amax coagulation analyser (Sigma/Amelung, Lemgo) on the basis of the coagulometric [4] and the chromogenic measuring principle. A native factor VIII deficient plasma, the test kit Immunochrom FVIII:C from Progen Immuno Diagnostika GmbH, Heidelberg and the aPTT reagent Platelin LS from Organon Teknika, Eppelheim were used.

For establishing human reference curves we prepared our own normal plasma by mixing citrated plasma from 40 clinically healthy subjects without coagulation disorders. Normal canine, feline and bovine plasmas were mixed plasmas prepared from citrated plasma from 12 clinically healthy individuals, respectively.

Determination of factor VIII inhibitors

The factor VIII inhibitor titers were determined by the Bethesda method [3, 5, 7]. In factor VIII inhibitor assays using animal plasma the plasma had to be prediluted before incubation because of the high factor VIII activities in animal plasma (Table 3).

Results

Determination of factor VIII activity in animal plasma

Table 1 shows the results of the measurement of factor VIII activity in 4 human plasmas using the coagulometric and the chromogenic method. Normal human plasma was used as reference plasma. The results of the two methods showed good agreement over the entire measuring range.

There was also good agreement between the two methods (correlation coefficient 0.939) with canine plasma provided a species-specific reference plasma was used for the calibration (Table 2).

Table 3 shows the results of determination of factor VIII activity in plasmas from different animal species using normal human plasma as reference plasma. With the exception of zebra plasma, the animal plasmas had to be prediluted to

Table 1. Factor VIII activity (%) in 4 human plasmas (Reference plasma: normal human plasma)

Human Plasma	Coagulometric Method	Chromogenic Method
1	101	98
2	41	43
3	18	17
4	2	3

Table 2. Factor VIII activity (%) in plasmas from 12 dogs (Reference plasma: normal canine plama)

Dog	Coagulometric Method	Chromogenic Method
1	96	98
2	89	85
3	103	109
4	128	138
5	100	94
6	108	114
7	90	96
8	101	92
9	122	120
10	95	88
11	97	99
12	77	78

Table 3. Factor VIII activity (%) in plasmas from 9 animals (Reference plasma: normal human plasma)

Plasma	Coagulometric Method	Chromogenic Method
Pig	635	600
Cattle	385	665
Dog	600	280
Cat	1710	615
Zebra	70	30
Llama	950	720
Leopard	1400	810
Kudu	260	560
Mink	1175	205

various degrees in order to reach activities in the measuring range of the reference curve prepared with human plasma. To obtain the values shown, the results were multiplied by the respective dilution factors. The factor VIII activities in all animals except the pig there were marked discrepancies between the results of the coagulometric and the chromogenic methods, although no systematic pattern was discernible.

Figures 1 and 2 show the reference curves for coagulometric and chromogenic factor VIII assays. In addition to normal human plasma, mixed canine, feline and bovine plasmas were used. With the coagulometric method the shortest clotting times were found for the cat, with all four calibration curves except for the 1:5 dilution showing a linear and parallel course. With the chromogenic method the highest absorbencies were in the cat and cattle. At high activities a linear and parallel course compared with the linear dilution curve of the human plasma was not found.

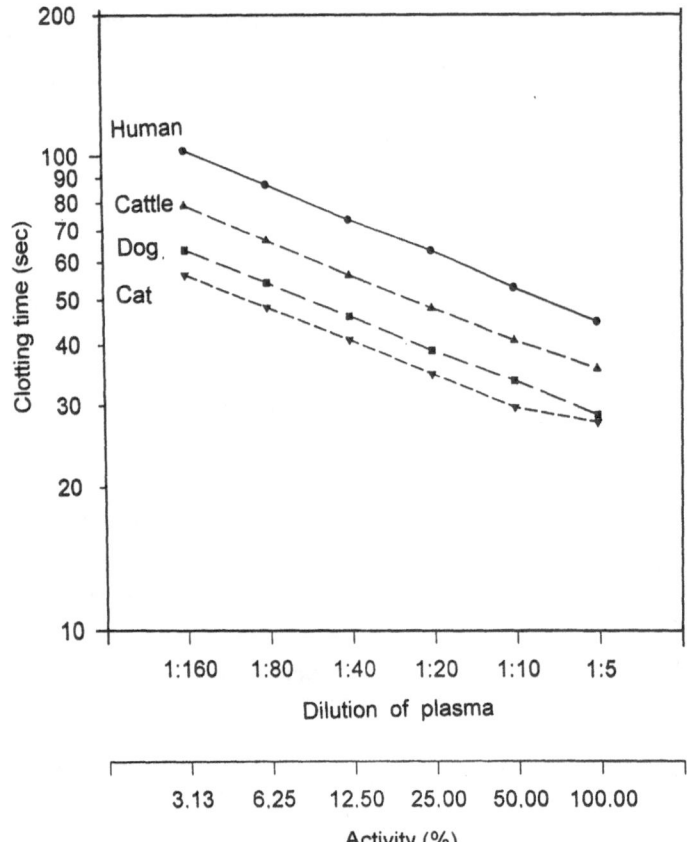

Fig. 1. Reference curves for the coagulometric factor VIII assay using normal human, canine, feline and bovine plasmas

Determination of factor VIII inhibitors using animal plasma as source of factor VIII

In inhibitor assays with animal plasma predilution was necessary. The predilution reduced the factor VIII to measurable activities in the range of the reference curve prepared with human plasma. The predilution was performed with imidazole buffer and with factor VIII deficient plasma from two different manufacturers. The characteristics of these factor deficient plasmas are shown in Table 4 where it can be seen that the factor VIII deficient plasma from manufacturer 2 did not contain any von-Willebrand factor.

Table 4. Factor VIII/vWF complex (%) in 2 commercial factor VIII deficient plasmas

Manufacturer	1	2
Factor VIII source	human, native	human, immune-adsorbed
Factor VIII activity	<1	<1
Ristocetin cofactor	180	<1
Willebrand factor antigen	170	<1

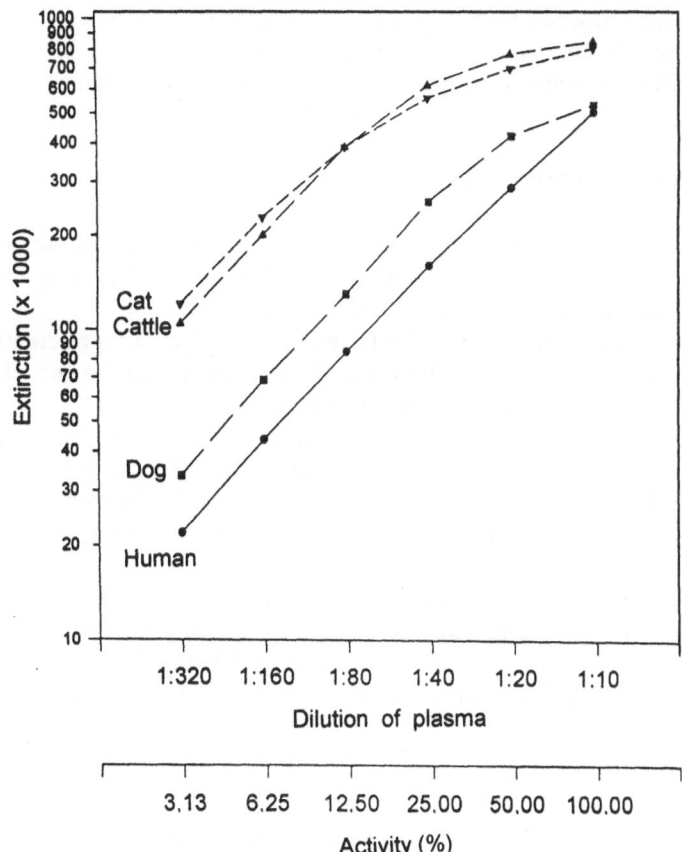

Fig. 2. Reference curves for the chromogenic factor VIII assay using normal human, canine, feline and bovine plasmas

Table 5 shows the results of inhibitor assays in which porcine, bovine and canine plasmas prediluted with imidazole buffer and factor VIII deficient plasmas from two manufacturers were used as source of factor VIII activity. The factor VIII inhibitor in the plasma from patient A.W., with a titer of 123 Bethesda units/ml against human factor VIII, also inactivated animal factor VIII but to a lesser extent. A factor VIII deficient plasma containing sufficient amounts of von-Willebrand factor (Manufacturer 1) was necessary for predilution of the animal plasmas. Predilution

Table 5. Determination of inhibitor activity in plasma from patient A.W. using animal factor VIII and three different predilution agents (values in Bethesda units/ml patient plasma)

Factor VIII source	Dilution with imidazole buffer	Dilution with factor VIII deficient plasma (Manufacturer 1)	Dilution with factor VIII deficient plasma (Manufacturer 2)
Pig	33	18	37
Cattle	54	42	57
Dog	109	60	–

with imidazole buffer or a factor VIII deficient plasma without von-Willebrand factor (Manufacturer 2) led to a stability-related loss of activity of animal factor VIII during incubation and thus to falsely high inhibitor values.

Summary and conclusions

– Determination of factor VIII activity in animal plasma can be performed by both the coagulometric and the chromogenic method provided that **species-specific** normal plasma is used as reference material.
– However, species-specific normal plasma from a representative number of individuals is either of limited availability because of the cost of preparation or unobtainable in the case of rare animal species.
– The precondition for the use of normal **human** plasma as reference material for factor VIII assays in animals is parallelism of the reference curves. This exists for factor VIII. Only the coagulometric method of factor VIII determination provided plausible results, although in most animal species considerably higher activities were observed than in humans.
– Determination of factor VIII inhibitors using animal plasmas as source of factor VIII is possible with the Bethesda assay provided predilution into measurable activity ranges is carried out. The predilution should be performed with factor VIII deficient plasmas containing von-Willebrand factor.

References

1. Gentry PA, Feldman BF, O'Neill SL. An evaluation of the effect of the reagent modification on routine laboratory coagulation tests. Equine Vet J 1992; 24: 30–32
2. Gopegui RR (ed). Hemostasis. In: Feldman BF, Zinkl JG, Jain NC (eds). Veterinary hematology. Lippincott Baltimore Philadelphia 2000; 517–593
3. Kasper CK. Laboratory diagnosis of factor VIII inhibitors. In: Kessler C, Garvey MB, Green D, Kasper C, Lusher J (eds). Acquired hemophilia. Excerpta Medica Princetown 1995; 9–23
4. Langdell RD, Wagner RH, Brinkhous KM. Effect of antihemophilic factor on one-stage clotting tests. J Lab Clin Med 1953; 41: 637–647
5. Lutze G, Breyer J, Naumann C, Zawta B. Useful facts about coagulation. Roche Diagnostics Mannheim 2000
6. Lutze G, Lutze GJR, Kutschmann K. Hämophilie A und B beim Hund. J Lab Med 2000; 24: 319–324
7. Lutze G, Schlote A, Mittler U. Untersuchungen zur Bestimmung des Gerinnungsfaktor VIII-Inhibitors. Z Ges Inn Med 1980; 35: 330–336
8. Lutze G JR. Untersuchungen zur Wirkung von Gerinnungsfaktor VIII-Inhibitoren bei angeborenem und erworbenem Faktor VIII-Mangel (Hemmkörperhämophilie A und spontane Hämophilie A) auf tierischen Faktor VIII. Otto-von-Guericke-Universität Magdeburg 2000; Inauguraldissertation
9. Mischke R. Optimization of coagulometric tests that incorporate human plasma for determination of coagulation factor activities in canine plasma. Am J Vet Res 2001; 62: 625–629
10. Stokol T, Trepanier L, Parry BW, Finnin BC. Pharmacokinetics of von Willebrand factor and factor VIII in canine von-Willebrand disease and haemophilia A. Res Vet Sci 1997; 63: 23–27
11. Wagenvoord RJ, Hendrix HH, Hemker HC. Development of a simple chromogenic factor VIII assay for clinical use. Haemostasis 1989; 19: 196–204

Inactivation of Animal Factor VIII by human Factor VIII Inhibitors: Investigation of Plasma from Patients with Inhibitors in congenital Hemophilia A and from Patients with acquired Hemophilia A

V. Aumann, G. Lutze (Jr.), G. Lutze (Sen.), D. Franke, and U. Mittler

Introduction

In a number of patients with congenital Hemophilia A the treatment is complicated by the presence of factor VIII inhibitors. These are alloantibodies which the patients only develop after receiving replacement therapy with factor VIII preparations.

Spontaneous factor VIII inhibitors, on the other hand, are antibodies to factor VIII which occur as a result of an autoimmune reaction in individuals with previously normal coagulation and lead to a usually severe acquired factor VIII deficiency with the associated clinical consequences. This disorder is known as spontaneous or acquired hemophilia A [1, 2, 5-7, 10, 13-17].

These allo- and autoantibodies are currently the object of particular interest as their presence represents a potentially life-threatening situation for all patients. Current investigations are focussed on both theoretical and clinical aspects, particularly on structure-effect relationships and possible therapeutic approaches.

With the exception of porcine factor VIII, we know practically nothing about the effect of the human factor VIII antibodies on animal factor VIII [12]. Porcine factor VIII is an exception as it is available as commercial product used for therapeutic purposes particularly in Anglo-American countries. In Germany, experience with porcine factor VIII is practically nil [4, 9, 11, 13].

The objectives of our investigations were
A. to determine the effects of human factor VIII inhibitors on animal factor VIII
B. to measure inhibitor formation after treatment with a porcine factor VIII concentrate
C. to determine the factor VIII inhibitor types (type I or type II kinetics).

Methods

Plasma tested

Nine patient plasmas were examined, four from patients with congenital hemophilia A and inhibitors and five from patients with acquired hemophilia A.

In addition to native animal plasmas from pig, cattle, dog, cat, zebra, llama, snow leopard, greater kudu and mink, Porcine Factor VIII:C Hyate:C® (Porton Speywood Ltd., Great Britain), currently the only commercially available therapeutic factor VIII concentrate obtained from porcine plasma, was used.

I. Scharrer/W. Schramm (Ed.)
32nd Hemophilia Symposion Hamburg 2001
© Springer-Verlag Berlin Heidelberg 2003

Definition of cross-reactivity

The cross-reactivity compares the activity of the factor VIII inhibitor from one and the same patient against animal and human factor VIII. It is calculated by dividing the Bethesda units per ml animal plasma by the Bethesda units per ml human plasma and is given as a percentage.

Results

Effects of human factor VIII inhibitors on animal factor VIII

Table 1 shows the inhibitor concentrations in two patients with severe hemophilia A who had previously developed factor VIII inhibitors after replacement therapy with factor VIII. In patient A.U. the inhibitor concentration after use of human factor VIII concentrates was 336 BU/ml plasma against human factor VIII, but only 67 BU/ml plasma against porcine factor VIII. However, the effect on factor VIII from other species was more marked. In patient U.K. there was a similar picture after administration of human factor VIII but with a lower level of inhibitor activity and thus of cross reactivity.

Table 2 shows the results of the examination of plasmas from patients with acquired hemophilia A before the beginning of treatment. It was striking that there was often only little activity against porcine factor VIII (patient W.P.) while, as in the patients in Table 1, the inhibitory activity against the factor VIII from other species was more marked. Thus both groups of patients showed a comparable picture with regard to the inactivation of animal factor VIII by human factor VIII inhibitors. The cross reactivity with porcine factor VIII was always least marked and there was usually an increase in the order cattle ⇒ dog ⇒ cat.

Figure 1 shows the inhibitory activity of the factor VIII antibodies in the plasma of a patient with acquired hemophilia A against the factor VIII from ten different animal species. The extent of inactivation presents a varied picture. With an inhi-

Table 1. Patients with severe hemophilia A and known factor VIII inhibitor formation

Inhibitor concentrations (BU/ml patient plasma) using human and animal plasma as factor VIII source

Patient	Human	Pig	Cattle	Dog	Cat
A.U.	336	67	99	179	287
U.K.	73	6	14	23	43

Cross reactivity (%) with animal factor VIII

Patient	Pig	Cattle	Dog	Cat
A.U.	19.9	29.5	53.3	85.4
U.K.	8.2	19.2	31.5	58.9

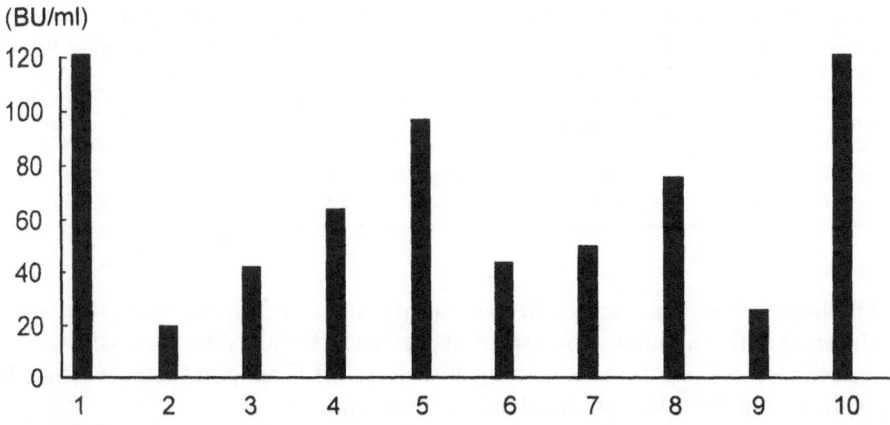

Fig. 1. Inhibitory activity of the factor VIII antibodies against the factor VIII from 10 different animal species in the plasma of a woman with acquired hemophilia (patient A.W.)
1 Human, *2* Pig, *3* Cattle, *4* Dog, *5* Cat, *6* Zebra, *7* Llama, *8* Snow leopard, *9* Greater kudu, *10* Mink

Table 2. Patients with spontaneous development of factor VIII inhibitors before beginning treatment (acquired hemophilia A)

Inhibitor concentrations (BU/ml patient plasma) using human and animal plasma as factor VIII source

Patient	Human	Pig	Cattle	Dog	Cat
A.W.	39	5	13	10	29
W.P.	30	0,6	5	24	29

Cross reactivity (%) with animal factor VIII

Patient	Pig	Cattle	Dog	Cat
A.W.	12.8	33.3	25.6	74.4
W.P.	2.0	16.7	80.0	96.7

bitor concentration of 123 BU/ml towards human plasma, the relatively low activity against porcine factor VIII (20 BU/ml) and the high activity against feline factor VIII (97 BU/ml) were not unexpected (Tables 1 and 2). The cross-reactivities with plasmas from zoo animals, however, also varied considerably. In the present example they were 21 % for the greater kudu, 36 % for the zebra, 40 % for the llama, 62 % for the snow leopard and 100 % for the mink.

Inhibitor formation after treatment with porcine factor VIII concentrate

Table 3 shows the activity of a spontaneous factor VIII inhibitor before and after treatment with porcine factor VIII (Hyate:C). In patient M.F., who had a very low

Table 3. Inhibitory activity of a spontaneous factor VIII inhibitor before and after treatment with porcine factor VIII (Hyate:C). Inhibitor concentrations (BU/ml patient plasma) using human and animal plasma as factor VIII source

Patient	Date	Human	Pig	Cattle	Dog	Cat
M.F.	21.03.	213	0.8	35	30	56
	10.04.	188	10	18	44	63

inhibitor titre to porcine factor VIII (0.8 BU/ml plasma) before treatment, there was an increase in the inhibitor activity against porcine factor VIII after successful treatment with Hyate:C, while the activity against factor VIII from other sources differed very little from the values obtained before treatment.

Determination of the inhibitor types

Two different types of factor VIII inhibitors are distinguished on the basis of their inactivation kinetics. Type I inhibitors possess a linear inactivation pattern with complete inactivation, type II inhibitors are characterized by a non-linear inactivation pattern with incomplete inactivation. The inhibitor kinetics and the division into type I and type II inhibitors are of practical significance as this is the only way to ensure genuinely correct determination of the inhibitor concentrations and comparability of the values, particularly in the case of type II inhibitors [3, 8, 12].

In the inactivation of animal factor VIII the pattern of occurrence of inhibitor types I and II was the same as in human plasma. Inhibitors in plasma from hemophilia A patients with inhibitors inactivated animal factor VIII with type I kinetics. In patients with acquired hemophilia A both type I and type II inhibitors occurred, a change in type sometimes being observed in the course of the illness.

Summary and conclusions

- The cross reactivity of human factor VIII inhibitors with porcine factor VIII in plasma from hemophilia A patients with inhibitors and particularly in plasma from patients with acquired hemophilia A was low (< 1 %–15 %). This finding supports the concepts about use of porcine factor VIII in these disease states.
- The cross reactivity of human factor VIII inhibitors with factor VIII from other animals was greater and particularly marked in the cat and the mink.
- Human factor VIII inhibitors inactivated animal factor VIII with the same inactivation patterns as human factor VIII (type I and type II kinetics).
- After treatment with porcine factor VIII, but also after human factor VIII, the antiporcine inhibitor titres usually increased. The inhibitor activity against the factor VIII from other species varied. Determination of the antiporcine inhibitor titre is essential before therapeutic use of a porcine factor VIII concentrate.
- The different patterns of behavior of human factor VIII antibodies towards animal factor VIII are evidence of the existence of different structures of the factor

VIII molecules. Structural elucidation of the animal factor VIII molecules could thus provide important information about the interactions between factor VIII and factor VIII inhibitors.

References

1. Gilles JGG, Jacquemin MG, Saint Remy JMR. Factor VIII inhibitors. Thromb Haemost 1997; 78: 641–646
2. Green D. Acquired factor VIII inhibitors and immunosuppression of autoantibodies. In: Kessler C, Garvey MB, Green D, Kasper C, Lusher J (eds). Acquired hemophilia. Excerpta Medica Princetown 1995; 25–40
3. Green D, Blanc J, Foiles N. Spontaneous inhibitors of factor VIII: kinetics of inactivation of human and porcine factor VIII. J Lab Clin Med 1999; 133: 260–264
4. Hay CR. Porcine factor VIII: past, present and future. Haematologica 2000; 85 (10 Suppl): 21–24
5. Hay CRM, Baglin TP, Collins PW, Hill FGH, Keeling DM. The diagnosis and management of factor VIII and IX inhibitors: A guideline from the UK Haemophilia Centre Doctor's Organization (UKHCDO). Brit J Haematol 2000; 111: 78–90
6. Hoyer LW. Inhibitors in hemophilia. In: Forbes CD, Aledort L, Madhok R (eds). Hemophilia. Chapman Hall London 1997; 213–227
7. Huhmann I, Lechner K. Spontane Faktor VIII-Inhibitoren. Hämostaseologie 1996;16: 164–170
8. Kasper CK. Laboratory diagnosis of factor VIII inhibitors. In: Kessler C, Garvey MB, Green D, Kasper C, Lusher J (eds). Acquired hemophilia. Excerpta Medica Princetown 1995; 9–23
9. Kessler CM. The treatment of acquired factor VIII inhibitors: Worldwide experience with porcine factor VIII. In: Kessler C, Garvey MB, Green D, Kasper C, Lusher J (eds). Acquired hemophilia. Excerpta Medica Princetown 1995; 71–89
10. Lechner K. Antikörperbildung – die derzeit gravierendste Komplikation der Substitutionstherapie bei Hämophilie. In: Scharrer I, Schramm W (eds). 26. Hämophilie-Symposion Hamburg 1995. Springer Berlin Heidelberg 1997; 61–67
11. Lutze G, Kutschmann K, Thomae K, Lutze GJR, Franke D. Erfolgreicher therapeutischer Einsatz von porcinem Faktor VIII bei der Hämophilie A des Hundes. Prakt Tierarzt 1999; 80: 664–670
12. Lutze G JR. Untersuchungen zur Wirkung von Gerinnungsfaktor VIII-Inhibitoren bei angeborenem und erworbenem Faktor VIII-Mangel (Hemmkörperhämophilie A und spontane Hämophilie A) auf tierischen Faktor VIII. Otto-von-Guericke-Universität Magdeburg 2000; Inauguraldissertation
13. Meili EO, Von Felten A. Bestimmt die Art der Blutstillung den klinischen Verlauf bei Patienten mit erworbener Hemmkörperhämophilie? In: Scharrer I, Schramm W (eds). 27. Hämophilie-Symposion Hamburg 1996. Springer Berlin Heidelberg 1998; 89–91
14. Moliterno A, Bell WR. Acquired coagulation inhibitors in the non-congenital factor deficient population: Clinical manifestations and management. In: Scharrer I, Schramm W (eds). 27. Hämophilie-Symposion Hamburg 1996. Springer Berlin Heidelberg 1998; 67–75
15. Scharrer I. Acquired inhibitors against factor VIII and factor IX. In: Hach-Wunderle V, Nawroth PP (eds). Life-threatening coagulation disorders in critical care medicine. Springer Berlin Heidelberg 1997; 51–59
16. Shapiro SS, Rajagopalan V. Hemorrhagic disorders associated with circulating inhibitors. In: Ratnoff OD, Forbes CD (eds). Disorders of hemostasis. W.B. Saunders Philadelphia London 1996; 208–227
17. Tuddenham EGD, McVey JH. The genetic basis of inhibitor development in haemophilia A. Haemophilia 1998; 4: 543–545

Factor VIII:C Measurement – Comparison between chromogenic and coagulometric Methods in Hemophilia A-Patients with the B-Domain depleted recombinant F VIII-Preparation ReFacto

A. Siegemund, T. Siegemund, U. Scholz, S. Petros, and L.Engelmann

Introduction

Moroctocog alfa (ReFacto, antihemophilic recombinant factor) is in use in the management of hemophilia A. It is a glycoprotein with 1438 amino acids and a molecular weight of 170 kDa. It is composed of the 90 and 80 kDa-parts of the human factor VIII with the B-domain deleted. According to the WHO standard the specific activity of this protein is 11.2-15.5 kIU.

The effect of this concentrate is very good. However, laboratory control of the plasma concentration requires some experience. The kinetic parameters of ReFacto are similar to those of the human factor VIII. In coagulometric tests for the determination of the F VIII-plasma concentration the values were underestimated. Only the determination of the concentration in an assay using the activator DAPPTIN (Progen Immuno) for the endogenous system gives consistent results.

This can be improved using the ReFacto-laboratory standard containing Moroctocog alfa with an activity range of about 10 IU.

The aim of our study was to show that in the case of using the ReFacto-laboratory standard for the calibration of the coagulometric tests the results are in good agreement with chromogenic assays that are the reference methods for the determination of factor VIII.

Materials and Methods

From two patients with hemophilia A under substitution with ReFacto blood samples were collected in a time range from 0 up to 24 hours (0 h, 30 min, 60 min, 120 min, 3 h, 6 h, 12 h, and 24 h) after injection of 2000 U of ReFacto. The factor VIII-activities were determined with the following methods:

Chromogenic Assays:
– Immunochrom Factor VIII   (Progen Immuno, Heidelberg, Germany)
– Berichrom Factor VIII   (Dade Behring Marburg GmbH, Marburg, Germany)
– COAMATIC Factor VIII   (Haemachrom Diagnostica GmbH, Essen, Germany)

Coagulometric Assays:
– Factor VIII-deficient Plasma   (Dade Behring)
– Pathromtin SL   (Dade Behring)
– DAPPTIN   (Progen Immuno)

I. Scharrer/W. Schramm (Ed.)
32nd Hemophilia Symposion Hamburg 2001
© Springer-Verlag Berlin Heidelberg 2003

Standards:
– ReFacto -Laboratory Standard   (Wyeth-Pharma GmbH, Münster)
– Standard Human Plasma   (Dade Behring)

For all assays the BCS Coagulation Analyzer (Dade Behring) was used.

Results

The determination of factor VIII with the different chromogenic assays gave a good comparability for the results ($r^2 > 0.96$, Fig. 1a-c, Table 1). There is a good correlation between chromogenic and coagulometric assays (for DAPPTIN $r^2 > 0.95$, and $r^2 > 0.82$ for Pathromtin SL, resp., Table 1). Using a plasma standard for factor VIII

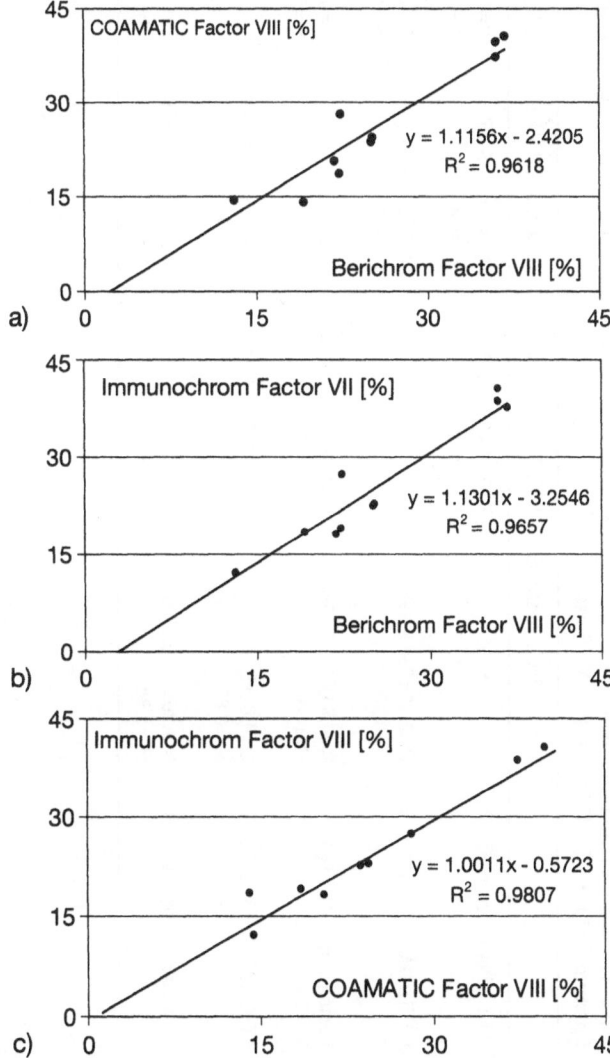

Fig. 1a–c. Comparison between Berichrom F VIII, Immunochrom F VIII, and COAMATIC F VIII

282 A. Siegemund et al.

Table 1. Determination of factor VIII – Comparison of coagulometric (Pathromtin SL, DAPPTIN) and chromogenic (Berichrom F VIII, Immunochrom F VIII, COAMATIC F VIII) assays

	F VIII / Pathromtin SL	F VIII / DAPPTIN	Berichrom F VIII	COAMATIC F VIII	Immunochrom F VIII
F VIII/Pathromtin SL (P)		P=1.10xD - 1.32% r^2 = 0.79	P=1.08xB - 5.96% r^2= 0.90	P=1.00xC - 5.90% r^2= 0.82	P=0.99xI - 5.75% r^2=0.93
F VIII/DAPPTIN (D)	D=0.72xP + 5.69% r^2=0.90		D=0.69xB + 0.18% r^2 = 0.95	D=0.79xC - 2.88% r^2=0.97	D=0.81xI - 3.77% r^2=0.98
Berichrom F VIII (B)	B=0.83xP + 7.15% r^2 =0.90	B=1.38xD + 1.15% r^2 =0.95		B=1.12xC - 2.42% r^2=0.96	B=1.13xI - 3.25% r^2=0.97
COAMATIC F VIII (C)	C=0.82xP + 8.87% r^2 =0.82	C=1.22xD + 4.34% r^2=0.97	C=0.86xB + 2.83% r^2=0.96		C=1.00xI - 0.57% r^2=0.98
Immunochrom F VIII (I)	I=1.20xP - 0.25% r^2 =0.94	I=1.22xD + 5.17% r^2=0.98	I=0.85xB + 3.45% r^2=0.97	I=0.98xC + 0.94% r^2=0.98	

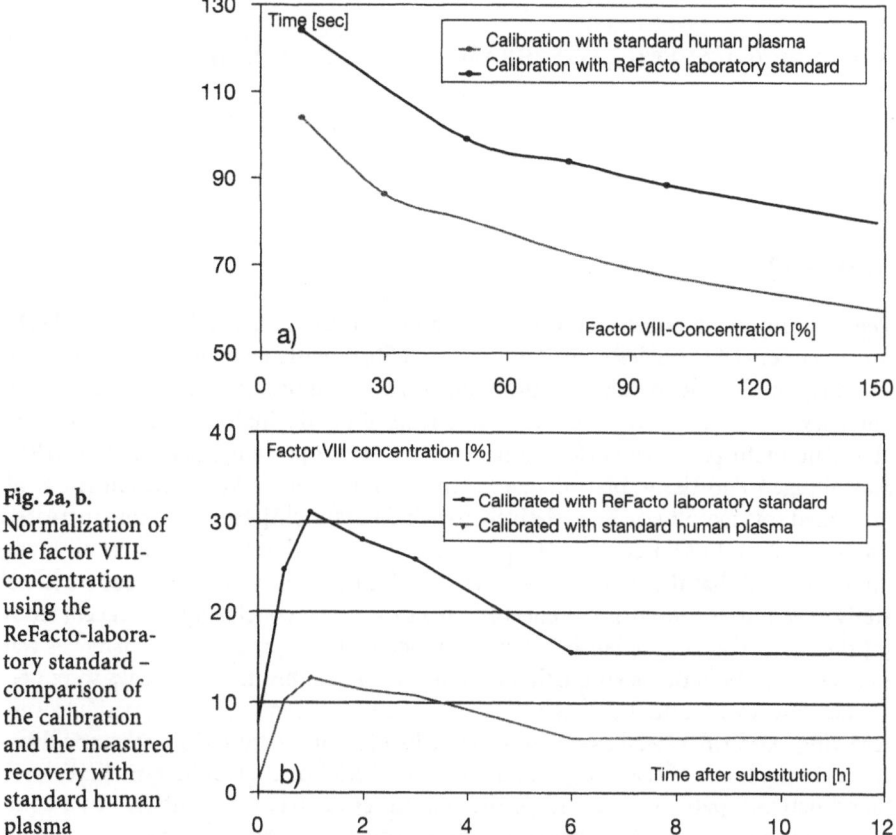

Fig. 2a, b. Normalization of the factor VIII-concentration using the ReFacto-laboratory standard – comparison of the calibration and the measured recovery with standard human plasma

the coagulometric tests show significantly underestimated results, which are normalized using the ReFacto-laboratory standard (Fig. 2a and b).

Conclusions

A plasma-based standard can not be used for monitoring the therapy with ReFacto, because the activities determined are too low. In this case it is necessary using the ReFacto laboratory standard or measuring the activity with a chromogenic assay. The cause of this effect is the changed activation by thrombin as a result of the depletion of the B-domain in the modified factor VIII-molecule and the origin of phospholipids [1] in the PTT reagent. For monitoring other factor VIII concentrates, plasma or WHO concentrate standards can be used.

Reference

1. Mikaelsson M, Oswaldsson U, Jankowski MA: Measurement of factor VIII activity of B-domain depleted recombinant factor VIII; Seminars in Hematology 2001; 38: 13–23

Functional Assessment of fibrinolytic Resistance in whole Blood

A. WERNI, A. CALATZIS, W. SCHRAMM, and M. SPANNAGL

Introduction

Venous thromboembolism represents a significant cause of morbidity worldwide [1]. Korninger et al. [2] suggested that an impaired fibrinolytic response to venous occlusion may predispose to recurrent thrombosis. Various immunochemical and functional assays for the assessment of the components of the fibrinolytic pathway are available. The main parameters determined are the tissue plasminogen activator (tPA), plasminogen and tissue plasminogen activator inhibitor I (PAI-1). Schulman et al. examined this hypothesis in a relatively large population [3]. He found that increased levels of tPA and PAI-1 correlated significantly with the development of recurrences, but concluded that the measurements were of limited utility. A large cross-sectional study of venous thrombosis patients [4] came to a similar conclusion. In a recent study [5] the value of a comprehensive fibrinolytic screening in predicting recurrences was evaluated in 319 patients with a first episode of venous thrombosis. Assays were performed four weeks after the diagnosis of deep venous thrombosis while patients were receiving warfarin as well as one week after its discontinuation. No systematic differences in the levels of tPA antigen and functional PAI-1 or euglobulin lysis times were found between patients who did, or did not, suffer recurrent thrombosis. In a commentary to this article [6] Bauer comes to the conclusion that these classical fibrinolysis parameters are not useful in the assessment of the thrombophilia risk of patients with an initial episode of venous thrombosis. However the author also states that other mechanisms involved in the downregulation of fibrinolysis such as the thrombin activatable fibrinolysis inhibitor might be involved in the pathogenesis of thrombosis and that new assay systems of fibrinolysis might lead to an improved definition of the clinical implications of fibrinolysis abnormalities in patients with venous thrombosis.

In recent time there is a rising insight into the interactions of cellular and plasmatic components in blood coagulation and fibrinolysis. New assays have been developed assessing these interactions in whole blood [7]. In this pilot study we examined the individual fibrinolytic response to a standardized stimulation of the lytic system in whole blood.

Methods

Citrated blood was drawn from 51 thrombophilia patients and 29 healthy volunteers. Whole blood coagulation and lysis were assessed in duplicate on the ROTEG coagu-

I. Scharrer/W. Schramm (Ed.)
32nd Hemophilia Symposion Hamburg 2001
© Springer-Verlag Berlin Heidelberg 2003

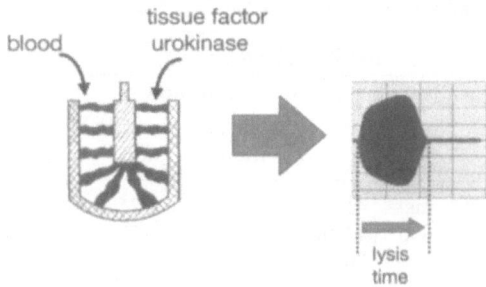

Fig. 1. Principle of the analysis: Citrated blood is clotted by the addition of tissue factor and $CaCl_2$. Fibrinolysis is triggered by the addition of a standardized dose of urokinase. The individual fibrinolytic response is characterized by the lysis time, i.e. the time from the onset of clotting until the lysis of the clot.

lation analyzer (Pentapharm, Munich), a novel thrombelastographic system with 4 channels and computer analysis [8]. Coagulation was triggered by the addition of 20 μl of 0.2 M $CaCl_2$ solution and 20 μl of recombinant tissue factor (2 μg/ml in barbitone buffer) to 300 μl of citrated blood. Fibrinolysis was triggered by the addition of 30 or 60 U urokinase/ml blood (Medac) (Fig.1). Fibrinolysis was characterized by the lysis time (time from the onset of clotting until the lysis of the clot).

Results

A typical fibrinolysis pattern during the analysis is shown in Figure 2. The mean lysis times which were determined by the two different fibrinolytic stimulations are shown in Table 1. The distribution of the lysis times in the two groups tested is shown in Figure 3. Significantly longer lysis times were found in the thrombophilia

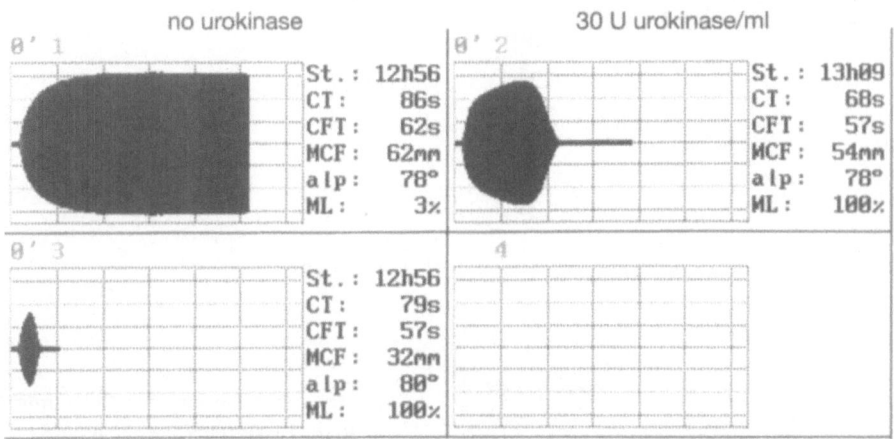

Fig. 2. Typical fibrinolysis pattern during the analysis: The analysis without urokinase shows no fibrinolysis. The higher urokinase stimulus results in much shorter lysis times when compared to the lower dose.

Table 1. Biometric data and lysis times in the two evaluated groups.

healthy volunteers					thrombophilia patients			
gender	age	lysis time			gender	age	lysis time	
	[years]	low uk [min]	high uk [min]			[years]	low uk [min]	high uk [min]
38% male	41.62	22.28	4.76	mean	37% male	47.94	23.79	5.42
62% fem	15.48	9.94	0.77	sd	63% fem	14.80	10.96	1.42
	70	41.5	6	max	1	84	54	10
	18	7	3	min	0	19	8	4
29	29	29	29	n	51	51	51	51

patients vs. the healthy volunteers when the high fibrinolysis stimulus was used but not when the low dose was applied. In Figure 4 the distribution of the lysis times is shown based on the percentiles. This figure shows that 20% of the thrombophilia patients had lysis times which were longer than that of any of the healthy volunteers. In order to exclude effects of the age of the patients and volunteers a correla-

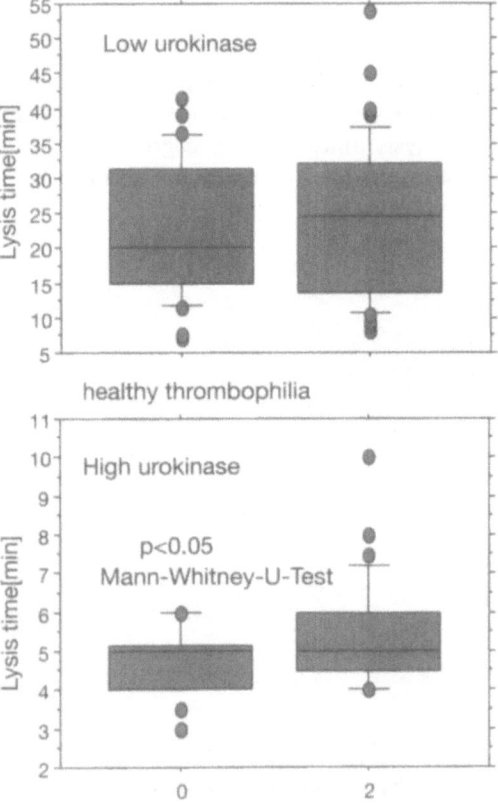

Fig. 3. Distribution of the lysis times in the two groups. For the high urokinase stimulus there were significantly longer lysis times in the thrombophilia group when compared to the healthy volunteers ($p < 0.05$, Mann-Whitney U-Test).

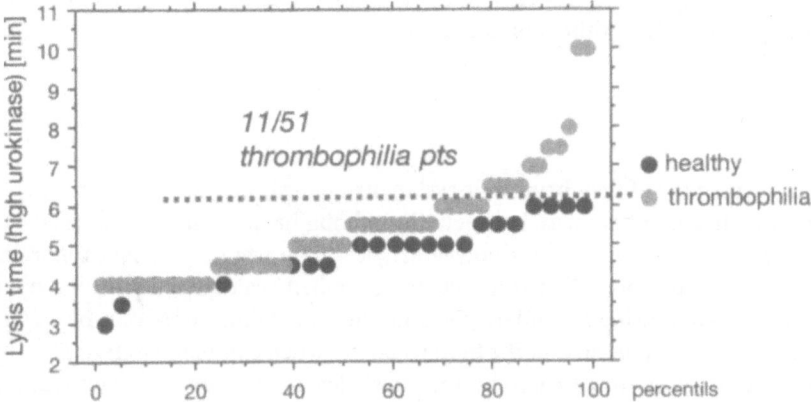

Fig. 4. Percentile diagram of the lysis times (using the high fibrinolysis stimulus) in the two groups.

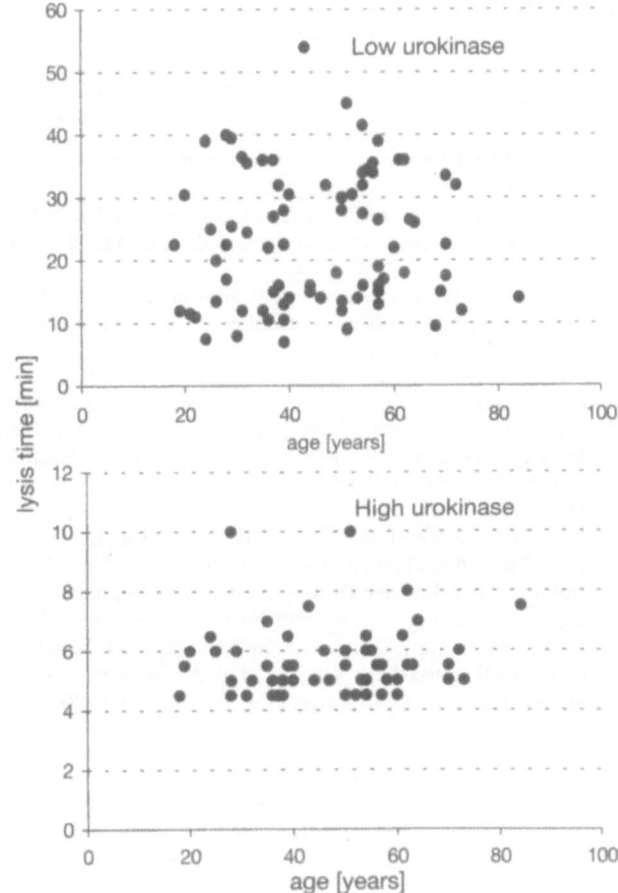

Fig. 5. Effect of the patient age on the lysis times

tion of the age of the subject and the lysis time was evaluated (Fig. 5). No effect of the age on the lysis time was found.

Conclusions

The assessment of the fibrinolytic system using the lower fibrinolytic trigger showed no significant differences between thrombophilia patients and normal subjects. However using the high fibrinolysis trigger there were significant differences between the two groups. The test system we applied evaluated the fibrinolytic system in whole blood using a standardized stimulus by a defined dose of urokinase. Urokinase was applied because of the better stability when compared to tPA. The approach to activate the clotting system by a relatively low amount of tissue factor and to trigger fibrinolysis by a defined stimulus mimics the in vivo situation, where fibrinolysis also only takes place when it is stimulated by tPA released by the endothelium.

This is a promising approach for a functional evaluation of the fibrinolytic system. Further evaluations with higher patient numbers are required in order to assess the clinical value of this method.

References

1. Martinelli I. Risk factors in venous thromboembolism. Thromb Haemost. 2001 Jul;86(1): 395–403.
2. Korninger C, Lechner K, Niessner H, Gossinger H, Kundi M. Impaired fibrinolytic capacity predisposes for recurrence of venous thrombosis. Thromb Haemost. 1984 Oct 31;52(2): 127–30.
3. Schulman S, Wiman B. The significance of hypofibrinolysis for the risk of recurrence of venous thromboembolism. Duration of Anticoagulation (DURAC) Trial Study Group. Thromb Haemost. 1996 Apr;75(4):607–11.
4. Malm J, Laurell M, Nilsson IM, Dahlback B. Thromboembolic disease—critical evaluation of laboratory investigation. Thromb Haemost. 1992 Jul 6;68(1):7–13.
5. Crowther MA, Roberts J, Roberts R, Johnston M, Stevens P, Skingley P, Patrassi GM, Sartori MT, Hirsh J, Prandoni P, Weitz JI, Gent M, Ginsberg JS. Fibrinolytic variables in patients with recurrent venous thrombosis: a prospective cohort study. Thromb Haemost. 2001 Mar;85(3):390–4.
6. Bauer KA. Conventional fibrinolytic assays for the evaluation of patients with venous thrombosis: don't bother. Thromb Haemost. 2001 Mar;85(3):377–8.
7. Holmes MB, Schneider DJ, Hayes MG, Sobel BE, Mann KG. Novel, bedside, tissue factor-dependent clotting assay permits improved assessment of combination antithrombotic and antiplatelet therapy. Circulation. 2000 Oct 24;102(17):2051–7.
8. Calatzis AN, Fritzsche P, Kling M et al: A new technique for fast and specific coagulation monitoring. European Surgical Research 28:S1 (89), 1996.

VIe. Miscellaneous

Quality Control of Platelet Concentrates during Storage using different Forms of Agitation measuring the Platelet Activation

M.K. Siemensen, V. Wilckens, F. Duka, M.M. Magens, P. Kuehnl, and K. Gutensohn

Introduction

In the past years prophylactic or therapeutic platelet transfusions have become a routine treatment. Therefore platelet storage prior to transfusion became necessary. One of the problems occurring during storage of platelet concentrates (PCs) is a decrease in platelet function, also known as platelet storage lesion [4]. It appears to be pronounced more with some forms of agitation of PCs during storage [1]. The platelet storage lesion is associated with an *in vitro* activation of platelets. The purpose of this study was to compare a new rotational storage device with the storage of PCs under routine conditions on a flat bed agitator. Quality control of PCs was performed measuring the P-selectin expression (CD62p), that is used as a predictor of platelet activation *in vitro*, on the platelet surface by flow cytometry [2,3].

Materials and methods

18 split PCs were obtained from 6 healthy donors by routine plateletpheresis procedures (Amicus™; Baxter Healthcare, USA; CobeSpectra; COBE BCT, Gambro, USA; MCS+; HAEMONETICS, USA). Half of the split PCs (n=18) were stored under routine conditions on a flat bed agitator (LPR1, Melco Engineering Corp., Glendale, USA) with an agitation rate of 60 shakes/minute at a constant temperature of 22±2°C. The other 18 PCs were stored in a rotational storage device (Gematron, Gematron Medical, Sweden) at 22±2°C. Storage time was set to 5 days for all products. Each day a sample of approximately 5 ml was taken. For flow cytometric analyses platelets were diluted to a concentration of 250/nl with platelet poor plasma (PPP) and stabilized. Then platelets were incubated with monoclonal antibodies in saturating concentrations at room temperature for 20 minutes. Analysis was performed using a FACScan® cytometer (Becton Dickinson, Mountain View, USA). CD62p positive platelets were detected using CD41a as tagging antibody (Beckman-Coulter, Glendale, USA). Results of flow cytometric analysis were expressed as mean channel fluorescence intensity (MCFI) in arbitrary units. MCFI of CD62p was positive, when it was higher than the unspecific IgG isotype control, calculated by subtraction.

I. Scharrer/W. Schramm (Ed.)
32nd Hemophilia Symposion Hamburg 2001
© Springer-Verlag Berlin Heidelberg 2003

Table 1. Mean values and standard deviation are expressed in MCFI; p-values for horizontal and rotational storage from day 1–5

	horizontal	rational	p-value
day 1	27.7 ± 5.4	28.1 ± 5.9	n.s.
day 2	31.7 ± 7.4	34.2 ± 7.7	< 0.05
day 3	35.7 ± 5.6	39.2 ± 7.4	< 0.05
day 4	38.0 ± 4.0	42.2 ± 5.7	< 0.05
day 5	35.8 ± 6.5	43.7 ± 6.6	< 0.05

Results

On the first day no significant difference in platelet activation could be detected comparing horizontally and rotationally stored PCs. On the following four days of storage platelets of the PCs stored on the flat bed agitator presented with a significantly lower degree of activation (see Table 1 and Fig. 1).

Discussion

In this study two different methods of platelet agitation during storage were compared to each other. CD62p expression on platelet surface was used as quality control for PCs. During the five days of storage the MCFI of CD62p expression was higher in PCs stored in the rotational storage device from days 2 to 4. Therefore PCs stored in this rotational storage device for more than one day display a higher degree of *in vitro* activation compared to PCs stored on the flat bed agitator used in this study under routine blood bank conditions.

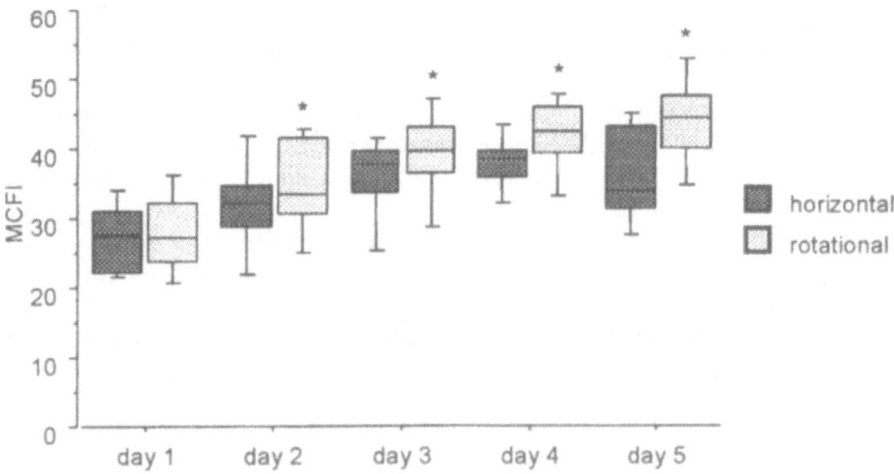

Fig. 1. PCs stored from day 1–5 either horizontally on a flat bed agitator or in the rotational storage device; significantly higher values are marked with a *.

Conclusion

The results of this study demonstrate that rotational storage with the Gematron device activates platelets to a significantly higher degree than horizontal storage. The increased platelet activation reduces quality of PCs, in addition a decrease of in vivo efficacy of these PCs can be expected. Thus, horizontal agitation and storage is recommended.

References

1. Holme S, Vaidya K, Murphy S: Platelet storage at 22°C: effect of type of agitation on morphology, viability and function in vitro. Blood 1978; 52: 425
2. Michelson AD: Flow cytometric analysis of platelets. Vox Sanguinis 2000; 78: 137–142
3. Rinder HM, Murphy M, Mitchell JG, Stocks J, Ault KA, Hillman RS: Progressive platelet activation with storage: evidence for shortened survival of activated platelets after transfusion: Transfusion 1991; 31: 409–414
4. Bode AP: Platelet activation may explain the storage lesion in platelet concentrates: Blood Cells 1990; 16: 109–126

Platelet Activation before and after Cryopreservation of Platelet Concentrates with a new Storage Solution

M.K. Siemensen, M.A. Brockmann, K. Geidel, A. Sputtek, P. Kuehnl, and K. Gutensohn

Introduction

Storage of regular platelet concentrates (PCs) is limited to 5 days, predominantly due to the risk of possible bacterial contamination. Alternative approaches for platelet storage may result in a prolonged storage period. In this study PCs were cryopreserved with a new storage solution (ThromboSol; LifeCell Corp., Branchburg, USA) [1, 2]. CD62p expression is a useful measure for quality control during platelet storage [3]. To verify platelet activation flow cytometric analyses was performed in the cryopreserved PCs [4]. For this purpose the expression of an activation-dependent neoepitope (CD62p) was analyzed on platelet surface in PCs before and after platelet cryopreservation.

Materials and methods

18 PCs were obtained with 3 different cell separators. The targeted yield in each PC was 5.0×10^{11} platelets per product (60 ml total volume). With the AMICUS™ cell separator (Baxter Healthcare, USA) PCs and plasma were collected separately. The PCs obtained by the cell separators from COBE Spectra (COBE BCT, Gambro, USA) and Haemonetics (Haemonetics, USA) were centrifuged to obtain the volume reduced product and separate the plasma. PCs were allowed to rest for 1h before further procession. The first sample was taken. PCs were transferred into special freezing containers (Baxter Healthcare, USA) and 1.2 ml of storage solution, ThromboSol (LifeCell Corp., USA) were added. Platelet products were placed into an aluminum cassette and directly put into the gas phase of a liquid nitrogen tank (–196°C) and stored for 7 days. The autologous plasma was frozen (–80°C) and thawed separately under routine blood bank conditions. PCs were thawed in a 37°C warm water bath for 3 min and resuspended in autologous plasma. The second sample was taken 1h after thawing. PCs were stored for further 24 hrs on a flat bed agitator (60 shakes/min, 22±2°C) before the third aliquot was taken for final analysis. To evaluate the degree of platelet activation flow cytometry was applied using a FACScan® cytometer (Becton Dickinson, USA). Platelet poor plasma was used to dilute platelet concentration in the samples to 250/nl. Platelets were stabilized and then incubated with monoclonal antibodies in saturating concentrations for 20 min. CD62p-positive platelets were detected using CD41a as tagging antibody (Beckman-Coulter,

I. Scharrer/W. Schramm (Ed.)
32nd Hemophilia Symposion Hamburg 2001
© Springer-Verlag Berlin Heidelberg 2003

Glendale, USA). Results were expressed as mean channel fluorescence intensity (MCFI) in arbitrary units.

Results

After thawing of cryopreserved PCs there was a significant increase ($p < 0.05$) in CD62p expression (before: 47.3 ± 19.7 MCFI; 1h: 50.2 ± 11.6 MCFI; 24hrs: 87.2 ± 27.0 MCFI).

PCs obtained with the COBE cell separator showed a significant increase in the CD62p expression after thawing (1h vs. 24 hrs; $p < 0.05$). PCs obtained with the Haemonetics cell separator only showed a significant increase in CD62p expression comparing the results prior to cryopreservation with those obtained 1h after thawing (before vs. 1h; $p < 0.05$). In PCs obtained with the cell separator from Baxter no significant changes occurred in CD62p expression during storage ($p = 0.07$). Before cryopreservation CD62p expression on platelet surface was highest in PCs obtained with the Baxter cell separator and lowest in PCs obtained with the cell separator from Cobe (Baxter: 62.0 ± 26.3 MCFI; Cobe: 35.7 ± 6.4 MCFI; Haemonetics: 44.2 ± 12.4 MCFI). 1h after thawing, platelets presented with a significantly higher MCFI of CD62p in PCs obtained with the Haemonetics cell separator compared to the Cobe cell separator (Baxter: 45.6 ± 10.7 MCFI; Cobe: 44.1 ± 8.5 MCFI; Haemonetics: 60.8 ± 7.9 MCFI; $p < 0.05$). 24 hrs after thawing there were no significant differences in platelet activation between the PCs obtained with the different cell separators (Baxter: 77.4 ± 30.6 MCFI; Cobe: 92.8 ± 18.1 MCFI; Haemonetics: 91.5 ± 32.4 MCFI).

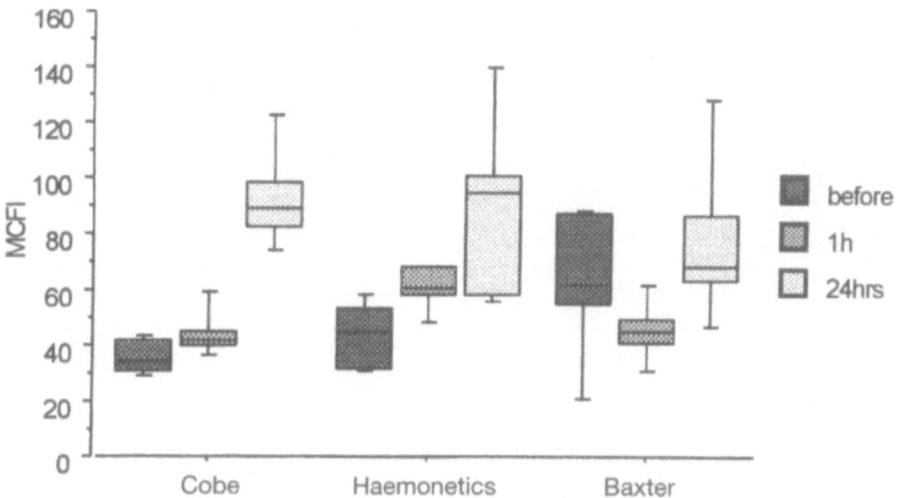

Fig. 1. MCFI values for PCs obtained by different cell separators (Cobe; Haemonetics; Baxter) before, 1h and 24hrs after cryopreservation for 7 days

Conclusion

This study was designed to investigate an alternative approach to storage of platelet concentrates. Cryopreserved PCs show a significant increase in MCFI of CD62p expression 1h after thawing to 24hrs after thawing. Compared to horizontally stored apheresis PCs obtained from the same donors platelets are moderately activated 1h after thawing (data not shown).

In conclusion platelet activation is higher in PCs after cryopreservation. However, briefly after thawing (1h) the increase in CD62p expression as a measure for platelet activation is moderate. Between PCs obtained with these three cell separators no relevant differences could be detected before and after cryopreservation. Cryopreservation of PCs with ThromboSol (LifeCell Corp., USA) as a storage solution may be an alternative to regular storage.

References

1. Currie LM, Livesey SA, Harper JR, Connor J. Cryopreservation of single-donor platelets with a reduced dimethyl sulfoxide concentration by the addition of second-messenger effectors: enhanced retention of in vitro functional activity. Transfusion 1998;38:160–167
2. Lozano M, Escolar G, Mazzara R, Connor J, White JG, DeLecea C, Ordinas A. Effects of the addition of second-messenger effectors to platelet concentrates separated from whole-blood donations and stored at 4°C or −80°C. Transfusion 2000;40:527–535
3. Michelson AD. Flow cytometric analysis of platelets. Vox Sanguinis 2000;78:137–142
4. Stohlawetz P. Flow Cytometric Evaluation of P-Selectin Expression on Platelets and P-Selectin Plasma Concentrations during Plateletpheresis. In: K. Gutensohn H-HS, F. Schunter, P. Kühnl, ed. Flow Cytometry in Transfusion Medicine. Heidelberg: Clin Lab Publications, pp. 67–73, 1998

Flow Cytometric Measurement of CD34+ Cells: How reliable are absolute Cell Counts generated by the Integration of Beads?

M.M. Magens, M.A. Brockmann, M. Siemensen, M. Weilandt, B. Bernien, P. Kuehnl, and K. Gutensohn

Introduction

For the reconstitution of hematopoiesis after myeloablative chemo-therapy the transplantation of peripheral blood progenitor cells (PBPC) is increasingly performed. The engraftment success is correlated with the number of infused CD34+ cells [2]. For the flow cytometric determination of these cells there are two main clinical applications: The timing of the stem cell harvest and the determination of the harvest yield.

Many recommendations have been given as to how the measurement should be performed [1,5,6]. Unfortunately, multicenter studies revealed that the lack of standardization causes the results to vary greatly between different laboratories [3,4]. Therefore, in 1996 the International Society for Hematotherapy and Graft Engineering (ISHAGE) published its »guidelines for CD34+ cell determination by flow cytometry« [7]. As this approach employs the WBC (white blood cell count) from a hematological analyzer to calculate the absolute CD34+ concentration, it is categorized as a **dual-platform method (DP)** (Fig. 1). The **single-platform method**

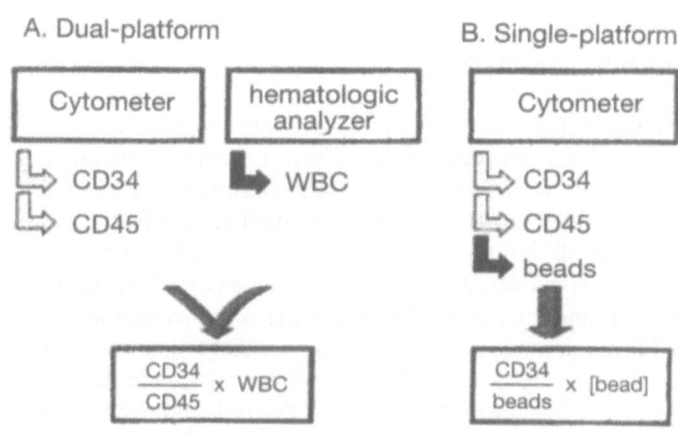

Key to Figure 1:
CD34   number of CD34+ cells counted
CD45   number of CD45+ cells counted
WBC   concentration of white blood cells (per µL)
beads   number of beads counted
[bead] given concentration of beads

Fig. 1. Calculating the CD34+ concentration

I. Scharrer/W. Schramm (Ed.)
32nd Hemophilia Symposion Hamburg 2001
© Springer-Verlag Berlin Heidelberg 2003

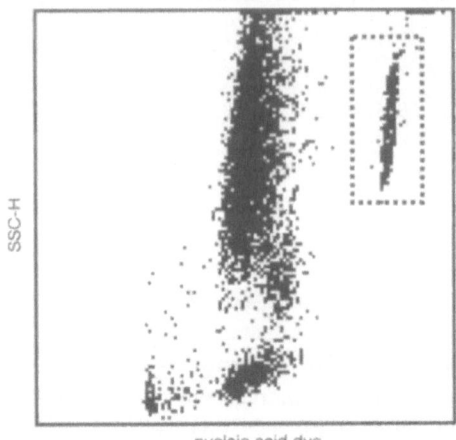

Fig. 2. In this dot plot from a SP analysis the bead-population is surrounded by a small rectangle. The number of acquired beads is used to calculate absolute concentrations of CD34+ cells as well as of CD45+ cells. The big rectangle (left side) was set to exclude debris.

(SP) on the contrary, allows the direct measurement of the absolute concentration (Fig. 1) on the flow-cytometer by the integration of plastic particles (beads) in a defined concentration (Fig. 2).

The purpose of this study was to compare the reliability of absolute cell counts generated by a commercially available SP-assay (ProCOUNT™, Becton Dickinson Immunocytometry Systems, BDIS, San Jose, USA) to the ISHAGE-guidelines, bearing in mind that the process of standardizing the flow cytometric CD34+ measurement has not come to an end, yet.

Material and methods

Methods: The study included 22 patients with Non-Hodgkin's Lymphoma (NHL) to whom G-CSF was administered after a chemotherapeutic treatment in preparation of a stem cell harvest. From the same peripheral blood sample, a measurement with each of the two methods was performed in parallel.

Over all, 116 samples (86 peripheral blood, 30 stem cell harvest aliquots) were analyzed on a FACSCalibur™ (BDIS). The CD34+ counts of both methods were correlated, and the mean difference in per cent was calculated for the concentrations of clinical relevance (i.e. counts below 10 CD34+ cells were not considered). In a similar way, the CD45+ data of the SP were compared to the WBC data of a hematologic analyzer (Sysmex SE-9000, Sysmex Deutschland GmbH, Norderstedt, Germany).

Results

The CD34+ cell concentrations from both techniques, the dual- and the single-platform (ISHAGE and ProCOUNT™), showed a correlation of r = 0.99 (Fig. 3). In average, the CD34+ concentration determined with the DP was 10.4% higher than that of the SP.

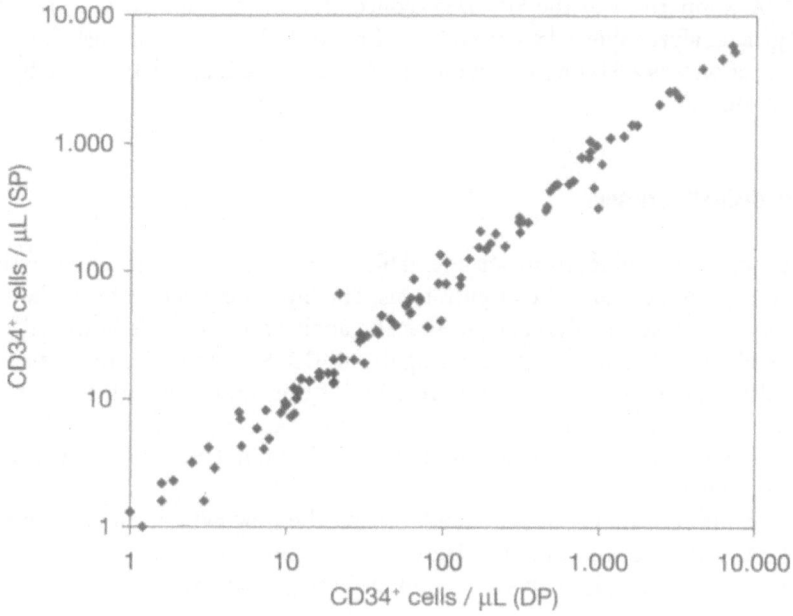

Fig. 3. Correlation CD34+ cells / µL

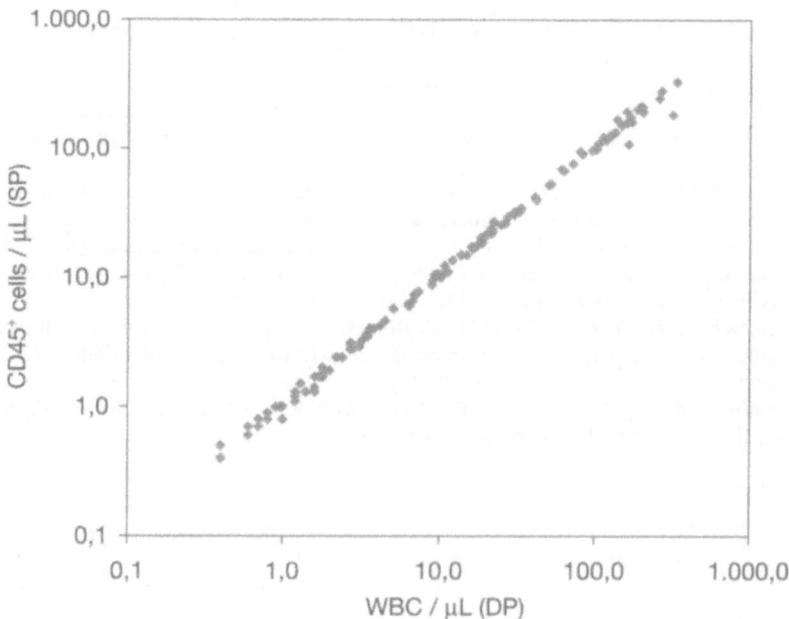

Fig. 4. Correlation SP-CD45+ / µL and WBC

A comparison of the SP-CD45$^+$ concentrations and the WBC from a hematological analyzer showed a correlation of r = 0.98 (Fig. 4). In average, the WBC concentration was 2.5% lower than the CD45$^+$ concentration as determined by the bead method.

Discussion/Conclusion

By including samples from peripheral blood and stem cell products, analysis of data covered a wide range of concentrations. The high coefficients of correlation found in both data-sets analyzed, show that the application of beads in the SP generates reliable results. Especially, comparing the SP-CD45$^+$ to the WBC of the hematologic analyzer demonstrates the high precision of this approach with an average difference of only 2.5%. The average difference of 10.4% calculated for the final concentrations of CD34$^+$ cells is a little bigger. This cannot be attributed to the bead-method itself.

In the process of further standardizing the flow cytometric determination of CD34$^+$ cells, the application of DP or SP is a minor issue. Instead, the main focus should be on sample-preparation and the gating-strategy.

References

1. Bender J, Unverzagt K (1993) Flow cytometric analysis of peripheral blood stem cells. J Haematother 2: 421–430
2. Bensinger W, Longin K, et al. (1994) Peripheral blood stem cells collected after recombinant granulocyte colony stimulating factor: an analysis of factors correlating with the tempo of engraftment after transplantation. Br J Hematol 87: 825–831
3. Chang A, Ma D et al. (1996) The influence of flow cytometric gating strategy on the standardization of CD34+ cell quantitation: an Australian multicenter study. J Haematother 5: 605–616
4. Lowdell M, Bainbridge D et al. (1996) External quality assurance for CD34 cell enumeration – results of a preliminary national trial. Bone Marrow Transplant 17: 849–853
5. Serke S, Säuberlich S, Huhn D (1991) Multiparameter flow-cytometrical quantitation of circulating CD34+ cells: correlation to the quantitation of circulating haemopoietic progenitor cells by in vitro colony-assay. Br J Haematol 77: 453–459
6. Siena S, Bregni M, et al. (1991) Flow cytometry to estimate circulating hematopoietic progenitors for autologous transplantation: comparative analysis of different CD34 monoclonal antibodies. Haematologica 76: 330–333
7. Sutherland D, Anderson L et al. (1996) The ISHAGE guidelines for CD34+ cell determination by flow cytometry. J Hematother 5: 213–226

An innovative Approach to Teach and Learn diagnostic Skills and therapeutical Management of Coagulation Disorders: CAMPUS – an interactive, Computer- and Case-based Program

K. Selke, B. Zieger, A. H. Sutor, R. Klar, L. B. Zimmerhackl,
and the consortium of CASEPORT [1]

Introduction

Up to now medical education mainly involves the teaching of theoretical knowledge about diseases. However, new teaching strategies as the problem- and case-based learning are becoming more and more important in the modern curriculum in medical school. The computer program CAMPUS was designed to present the student a more practical training using virtual scenarios. Aim of this new learning approach is to give students a better possibility to apply their knowledge and to correctly diagnose the patient's disease.

New technologies like multimedia, the World Wide Web and computer-based training systems provide advantages and new possibilities for establishing these up-to-date learning strategies. In this context case-based training systems are an important supplement to traditional medical education. Therefore, the MediCase working group [2] in the laboratory for Computer-Based Training in Medicine of the University of Heidelberg/Heilbronn (Prof. F.J. Leven et al.) developed CAMPUS, an interactive, computer- and case-based, multimedial learning system.

CAMPUS – an interactive, computer- and case-based program

With CAMPUS, authentic medical cases can be used for medical training in an interactive and almost realistic way. All cases have the same structure: First the student has to take the patient's history, then to examine the patient »physically«. After these steps he has to determine differential diagnoses. To confirm the correct diagnosis the student can use one or several diagnostic loops in the program for further investigations. These loops include lab work, ultrasound, x-ray etc. After the student has identified the correct diagnosis he has to initiate the adequate therapy. At the end, the program provides the student an overview of the medical case including information about the prognosis of the patient.

At all these steps the users can get help via expert comments or context-sensitive systematic knowledge which is available in addition to the case data on demand.

[1] Supported by CASEPORT a project of the Bundesministerium für Bildung und Forschung (BMBF), Förderkennzeichen 08NM111A

I. Scharrer/W. Schramm (Ed.)
32th Hemophilia Symposion Hamburg 2001
© Springer-Verlag Berlin Heidelberg 2003

Questions can be defined by the author to enhance active knowledge processing and interactivity. By using different multimedia components like text, picture, sound or animation complex medical interactions can be better understood.

Demonstration of a CAMPUS-case: presenting a patient with a coagulation disorder

We designed an interactive case report to introduce the student to an efficient diagnostic and therapeutic proceeding in a medical case with a patient who presents a coagulation disorder. Further aims of this interactive case-report include teaching the student about the pathophysiology of the coagulation system. A variety of laboratory tests in hemostaseology and the differential diagnoses in a case with bleeding symptoms are explained. Furthermore, therapy and complications of hemophilia are described.

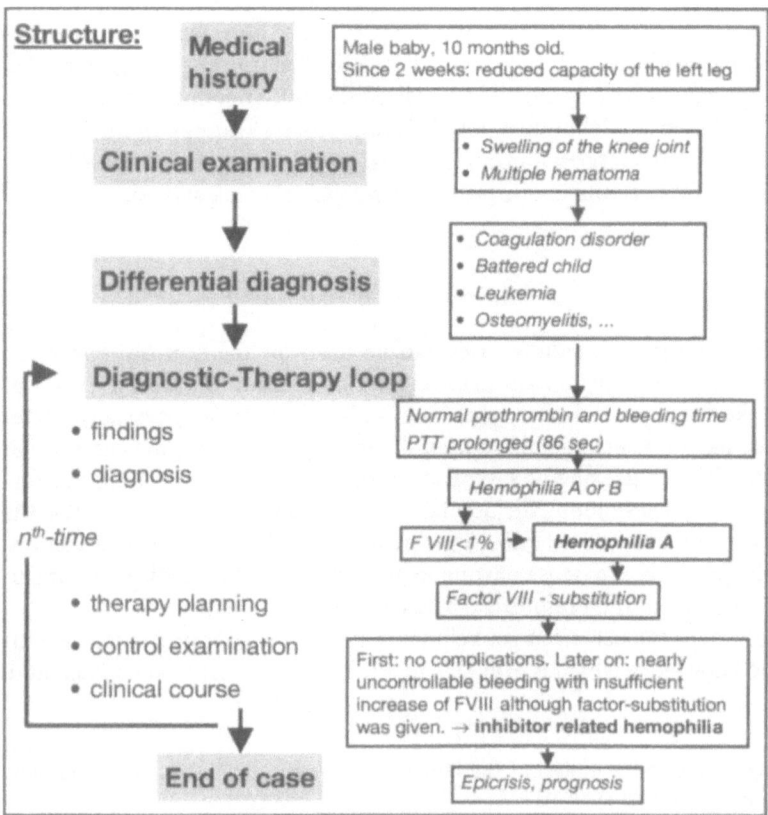

Fig. 1. Schema of general and specific case handling

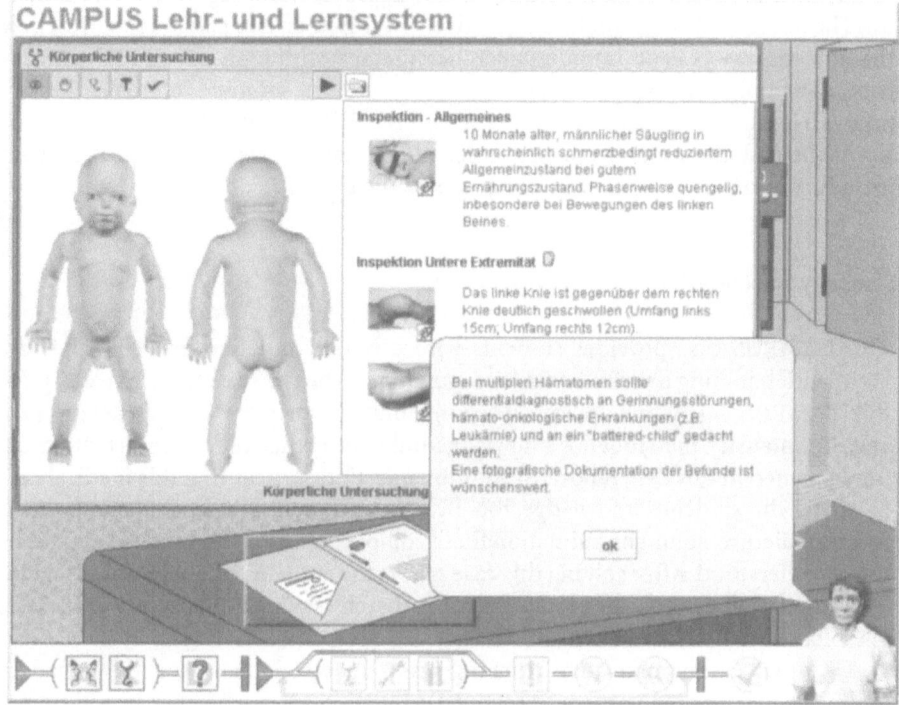

Fig. 2. Screenshot of the physical examination

We present a 10-months old male baby who has favoured his right leg for the past two weeks. The physical examination shows a significant swelling of the left knee and multiple hematomas on both legs, arms and on the back.

Based on this information, the student must determine differential diagnoses such as e.g. coagulation disorder, battered child, leukemia or osteomyelitis. These differential diagnoses should be excluded or confirmed step by step by a systematic, diagnostic approach: After a detailed tracking of the medical history, the student should first initiate the routine coagulation test. Then, depending on the appropriate results, the student must initiate the extended and more specific diagnostic coagulation tests. In our case prothrombin time and bleeding time was normal, however the partial thromboplastin time was prolonged (86 sec).

These results are characteristic of a disorder in the intrinsic coagulation system (e.g. factor VIII or factor IX deficiency). The following analysis of the factor VIII-activity showed a factor VIII-activity under 1%. This result confirms the diagnosis of hemophilia A. Now the student has to determine the adequate therapy. In the following the program shows that the patient was successfully treated with a factor VIII-concentrate. However, two months later the boy suddenly develops a mucosal bleeding which does not stop although FVIII-concentrate has been applied first at prophylactic and then at therapeutic levels. The student is asked for an explanation of this phenomena. The student now has to suggest a screening for a FVIII-inhibitor. The test for a FVIII-inhibitor is positive. These new circumstances require a new therapy strategy (e.g. an immune tolerance therapy with high-dose FVIII-concentrate). The program shows that after several months of immune tolerance therapy no FVIII-inhibitor is measured anymore and the FVIII-recovery is back to normal.

At the end, the program provides the student an overview of the medical case including information about the prognosis of the patient.

Summary and outlook

This CAMPUS-case provides students with a virtual situation in which they are faced with handling a patient with a coagulation disorder. The interactive design of this CAMPUS-case avoids passive learning, but supports the active learning process. To intensify the student's knowledge links to further related information are implemented in this case report. In addition questions concerning this medical case enhances the student's knowledge, too. By using different multimedia components like text, picture, sound or animation these complex medical interactions should be better understood. After solving this case report the student should be able to handle a coagulation disorder in a logical manner thereby saving unnecessary costs, tests and blood.

CAMPUS is an innovative teaching program which has been developed to improve education in the medical school. CAMPUS cases can be used in addition to conventional medical text books, but are not intended to replace bed side clinical training. Main topics of interests of our cases are an improvement of problem-solving ability, a better knowledge-management and a higher motivation for life-long-learning. Moreover, using a web-based training system like CAMPUS allows the student to access the teaching and learning system at any time or location.

Our first efforts to implement CAMPUS cases in the curriculum showed a high acceptance from the students. The specific use of CAMPUS seems to supplement and enrich the medical curriculum efficiently. Scientific studies are planned to evaluate the effectiveness of problem based teaching using CAMPUS cases.

References

1. http://www.caseport.de
2. http://www.medicase.de

Expression of Protease-activated Receptors in Neuroblastoma Cells

C. Wermes, A. Siebke, C. Wilhelm, K.W. Sykora, S. Glueer, A. Ganser, and M. von Depka Prondzinski

Background

Children with cancer are on high risk to develop thrombosis. The underlying pathophysiological mechanisms are not completely understood. Most coagulation factors are expressed in liver or endothelial cells. Some of them, e.g. thrombin, Plasminogen activator inhibitor-1 and tissue factor, have been detected in neuroblastoma cells as well, suggesting that tumor cells directly take part in thrombogenesis [5,9].

Protease activated receptors are a recently described, novel family of seven transmembrane G-proteine-coupled receptors. Their activation is initiated by cleavage of the N-terminus of the receptor by serine-proteases. Classically, serine proteases have been shown to play important roles in diverse biological functions, particularly in relation to clot formation and wound healing [6]. To date, four protease activated receptors (PAR1–4) have been identified, with distinct N-terminal cleavage sites and tethered ligand pharmacology. PAR2 was found in vascular, airways, and intestinal smooth muscle cells, neuronal tissue, leucocytes, osteoblasts, lymphoid tissues and endothelial cells [7]. PAR3 was found to be expressed in a variety of tissues, including heart, small intestine, bone marrow, airway smooth muscle cells, vascular endothelium and astrocytes. The tissue distribution of PAR4 was found to be distinct from the other PAR-family members, with the highest levels of receptor-mRNA detected in lung, pancreas, thyroid, testis, and small intestine. PAR2 activation may play a role in regulation of some forms of cancer, especially of gastrointestinal forms [8]. The expression and function of PAR2, PAR3 and PAR4 in neuroblastoma is unknown.

Materials and methods

Cell culture

Human neuroblastoma cells of the cell line NB-11 MHH were grown with RPMI 1640 medium containing 10% heat-inactivated FCS and 1% penicillin/streptomycin. The medium was changed every second day and cells were passaged weekly. To differentiate the NB-11-cells into neuron-like NB+-cells, they were grown in the presence of 1 µl/ml of a 10 µm suspension of retinoic acid in DMSO for 8 days [4].

I. Scharrer/W. Schramm (Ed.)
32th Hemophilia Symposion Hamburg 2001
© Springer-Verlag Berlin Heidelberg 2003

HUVEC cells, which served as controls, were isolated from fresh human umbilical cord by incubation with cord buffer containing 0.01% collagenase, and grown with RM-medium containing 10% heat-inactivated FCS, 1% penicillin/streptomycin and 1% L-glutamine.

RNA extraction and reverse transcription

The RNA was isolated with the TRIzol method, an improvement to the single step RNA isolation method developed by Chomczynski et al. [2]. The reverse transcription was performed using superscript reverse transcriptase (GIBCO BRL).

TaqMan Analysis

Quantitative analysis was performed using the quantitative real-time PCR (TaqMan®-PCR).

The probes and primers were as follows:

PAR2:	sense primer:	5' - TTC CCA CTC GTT CCC CTC - 3'
	antisense primer:	5' - GCC GAT GAG TAC AGG CCT T - 3'
	probe:	5' - TCT TCC GAG CTG CCT TGT GGG C - 3'
PAR3:	sense primer:	5' - AGT TTT GAG CAA CCC TGG CC - 3'
	antisense primer:	5' - GGA CAC CGA GTG TCG CCC - 3'
	probe:	5' - AAC GCA CGG CCG GCG ACG - 3'
PAR4:	sense primer:	5' - GGA AGG CTG TAC TGG GTC G - 3'
	antisense primer:	5' - TCT GAG GTC CCA GGA AGG A - 3'
	probe:	5' - CAG GGT CCC TTC CCC CAC TCC - 3'

As positive controls we used Annexin II (for PAR2) and PAI-1 (for PAR3 and 4). Negative controls were performed without template.

Results

PAR2 mRNA was expressed in neuroblastoma cells (NB-11 MHH), in differentiated nerval cells (NB+) and in HUVEC as demonstrated in Figure 1. In addition positive (Annexin II) and negative controls are shown (Fig. 4).

PAR3 mRNA was also found in neuroblastoma cells, in differentiated nerval cells and in HUVEC (Fig. 2). Here PAI-1 served as positive control (Fig. 4).

PAR4 mRNA was expressed in differentiated nerval cells and in HUVEC, but **not** in neuroblastoma cells (Fig. 3).

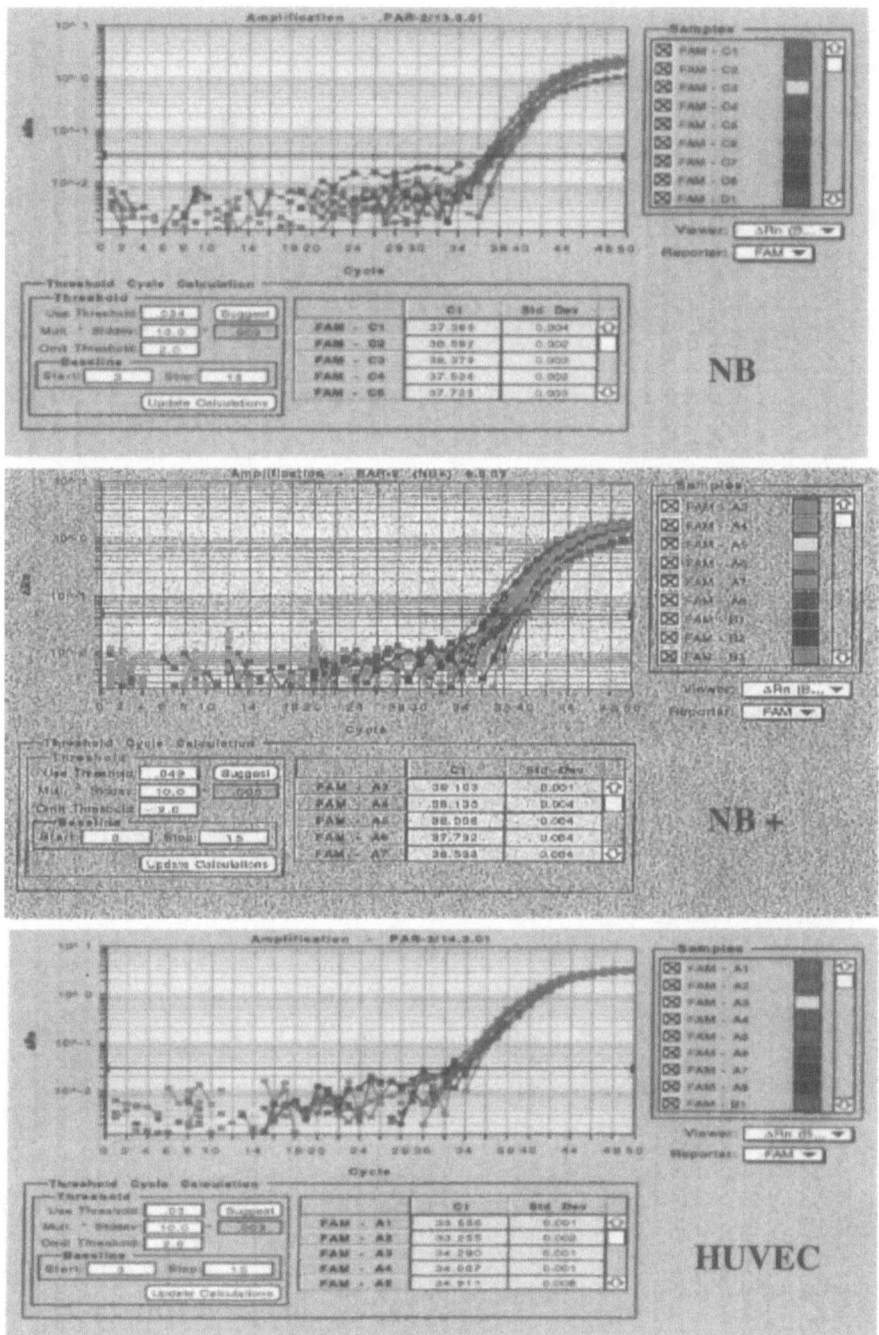

Fig. 1. PAR2 mRNA expression in neuroblastoma cells, differentiated nerval cells (NB+) and HUVEC

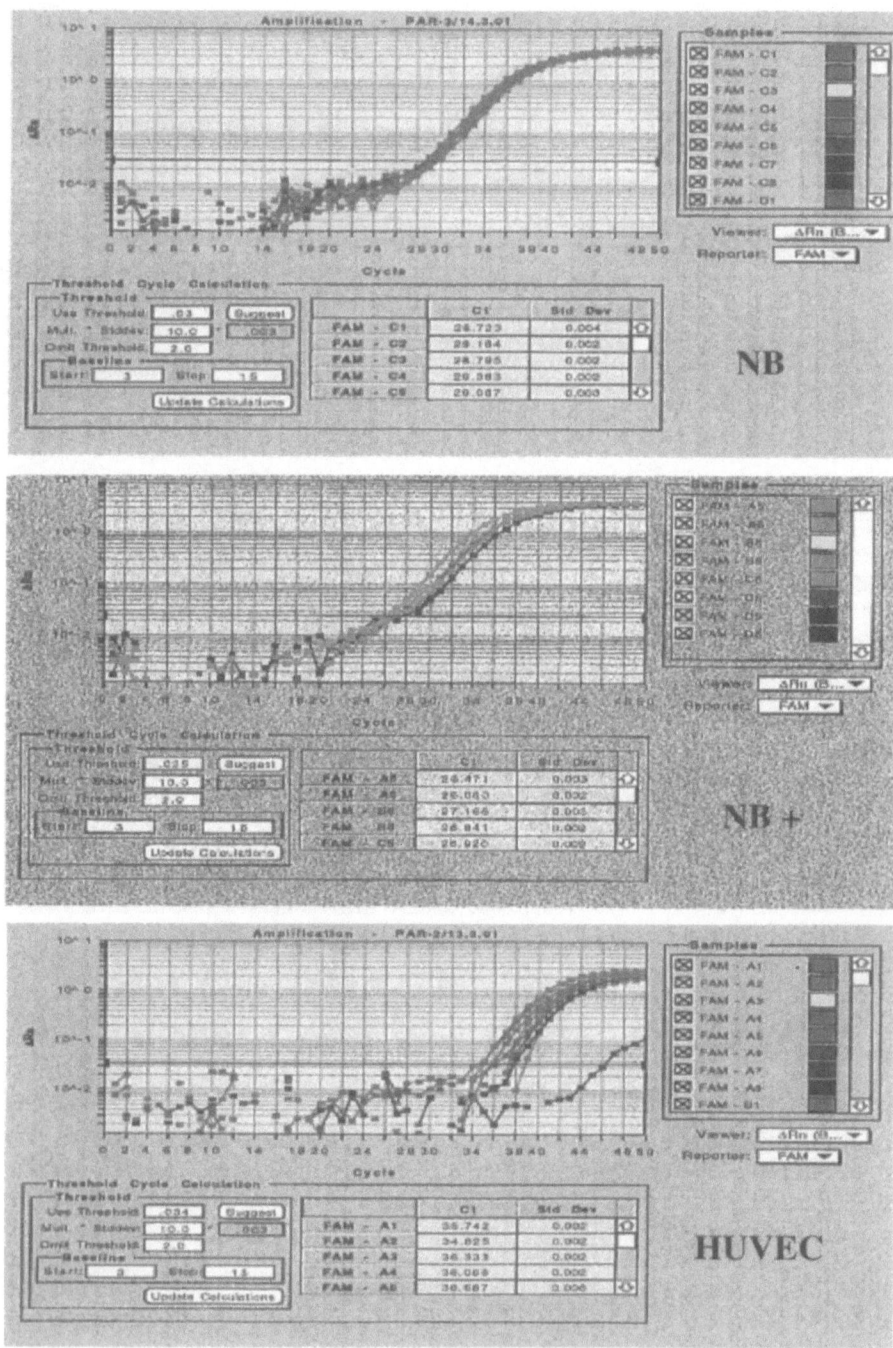

Fig. 2. PAR3 mRNA expression in neuroblastoma cells, differentiated nerval cells (NB+) and HUVEC

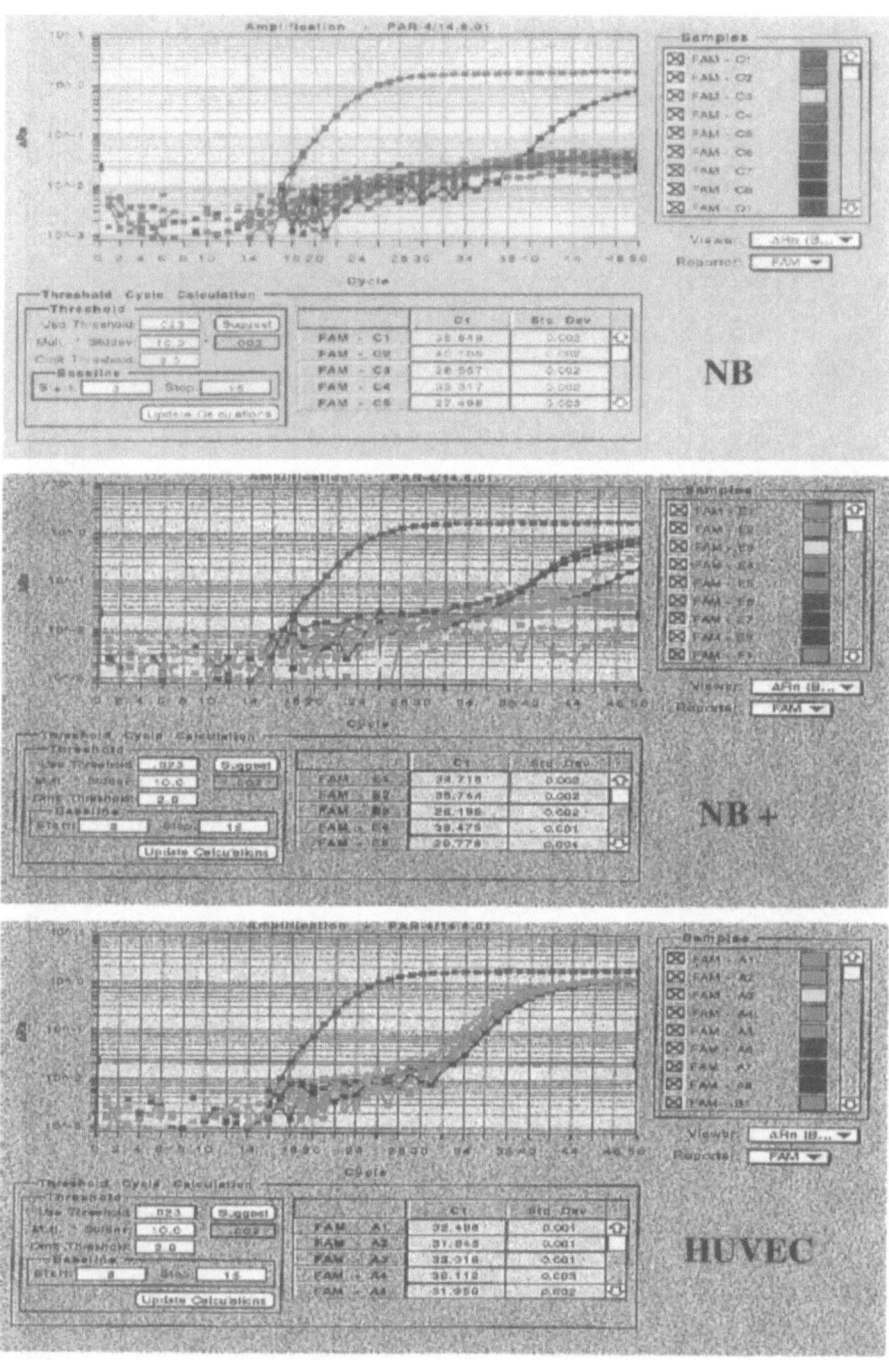

Fig. 3. PAR4 mRNA expression in neuroblastoma cells, differentiated nerval cells (NB+) and HUVEC

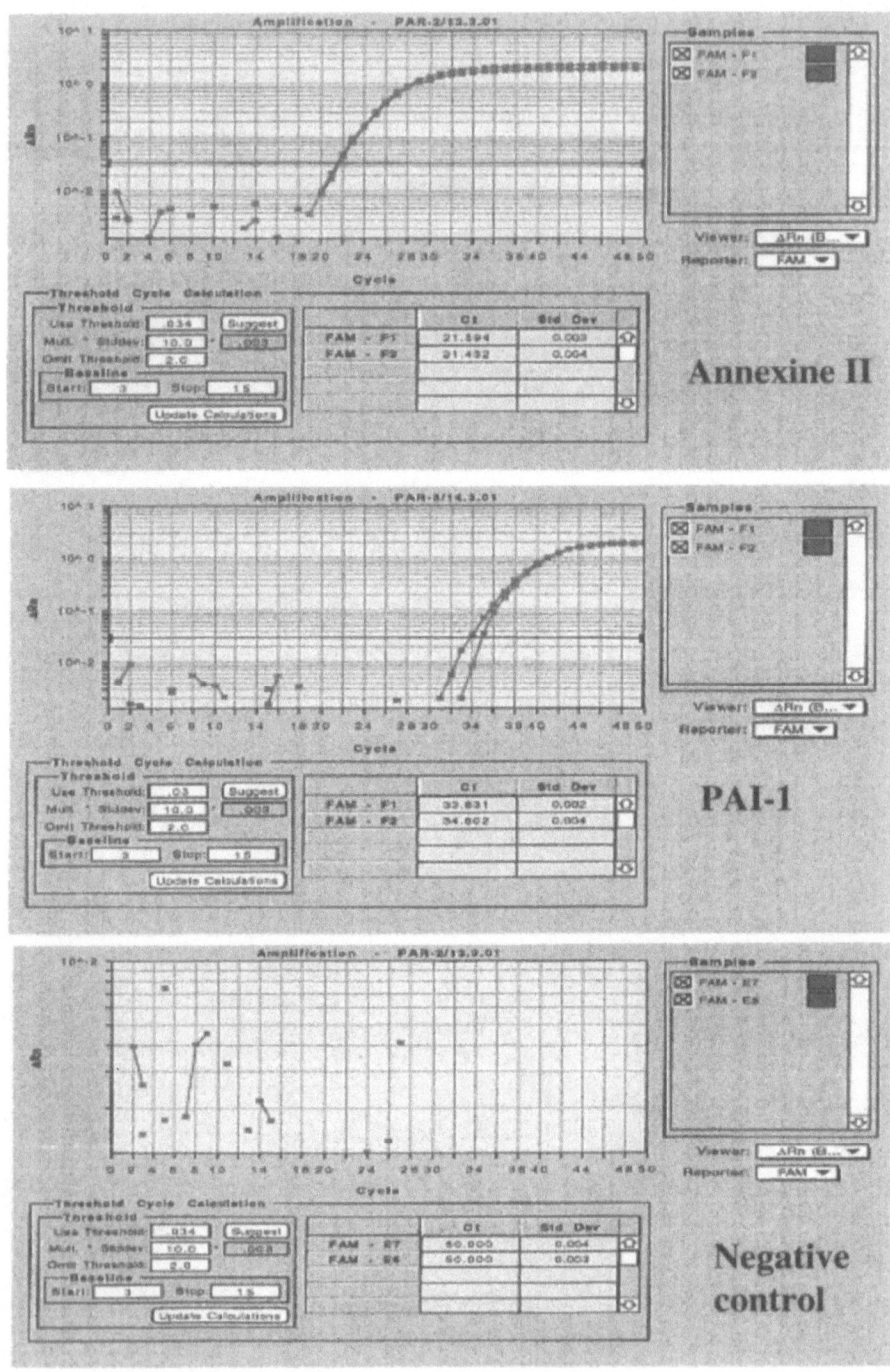

Fig. 4. Positive and negative controls

Discussion

We, for the first time, describe mRNA expression of PAR2 and PAR3 in neuroblastoma cells.

There are no investigations concerning neuroblastoma, PARs, and thrombus generation in children but it is known that PARs take part in blood coagulation by platelet aggregation (PAR1 and PAR4) (6) and formation of tissue factor in endothelial cells (PAR2) [1]. PAR1, PAR3 and PAR4 can be activated by thrombin. PAR2 can be activated by trypsin and tryptase as well as by coagulation factors VIIa and Xa but not by thrombin [3].

Only PAR1 is discussed to be involved in development of neuroblastoma [10]. The other PARs are not yet investigated. Possibly PAR2 and PAR3 play a similar role inhibiting neural outgrowth in neuroblastoma, although PAR2 is stimulated by trypsin and trypsin-like proteases and not by thrombin.

Protein expression and the clinical relevance of our findings have to be examined in further experiments.

References

1. Alm AK, Norstrom E, Sundelin J, Nystedt S (1999) Stimulation of proteinase activated receptor-2 causes endothelial cells to promote blood coagulation in vitro. Thromb Haemost 81(6):984-8
2. Chomczynski P, Sacchi N (1987) Single-step method of RNA isolation by acid guanidinium thiocyanate-phenol-chloroform extraction. Anal Biochem 162:156
3. Coughlin SR (2001) Protease-activated receptors in vascular biology. Thromb Haemost; 86:298-307
4. Hildebrandt et al. (1998) Polysialic acid on the neural cell adhesion molecule correlates with expression of polysialyltransferases and promotes neuroblastoma cell growth. Cancer Res. 58(4):779
5. Inuyama H, Saito T, Takagi J, Saito Y (1997) Factor X-dependent, thrombin-generating activities on a neuroblastoma cell and their disappearance upon differentiation. J Cell Physiol 173(3):406
6. Macfarlane SR, Seatter MJ, Kanke T, Hunter GD, Plevin R (2001) Proeinase-activated receptors. Pharm Rev 53(2):245
7. Mirza H, Yatsula V, Bahou WF (1996) The proteinase activated receptor-2 (PAR-2) mediates mitogenic responses in human vascular endothelial cells. J Clin Invest 97(7):1705
8. Miyata S, Koshikawa N, Higashi S, Miyagi Y, Nagashima Y, Yanoma S, Kato Y, Yasumitsu H, Miyazaki K (1999) Expression of trypsin in human cancer cell lines and cancer tissues and its tight binding to soluble form of Alzheimer amyloid precursor protein in culture. J Biochem (Tokyo) 125(6):1067-76
9. Sugiura Y, Ma L, Sun B, Shimada H, Laug WE, Seeger RC, DeClerk YA (1999) The plasminogen activator (PA) system in neuroblastoma: role of PA inhibitor-1 in metastasis. Cancer Res 59(6):1327
10. Turgeon VL, Lloyd ED, Wang S, Festoff BW, Houenou LJ (1998) Thrombin pertubs neurite outgrowth and induces apoptotic death in enriched chick spinal motoneuron cultures through caspase activation. J Neurosci 18(17):6882-91

Subject Index